Disorders of Human Learning, Behavior, and Communication

Ronald L. Taylor and Les Sternberg
Series Editors

Michael G. Aman Nirbhay N. Singh *1988*
Editors

Psychopharmacology of the Developmental Disabilities

Springer-Verlag
New York Berlin Heidelberg
London Paris Tokyo

Michael G. Aman, Nisonger Center for Mental Retardation, The Ohio State University, Columbus, Ohio, 43210-1205 USA

Nirbhay N. Singh, Educational Research Services Center, De Kalb, Illinois, 60115 USA

Library of Congress Cataloging-in-Publication Data
Psychopharmacology of the developmental disabilities
      p. cm.—(Disorders of human learning, behavior, and communication)
    Includes bibliographies.
      1. Developmentally disabled children—Medical care. 2. Pediatric
psychopharmacology. I. Aman, Michael G. II. Singh Nirbhay N.
III. Series.
    [DNLM: 1. Child Development Disorders—drug therapy. 2. Mental
Retardation—drug therapy. 3. Psychopharmacology. 4. Psychotropic
Drugs—pharmacology. WM 300 P9753]
RJ507.D48P79   1988
618.92′8588—dc19
DNLM/DLC
for Library of Congress   88-1858
                                                        CIP

Typeset by Asco Trade Typesetting Ltd., Hong Kong.
Printed and bound by R.R. Donnelley and Sons, Harrisonburg, Virginia.
Printed in the United States of America.

9 8 7 6 5 4 3 2 1

ISBN 0-387-96679-X   Springer-Verlag New York Berlin Heidelberg
ISBN 3-540-96679-X   Springer-Verlag Berlin Heidelberg New York

Preface

Purpose and Scope

The purpose of this book is to make the considerable developments in psychopharmacology of the developmental disabilities readily available in one source. We have defined developmental disability as a significant shortfall in intellectual ability, academic achievement, or adaptative behavior relative to age expectations (Matson & LaGrow, 1983). The book sets out to provide coverage of the major classes of medication currently in use, newer drugs being explored, and major areas of concern as they relate to drug treatment. In doing this, we have been extremely fortunate in being able to involve distinguished international experts in the field so that the book should contain a truly authoritative summary of the current state of psychopharmacology in this field.

This book is for all workers in developmental disabilities, not just those with medical or nursing responsibilities or a particular interest in pharmacotherapy. A knowledge of medication effects is of importance because psychoactive drugs may influence (either for better or worse) the effectiveness of other nonmedical forms of therapy such as behavior modification, special education, and so forth. As shown in Chapter 1, drug therapy is an extremely prevalent form, perhaps the single most common mode, of therapy in the developmental disabilities. Given that drugs can have far-reaching effects, both in terms of their therapeutic actions and in terms of adverse effects, some familiarity with the state of psychopharmacology is of obvious relevance to all in this field.

This is a timely point for such a book, because the level of research activity and general interest in psychoactive drugs has been high in recent years, due to several vigorous programs of drug research over the last decade. In addition, at the National Strategy Conference on Mental Retardation and Mental Health in Washington, D.C. (1985), major sections of the program were reserved for discussions of pharmacological and other therapies. Another reflection of this interest can be seen in *Psychopharmacology Bulletin*, which devoted a section to research on mentally retarded/developmentally disabled individuals (Reatig, 1985). In 1986, a special workshop was sponsored by the U.S. National Institute of Mental Health (NIMH) to consider the methodological problems in arriving at accurate and valid psychiatric/psychological diagnoses when conducting treatment research with mentally retarded populations (Special Workshop, 1986). In 1987, the NIMH and the National Institute of Child Health and Human Development put out a joint Request for Proposals (MH 87-11) which specified psychopharmacology of mentally retarded people as a high priority area for funding. Finally, there has also been greatly increasing legal activity of late in the United States with regard to drug treatment (see Chapter 2), and this may have major implications for the utilization of such therapy.

This book is largely concerned with the psychopharmacology of mentally retarded people. Research with autistic children is also reviewed and, to a lesser extent, various authors have discussed research with seizure disorders (insofar as they are often associated with lower functional levels), Tourette syndrome, hyperactivity (Attention Deficit Disorder), and childhood psychosis. However, the emphasis has consistently been placed on drug research carried out with people having subaverage intellectual functioning.

In selecting material we were guided by the following considerations. First, we wished to cover all of the major psychotropic drug groups used with this population. This resulted in separate chapters on neuroleptic drugs, antiepileptic drugs, other traditional psychotropic drugs (e.g., cerebral stimulants, antidepressants), and novel psychotropic agents (e.g., fenfluramine, clonidine). There is also a chapter on vitamin and dietary treatments for behavioral control. Second, there is a need for material on drug effects in their natural context and how to study their effects there, leading to a chapter on drug prevalence, patterns of drug use, methodological considerations, measures of drug change, and likely future directions. Third, the use of medication with this socially disadvantaged group raises a number of ethical and legal issues, resulting in a chapter summarizing the latest litigation relating to pharmacotherapy in the developmental disabilities. Fourth, there has been much concern about the neurological syndrome of tardive dyskinesia as a sequel to therapy with neuroleptics, and a separate contribution reviews this topic in detail. Fifth, advances in measuring drug concentrations in blood and related theoretical and technical problems quantifying and interpreting these concentrations are discussed in a separate chapter. Sixth, we felt that there has been a general failure in the past to relate the substantial body of animal drug research to this field. A chapter on behavioral pharmacology attempts to establish the relevance of this information to the treatment of the developmental disabilities and to show how its methods and findings might be extended to the field. Finally, this material is brought together and discussed in a separate chapter in terms of how psychopharmacological drug research with developmentally disabled persons relates to the broader area of psychopharmacology in general.

Drug Use Often a Matter of Controversy

The use of drugs to treat maladaptive behavior in developmentally disabled persons can be an emotive topic, especially to those who advocate the use of alternative methods (see Aman, 1985; Aman & Singh, 1986), and it can be seen as one way of arbitrarily defining the field as "medical." Hersen (1979) has discussed a problem which occurs when workers are so committed to a particular form of therapy that they reject all other approaches, such as pharmacotherapy. Elsewhere (Aman & Singh, 1986), we have suggested that there has been a prevalent "anti-drug" sentiment in the field in recent years. Workers cannot afford to make up their minds before the data are available, nor is it appropriate to design drug studies in such a way that a therapeutic outcome is unlikely. Although drugs appear to have been overused in the past (often as the *only* form of treatment), we believe that pharmacotherapy still has a legitimate and potentially valuable place in the treatment of developmentally disabled people. It is hoped that the discussions which appear in this book will help to give an objective summary of the potential and limitations of pharmacotherapy with this population.

Caveat—The Breuning Studies

In the early 1980s, a young researcher named Stephen E. Breuning published a large number of reports and reviews relating to drug effects in mentally retarded individuals. Many of the studies reported the use of large groups of subjects, extensive sampling of maladaptive and adaptive behavior, and often elegant and complex methological designs. Most of these investigations showed marked and clear-cut detrimental effects due to neuroleptic drugs in this population, and they were widely cited in the mental retardation literature (Aman & Singh, 1986). This work had a marked effect on the field, to the extent that at least one state modified its guidelines regarding the use of psychotropic drugs to be consistent with Breuning's findings (Holden, 1987).

In 1983, Robert L. Sprague, Ph.D. (a senior colleague of Dr. Breuning) noted irregularities in Breuning's reported results. In a detailed and lengthy letter, Sprague reported his concern about Breuning's research to the National Institute of Mental Health (NIMH). As a result of Sprague's action, the NIMH convened a panel of senior scientists to investigate possible scientific misconduct on the research grants with which Dr. Breuning was associated. On April 20, 1987, the investigative panel released its findings (Panel to Investigate Allegations of Scientific Misconduct, 1987). Among the panel's more important findings were the following:

> . . . that Stephen E. Breuning knowingly, willfully, and repeatedly engaged in misleading and deceptive practices in reporting results of research . . . that he did not carry out the described research; that only a few of the experimental subjects described in publications and progress reports were ever studied; and that the complex designs and rigorous methodologies reported were not employed. Dr. Breuning also misrepresented, implicitly or explicitly, the locations at which research was supposedly conducted (pg. 30).
> The Panel unanimously concludes, on the basis of all the facts, that Dr. Stephen E. Breuning has engaged in serious scientific misconduct (pg. 37).

Others have also commented on the scandal and the events surrounding it. Interested readers are referred to articles and/or letters by Aman (1987), Ferguson, Cullari, and Gadow (1987), Gualtieri (1987), Holden (1986, 1987), Hostetler (1987a, 1987b), Mulick (1987), and Sprague (1987). It is clear that great caution must be exercised in interpreting these studies—indeed, the NIMH panel concluded that most of Breuning's drug studies in this field were never actually carried out. Obviously, replication of these studies by independent and responsible workers should be a high priority for the field.

We, the editors, and most of the contributors were aware of the Breuning controversy when preparing chapters for this book. Therefore, we avoided citing the questionable material so as not to promulgate further what may be fabricated results. On one or two occasions, reference is made in the book to Breuning's research to place in context the impact his reports had on the field. However, it is important that workers new to the field (or not already aware of the alleged fraud) be cognizant of the episode so that they do not inadvertently adopt Breuning's numerous reports as the basis for further research or to guide clinical practice. This is clearly a danger which we must try to avoid.

Michael G. Aman
Nirbhay N. Singh

References

Aman, M.G. (1985). Drugs in mental retardation: Treatment or tragedy? *Australian and New Zealand Journal of Developmental Disabilities*, *10*, 215–226.

Aman, M.G., & Singh, N.N. (1986). A critical appraisal of recent drug research in mental retardation: The Coldwater studies. *Journal of Mental Deficiency Research*, *30*, 203–216.

Aman, M.G. (1987). Overview of pharmacotherapy: current status and future directions. *Journal of Mental Deficiency Research*, *31*, 121–130.

Ferguson, D.G., Cullari, S., & Gadow, K.D. (1987). Comment on the "Coldwater" studies. [Letter to the editor]. *Journal of Mental Deficiency Research*, *31*, 219–220.

Gualtieri, C.T. (1987). Re: M.G. Aman & N.N. Singh, "A critical appraisal of recent drug research in mental retardation: the Coldwater studies." [Letter to the editor]. *Journal of Mental Deficiency Research*, *31*, 222–223.

Herson, M. (1979). Limitations and problems in the clinical application of behavioral techniques in psychiatric settings. *Behavior Therapy*, *10*, 65–80.

Holden, C. (1986). NIMH review of fraud charge moves slowly. *Science*, *234*, 1488–1489.

Holden, C. (1987). NIMH finds a case of "serious misconduct." *Science*, *235*, 1566–1567.

Hostetler, A.J. (May, 1987a). Investigation fraud inquiry revives doubt: can science police itself? *American Psychological Association Monitor*, *18* (No. 5), 1, 12.

Hostetler, A.J. (July, 1987b). NIMH sends fraud case to Justice. *American Psychological Association Monitor*, *18* (No. 7), 18.

Matson, J.L. & La Grow, S.J. (1983). Developmental and physical disabilities. In M. Hersen, V.B. Van Hasselt, & J.L. Matson (Eds.), *Behavior therapy for the developmentally and physically disabled*, (pp. 3–24). New York: Academic Press.

Mulick, J.A. (1987). Editorial: Scientific misconduct and trust of science. *Psychology in Mental Retardation*, *13* (No. 1), 5–6, 9.

Panel to Investigate Allegations of Scientific Misconduct under Grants MH-32206 and MH-37449. (April 20, 1987). *Final report. Investigation of alleged scientific misconduct on grants MH-32206 and MH-37449*. Washington, D.C. Public Health Service.

Reatig, N. (1985). Workshop on pharmacotherapy and mental retardation. *Psychopharmacology Bulletin*, *21*, 248–333.

Sprague, R.L. (1987). [Letter to the editor]. *Journal of Mental Deficiency Research*, *31*, 223–225.

Special Workshop on *Methodological problems in treatment research with mentally retarded populations who are also mentally ill*. (May, 1986). 26th Meeting of the New Clinical Drug Evaluation Unit (NIMH), Key Biscayne, FL.

Acknowledgments

Work on this book was supported in part by a Senior Research Fellowship grant to Dr. M. Aman from the Medical Research Council of New Zealand. We are grateful to Mrs. Marsha Aman for extensive typing entailed in preparing correspondence and manuscripts. Most of the chapters were reviewed by two or more external authorities, and we would like to thank these workers for their helpful comments. The external reviewers were as follows:

John Birkbeck, M.B.Ch.B., F.R.A.C.P., Department of Medicine, University of Auckland.

Dennis Cantwell, M.D., Neuropsychiatric Institute, University of California, Los Angeles.

Edwin Cook, Jr., M.D., Division of Child and Adolescent Psychiatry, University of Chicago Hospital.

John Dawson, B.A. (Hons.), L.L.M., Legal Officer, Mental Health Foundation of New Zealand, Auckland.

George Ellman, Ph.D., University of California, San Francisco.

Kenneth D. Gadow, Ph.D., Department of Psychiatry & Behavioral Science, State University of New York at Stony Brook.

William C. Hodge, A.B., J.D., School of Law, University of Auckland.

Robert Hughes, Ph.D., Department of Psychology, University of Canterbury.

John Kalachnik, M.Ed., Cambridge State Hospital, Cambridge, Minnesota.

Richard Kern, M.D., The Nisonger Center for Mental Retardation, Ohio State University.

Marcel Kinsbourne, M.D., Department of Behavioral Neurology, Shriver Center.

Betty Kozlowski, Ph.D., The Nisonger Center for Mental Retardation, Ohio State University.

Gordon L. Lees, Ph.D., Department of Psychiatry & Behavioural Science, University of Auckland.

Neil McNaughton, Ph.D., Department of Psychology, University of Otago.

James W. Paxton, Ph.D., Department of Pharmacology & Clinical Pharmacology, University of Auckland.

Andrew Reid, Consultant Psychiatrist, Royal Dundee Liff Hospital, Dundee.

Charles Silverstein, Ph.D., Brain-Behavior Research Center, Sonoma Developmental Center, Eldridge, California.

Robert L. Sprague, Ph.D., Institute for Child Behavior & Development, University of Illinois, Champaign, Illinois.

Michael R. Trimble, M.D., Institute for Neurology, National Hospital for Nervous Disease, London.

G. John Turbott, M.B.Ch.B., F.R.A.C.P., Department of Psychiatry & Behavioural Science, University of Auckland.

John S. Werry, M.D., Department of Psychiatry & Behavioural Science, University of Auckland.

Contents

Contributors

Michael G. Aman, Ph.D., Director of Research, The Nisonger Center for Mental Retardation, and Department of Psychology, The Ohio State University, Columbus, Ohio 43210-1205, U.S.A.

Henry A. Beyer, J.D., Director, Pike Institute for the Handicapped, Boston University School of Law, Boston University, Boston, Massachusetts 02215, U.S.A.

Magda Campbell, M.D., Director, Division of Child and Adolescent Psychiatry, Department of Psychiatry, New York University Medical Center, New York, New York 10016, U.S.A.

Mark Chandler, M.D., Department of Psychiatry and Biological Sciences Research Center, University of North Carolina, Chapel Hill, North Carolina 27514, U.S.A.

John L. Evenden, Ph.D., Department of Experimental Psychology, University of Cambridge, Cambridge CB2 3EB England

Jeffrey J. Fahs, M.D., Department of Psychiatry, University of Alabama, Birmingham, Alabama 35294, U.S.A.

Gerald S. Golden, M.D., Director, Child Development Center, College of Medicine, University of Tennessee, Memphis, Memphis, Tennessee 38119, U.S.A.

C. Thomas Gualtieri, M.D., Division of Health Affairs, Department of Psychiatry, School of Medicine, University of North Carolina, Chapel Hill, North Carolina 27514, U.S.A.

Mark H. Lewis, Biological Sciences Research Center and Department of Psychiatry, University of North Carolina, School of Medicine, Chapel Hill, North Carolina 27514, U.S.A.

Richard B. Mailman, Ph.D. Biological Sciences Research Center and Department of Psychiatry, University of North Carolina, School of Medicine, Chapel Hill, North Carolina 27514, U.S.A.

Stephen R. Schroeder, Ph.D., Director, The Nisonger Center for Mental Retardation, The Ohio State University, Columbus, Ohio 43210-1205, U.S.A.

Nirbhay N. Singh, Ph.D., Senior Research Psychologist, Educational Research Services Center, DeKalb, Illinois 60115, U.S.A.

Mae S. Sokol, M.D., Instructor in Psychiatry, Cornell University Medical College, New York, New York 10021, U.S.A.

Gregory Stores, M.D., F.R.C.P., University Department of Psychiatry and National Centre for Children with Epilepsy, Park Hospital for Children, Oxford OX3 7LQ, England

John S. Werry, M.D., Department of Psychiatry, School of Medicine, University of Auckland, Auckland 1, New Zealand

1
Patterns of Drug Use, Methodological Considerations, Measurement Techniques, and Future Trends

MICHAEL G. AMAN AND NIRBHAY N. SINGH

Abstract

The prevalence of psychotropic and antiepileptic drug use with developmentally disabled people is comprehensively reviewed. Pharmacotherapy has been documented to be very common with mentally retarded individuals (especially those in institutions) but has not been well studied in other forms of developmental disabilities. Demographic, medical, and behavioral variables are examined with respect to medication use in an effort to indentify patterns of drug prescription. A number of programs which succeeded in reducing inappropriate medication use are also described. Some of the more frequently used measures for assessing drug change in this field are outlined. Future needs and trends, such as more attention to dual diagnosis, more work with noninstitutionalized populations, and greater attention to the quality-of-care dimension are addressed. In addition, more work in the areas of neurochemistry, pharmacokinetics, and psychophysiology is expected, with the inevitable consequence of a more interdisciplinary approach to the field.

This chapter begins with a section on prevalence and patterns of drug use to acquaint readers with the scope of medication use among developmentally disabled individuals. This is followed by short sections on methodology and measurement of drug effects, to provide some indication of strategies that either have been used or are available. Then a discussion of promising future directions for research in psychopharmacology is presented, followed by overall conclusions. In this chapter, *psychotropic drug* is defined as any substance that is administered for the purpose of producing behavioral, emotional, or cognitive changes. *Psychoactive drug* is defined as any agent that has such effects, regardless of the purpose of prescribing that medication.

Prevalence and Patterns of Drug Use

Prevalence

In Table 1.1, a large number of surveys of drug use have been summarized. Antiepileptic drugs are included because they are increasingly being recog-

TABLE 1.1. Prevalence of psychoactive drug use with developmentally disabled persons.

Authors	Number of persons surveyed	% Receiving psychotropic medication	% Receiving anticonvulsant drugs	Total percentage	Most common drugs prescribed
A. Public residential facilities for mentally retarded persons					
Lipman, 1970	Residents of 109 institutions	51[a]	NR[b]	NR	Thioridazine, chlorpromazine, trifluoperazine, diazepam, chloridiazepoxide
Spencer, 1974	585	22+ (only antipsychotics surveyed)	24	51+	Phenobarbital, haloperidol, chlorpromazine, phenytoin, thioridazine
Bullmore (in Kirman, 1975)	617	NR	27	60	NR
DiMascio, 1975 (2 facilities)	1,232	26	21	NR	Phenobarbitone, phenytoin, thioridazine, chlorpromazine primidone, diazepam
	785	53	90	NR	
Sewell & Werry, 1976	254	40	NR	NR	Thioridazine, chlorpromazine, methotrimeprazine, nitrazepam
Cohen & Sprague, 1977	1,924	51	36	66	Thioridazine, phenytoin, phenobarbital, diazepam, primidone, mesoridazine
Hughes, 1977	219	NR	NR	68	Phenobarbital, phenytoin, diazepam, chlorpromazine, thioridazine, haloperidol
Pulman, Pook, & Singh, 1979	435	47	34	60	Phenytoin, diazepam, carbamazepine, trimeprazine, haloperidol, phenobarbital
Silva, 1979	260	NR	24	66	Phenytoin, phenobarbital, thioridazine, hydroxyzine, primidone
Tu, 1979	2,238	42	27	58	Thioridazine, chlorpromazine, mesoridazine, diazepam, thioxanthene
Craig & Behar, 1980 In 1970	161	83	NR	NR (83+)	Piperidine, aliphatic, & piperizine neuroleptics; tricyclic antidepressants

Study	N				Drugs
In 1977	92	86	NR	NR (86+)	Aliphatic, piperidine, & butyrophenone neuroleptics
Jonas, 1980	596	NR	NR	70	Chloral hydrate, carbamazepine, thioridazine, diazepam, haloperidol
Errickson, Bock, Young, & Silverstein, 1981					
Public residential facility	2,808	30	NR	NR	
Intermediate care	3,004	23	NR	NR	
White, 1983	415	19	36	51	Carbamazepine, thioridazine phenytoin, sodium valproate, haloperidol
Radinsky, 1984					
Public residential facility	1,687	27+	48	51	Phenytoin, phenobarbital, thioridazine, carbamazepine
Intermediate care	388	23+	56	67	Chlorpromazine, haloperidol
Hill, Balow, & Bruininks, 1985	992	30	36	51+	Anticonvulsants (unspecified), phenothiazines, hypnotics
Intagliata & Rinck, 1985	171	54	42	76	Phenytoin, phenobarbital, thioridazine, diazepam, chlorpromazine
Aman, Richmond, Stewart, Bell, & Kissel, 1987					
U.S.A.	531	37+	41	58	NR
New Zealand	937	39+	28	60	NR
B. Mentally retarded persons living in the community					
Hansen & Keogh, 1971	229 EH Pupils[b]	31	NR	NR	CNS sedatives/tranquilizers, CNS stimulants, antihistamines
Gadow & Kalachnik, 1981	3,306 TMR pupils[b]	7	12	18	Phenytoin, phenobarbital, methylphenidate, primidone, thioridazine, diazepam
Radinsky, 1984	575 CRF[b]	36	33	36	Thioridazine, phenytoin, phenobarbital, haloperidol, carbamazepine
Martin & Agran, 1985	178 CRA[b]	32+	24	48	Phenytoin, thioridazine, phenobarbital, haloperidol, chlorpromazine

(continued)

TABLE 1.1. (continued)

Authors	Number of persons surveyed	% Receiving psychotropic medication	% Receiving anticonvulsant drugs	Total percentage	Most common drugs prescribed
Aman, Field, & Bridgman, 1985					
Preschool children	126	2	31	33	Carbamazepine, phenytoin, thioridazine, sodium valproate, phenobarbital, haloperidol
Special schools	356	3	17	21	
Adult centers	530	14	18	29	
Hill et al., 1985	962 CRF[b]	26	22	40+	Anticonvulsants (unspecified), phenothiazines, benzodiazepines
Intagliata & Rinck, 1985	295 CRF[b]	36	21	48	Thioridazine, phenytoin, phenobarbital, primidone, chlorpromazine
Gowdey, Zarfas, & Phipps, 1987	1,389 GH[b]	20	23	40	Phenytoin, phenobarbital, carbamazepine, thioridazine, chlorpromazine
C. Other clinical populations					
Gadow, 1976	2,559 ECSE[b]	8	7	14	Methylphenidate, phenytoin, phenobarbital, primidone, thioridazine
Krager, Safer, & Earhart, 1979	3,867	15+	NR	NR	NR
Ahsanuddin, Ivey, Schlotzhauer, Hall, & Prosen, 1983	100 Psych[b]	66	NR	NR	Thioridazine, chlorpromazine, others unspecified
Gualtieri & Schroeder, 1985	1,467 CAS[b]	17	6	NR	Antipsychotics (unspecified), antiepileptics, antidepressants

Note. This table has been adapted and extended from an earlier publication (Aman, M.G. [1983]. Psychoactive drugs in mental retardation. In J.L. Matson & F. Andrasik (Eds.), *Treatment issues and innovations in mental retardation* [pp. 445–513]. New York: Pergamon Press) and is reproduced by permission.

[a]This figure may overestimate point prevalence as the survey asked how many residents had been, or were currently being, treated with psychotropic medication.

[b]NR = Not reported; EH = educationally handicapped; TMR = trainable mentally retarded; CRF = community residential facility; CRA = community residential agency; GH = group home; ECSE = Early Childhood Special Education Program (Illinois) for developmentally handicapped children, 3–5 years; CAS = children included in a Class Action suit (North Carolina) for children with behavior, developmental, and neurological handicaps.

nized as having psychoactive effects (see Chapter 5; Aman, 1983; Stores, 1978; Trimble & Reynolds, 1976). Studies in Table 1.1 are grouped by setting: institutions for mentally retarded residents, community placements (again with retarded persons), and an "Other" series involving mixed psychiatric populations. This type of classification is somewhat crude and not completely satisfactory for a variety of reasons but, in the interests of simplifying a large amorphous body of data, some classification scheme is needed. We have not summarized surveys among hyperactive (Attention Deficit Disorder) children of normal IQ. For the interested reader, these have been discussed in detail by Gadow (1981).

INSTITUTIONS FOR MENTALLY RETARDED PERSONS

In the present scheme, intermediate care facilities (ICFs) and psychiatric facilities caring for mentally retarded individuals have been categorized under this heading. Surveys within institutions for mentally retarded persons have found a wide variation of prevalence of psychotropic drugs ranging from 19% (White, 1983) to 86% (Craig & Behar, 1980). This latter figure may be misleading, however, as the survey was carried out in a psychiatric center that included mentally retarded residents. On average, rates of psychotropic drug use range from approximately 30% to 50%. Antiepileptic drugs were also frequently employed in such institutions, with a range of 24% (Spencer, 1974) to 56% (Radinsky, 1984). (One facility, surveyed by DiMascio [1975], is not considered representative because it exclusively cared for individuals having documented epilepsy.) Typical prevalence figures of antiepileptics ranged from 25% to 45%. Total prevalence of psychotropic and antiepileptic medication in these institutions ranged from 51% to 86% (Craig & Behar, 1980). If one excludes the latter, atypical study, the large majority of surveys have reported total prevalence figures between 50% and 70%.

MENTALLY RETARDED INDIVIDUALS IN THE COMMUNITY

There have been far fewer surveys of medication use in the community, and the populations being serviced tended to be more varied, so that the available data base is less complete. Among mentally retarded children, a range of 2% (Aman, Field, & Bridgman, 1985) to 7% (Gadow & Kalachnik, 1981) receiving psychotropic drugs has been reported. The figure of 31% reported by Hansen and Keogh (1971) is difficult to assess owing to a lack of information about survey methods and the drugs concerned. The prevalence of antiepileptic drugs was reported to vary from 12% (Gadow & Kalachnik, 1981) to 31% (Aman et al., 1985), and the combined rate of psychotropic and antiepileptic drug use ranged from 18% to 33%. However, the studies are so few and the classification of the children involved is so varied that little in the way of generalization is possible.

Surveys conducted of drug use with mentally retarded adults have reported a range from 14% (Aman et al. 1985) to 36% (Intagliata & Rinck, 1985; Radinsky, 1984). Excluding the lower figure, which was derived in New Zealand, most studies have reported medication rates in the range of 26% to 36% (Table 1.1). The reported prevalence of antiepileptic drug prescription has been quite consistent, ranging between 18% and 24% for most surveys. Finally, the prevalence of combined psychoactive medication has tended to fall into a fairly narrow range of 36% to 48% for most studies (Table 1.1).

OTHER POPULATIONS

Surveys with a variety of other clinical populations have been summarized in the last part of Table 1.1. As is readily apparent, the rates differed widely, no doubt reflecting the fact that markedly different populations were studied. We were unable to locate any drug surveys with autistic children.

SUMMARY

To recap, the following percentages have typically been found to be receiving psychotropic drugs: institutionalized mentally retarded persons, 30–50%; children in the community, 2–7%; and adults in the community, 26–36%. The figures for antiepileptic medication have predominantly been as follows: mentally retarded residents, 25–45%; children in the community, 12–31%; and adults in the community, 18–24%. Finally, typical ranges reported for total psychoactive drug use were: institutionalized populations, 50–70%; children in the community, 18–33%; and adults in the community, 36–48%.

It is quite clear that psychoactive drugs represent a prevalent mode, perhaps the single *most* common mode, of treatment with developmentally disabled children and adults. Furthermore, most of these studies assessed medication rates at only one point in time, and the absolute percentage of individuals who would receive medication at some time in their lives is higher still. We feel that these figures speak for themselves, and no serious professional in this field can afford to ignore major developments in psychopharmacology.

Patterns

Recently, a number of studies have examined factors associated with the use of psychotropic and antiepileptic drugs, but they mainly concern populations of mentally retarded individuals. In terms of *demographic* variables, the large majority of studies have found no relationship between sex and the use of psychotropic drugs (Aman et al., 1985; Gadow & Kalachnik, 1981; Hill et al., 1985; Intagliata & Rinck, 1985), although Tu and Smith (1979, 1983) noted a higher prevalence among female residents. Age has been found to be positively associated with psychotropic drugs in a number of studies, with older subjects typically receiving more medication (e.g., Aman et al., 1985; DiMascio, 1975; Errickson et al., 1981; Hill et al., 1985; Intagliata & Rinck, 1985). Most studies that have examined level of mental retardation (or functional level) in relation to psychoactive drug use have found significantly higher rates of antiepileptic drugs among more severely impaired subjects (Aman et al., 1985; Intagliata & Rinck, 1985; Zimmerman & Heistad, 1980). Two studies have looked at residential placement and found markedly higher rates of psychotropic medication in larger and/or more restrictive residential placements in the community (Aman et al., 1985; Martin & Agran, 1985).

Aman et al. (1985) have examined a variety of *physical* variables (blindness, deafness, cerebral palsy, and epilepsy) in relation to prescription patterns. Blindness and deafness bore no relationship to either antiepileptic or psychotropic drugs, but a diagnosis of either epilepsy or cerebral palsy was associated with lower rates of psychotropic medication use. Last, some investigators have looked at *social/behavioral* variables in relation to psychotropic medication and found that higher ratings of social, behavioral, and sleep problems are associated with greater usage of psychotropic drugs (Aman et al., 1985; Zimmerman & Heistad, 1980). Tu and Smith (1983) have surveyed five institutions and identified behavioral and psychiatric problems associated with pharmacotherapy. The six most common problems and their prevalences among medicated individuals were as follows: aggressivity (29%), hyperactivity (24%), self-injury (19%), "excitability" (12%), screaming (10%), and anxiety (8%). Intagliata and Rinck (1985) examined behavior problems most associated with neuroleptic drugs in community residential facilities (CRFs) and public residential facilities (PRFs) and found that hyperactivity appeared to be tied to medication use in CRFs, whereas violent/destructive behavior was the strongest predictor in PRFs.

Bates, Smeltzer, and Arnoczky (1986) attempted to assess the appropriateness of psychotropic drug prescription in several institutions by comparing medication type with diagnosis. A sample of 242 residents was selected from a much larger group because these patients had been assigned a unanimous psychiatric diagnosis by a multidisciplinary team. Each combination of diagnosis and medication was rated according to generally recommended standards of drug treatment. Bates et al. found that 94 of these diagnosis/drug combinations were appropriate, 32 uncertain, and 81 probably inappropriate. In percentage terms, 45% were rated appropriate, 16% as uncertain, and 39% as probably inappropriate. Bates et al. described their judgments as conservative, and they remarked that the extent of inappropriate medication use (perhaps as high as 55%) was extremely high.

Recently, we conducted a survey among nursing staff, who are largely responsible for the day-to-day care of mentally retarded residents, in two institutions (Aman, Singh, & White, 1987; Aman, Singh, & Fitzpatrick,

1987). Drug use appeared to be largely governed by senior nursing staff and ward doctors, whereas other professionals had little input into drug decisions. Furthermore, greater age, status, qualifications, and male sex tended to covary among nurses and, although these traits were associated with greater influence on medication decisions, they were often not correlated with knowledge needed for such a role.

Comments

Finally, some comments seem in order regarding these drug prevalence and pattern studies. First, there is an abundance of surveys of drug prevalence in institutions for mentally retarded persons, although the same cannot be said of community surveys or studies with other clinical populations. It seems to us that there is little need for more prevalence studies in institutions unless they focus on *new* issues such as the success of drug reduction programs, appropriateness of medication, and so forth. Second, many have concluded from prevalence data alone that prescription rates are excessive. Although this may well be correct, such conclusions cannot be drawn without relevant data on the costs and clinical benefits derived (see Aman, 1985). The study by Bates et al. (1986), for example, is one of the few to address the issue of appropriateness of these treatments. The issues surrounding drug use are complex and the role of medication can only be resolved by the collection of valid and reliable data relating to the actual effects and costs associated with such treatment.

Programs to Reduce Medication Use

Recently, reports have appeared describing programs to reduce the prevalence of psychotropic drug use in facilities for mentally retarded people. The strategies have varied greatly, but several programs were based on an active commitment by pharmacy, psychology, or other staff to reduce unnecessary use of medication, to minimize polypharmacy, and to base treatment on widely accepted principles of drug use (Berchou, 1982; Ellenor & Frisk, 1977; Gerard, Podboy, & Boldt, 1981; Inoue, 1982; James, 1983; LaMendola, Zaharia, & Carver, 1980). Briggs, Hamad, Garrard, and Wills (1985) described a medication reduction program calling for objective identification of subject behaviors requiring treatment, baseline data, and regular multidisciplinary assessments. Another program adopted what appear to be objective subject criteria and determined drug reductions and increases on frequency counts of maladaptive behavior (Fielding, Murphy, Reagan, & Peterson, 1980).

It is difficult to characterize the extent of reduction achieved across these studies because the initial drug prevalence rates differed widely, and the drugs were classified in markedly different ways. Nevertheless, substantial reductions were achieved, ranging from an 18% drop in neuroleptic use in one study (Ellenor & Frisk, 1977) to a 57% decrease in another (Fielding et al., 1980). Where the data were available, total psychotropic prevalence rates were reported to range from 21% (LaMendola et al., 1980) to a high of 33% (Inoue, 1982) after institution of the programs, levels well below most of those reported in Table 1.1 for similar populations.

All of these programs were committed to reductions in the prevalence of drug use, smaller doses, and decreased polypharmacy, and it is likely that a prevailing sentiment existed in these facilities that medication is undesirable. Nevertheless, large reductions were widely achieved without obvious repercussions, such as deterioration in resident behavior. This suggests that much of the previous medication was in fact unnecessary. Unfortunately, only three of these studies (Ellenor & Frisk, 1977; Fielding et al., 1980; Gerard et al., 1981) reported any attempt to monitor objectively resident *behavior* while drugs were being phased out. Two of these reports suggested that drug reductions did not come at the expense of behavioral control, although the ways in which the data were collected make it impossible to reach such a conclusion firmly. In contrast, Gerard et al. (1981) found a significant correlation between medication reduction and both frequency ($r = -.53$) and amount ($r = -.46$) of restrictive procedures used to control disturbed behavior, which suggests that some behaviors did deteriorate as a result of drug withdrawal. This question of the interplay between behavioral effects and drug reduction and alternative behavioral control methods is important and worthy of much more attention in future attempts to minimize medication use.

Finally, there have been several studies looking at the success with which patients can be weaned off antiepileptic drugs after a period of seizure control. The issues are different here as (unlike the case with psychotropic drugs) there is little argument about the need for pharmacotherapy where a bona fide seizure disorder exists. In one study, Holowach, Thurstone, and O'Leary (1972) attempted to phase out antiepileptic medication in a mixed diagnostic group of 148 epileptic children (generally of normal IQ) who had been seizure-free for 4 years. Medication was tapered off over 3-month intervals and, when more than one drug was prescribed, only one medication was discontinued at a time. Thirty-six children (24%) relapsed, but the remainder (76%) continued to be seizure-free after drug withdrawal over a period of 5 to 12 years. Emerson et al. (1981) conducted a similar evaluation with 68 children who had also been seizure-free for 4 years. Fifty of the subjects (74%) were seizure-free after drug withdrawal, and statistical projections suggested that the probability of remaining free of seizures for 4 years after discontinuance was 69%. It is pertinent to point out here that both studies found that mental retardation and other "organic" factors were prognostic indicators associated with higher relapse rates.

Holowach et al. (1972) also surveyed other studies that phased out antiepileptic medication and assessed the rates of relapse. Most of these began to taper off medication after 2 seizure-free years, and the clinical populations were often unrepresentative of the greater epileptic population. Medication was successfully withdrawn from 54% to 79% of the patients in these studies. Although the rates of relapse in some investigations exceeded those in the above reports, these figures indicate that it is possible eventually to discontinue antiepileptic therapy for a large proportion of epileptic patients when they have been seizure-free for 2 or more years.

To summarize, these studies of psychotropic and antiepileptic drug discontinuation are noteworthy because they parallel a widespread movement to minimize or reduce the use of psychoactive drugs. The studies of psychotropic drug withdrawal indicated little in the way of clinical repercussions, suggesting that much of the medication was unnecessary either originally or at the time of the reduction programs. Given increasing pressures to justify ongoing medication use, these investigations may serve as models for monitoring and reducing medication, although in future endeavors we would like to see a much greater commitment to the concomitant measurement of behavior changes than has been evident in the past. Only in this way can any trade-off (e.g., increases in physical restraint) be determined as a consequence of such reduction programs.

Methodological and Dosage Considerations

Sprague and Werry (1971) are generally credited with first pointing out six minimal requirements for a scientifically controlled study in this field. These include provision of placebo controls, random assignment of subjects to drug groups, blind evaluations of drug effects to minimize bias, standardized doses, the use of standardized (i.e., valid and reliable) measures of drug effect, and appropriate use of inferential statistics to assess the significance of drug-related changes. We have suggested adding another criterion, namely that, where possible, trials should be free of other drugs that could potentially confound the actions of the agent under study (Aman & Singh, 1980). Readers not familiar with these methodological issues should consult Sprague and Werry's original review or one of the many methodological reviews that are available (e.g., Wysocki & Fuqua, 1982).

It is unfortunate but correct to say that the large majority of drug studies of earlier (pre-1975) years in this field violated one or more of these criteria (Aman & Singh, 1980; Lipman, DiMascio, Reatig, & Kirson, 1978; Sprague & Werry, 1971). More recently, the level of sophistication has risen markedly, such that the number of adequately controlled studies probably exceeds that of uncontrolled reports. This is a trend that is greatly to be encouraged, although we must also acknowledge that the difficulties in working with developmentally disabled people often make it particularly challenging to conduct elaborate research in this field (Aman, 1987).

To change gears slightly, the selection of the optimal dosage regimen for research, with this and other clinical populations, has been a vexing problem. Many researchers point to the widely differing blood concentrations that are observed when a standardized dose (i.e., based on body weight) of a drug is given to a group of subjects. For this reason, many researchers prefer to titrate dosage separately for each individual in the study. Usually, this entails increasing the dosage until the "optimal" clinical effect is seen or until side effects begin to interfere with desired changes. Although this appears to cope with the problem of wide individual differences of response, the use of titration poses a number of research dilemmas as well. First, the reliability of the procedure is unknown (and unresearched) and it is, therefore, likely that different clinicians would titrate to entirely different doses for the same patients. This means that the magnitude of the independent variables may be essentially uncontrolled and not amenable to comparison across studies. Second, it seems to us that titration of this type may introduce additional problems of control, insofar as the clinician is very likely to witness side effects with active drug and none with placebo. There are also potential problems relating to interpretation, as the subject may improve because of a recent increase in dosage or because of circumstances unknown to the experimenter. In a similar vein, higher doses may be confounded with greater time on medication. Third, the procedure *seems* tautological in that the use of titration is tantamount to prejudging the nature of drug-related changes. As we argued elsewhere (Aman, 1983), it assumes that the investigator can reliably forecast the optimal dosage level before having access to the results of the study.

The most common alternative to the use of titrated doses is to employ standardized doses based on the subject's body weight. This has the advantage of being objective and, therefore, allowing comparisons across studies. Its major disadvantage is that the concentration of drug in the central nervous system may differ markedly across subjects. However, some workers have employed standardized doses of neuroleptic drugs and obtained results as favorable as those derived with titration (Singh & Aman, 1981). Others have observed characteristic dose response curves with neuroleptics in hyperactive children, in which different types of behavior changed with different doses (Werry & Aman, 1975; Werry, Aman, & Lampen 1975). Sprague & Sleator (1975, 1977) have carried out an important series of dose studies with methylphenidate (Ritalin) in hyperactive children of normal IQ and found that learning performance peaked at low to moderate doses and worsened thereafter, whereas behavioral compliance improved steadily with dose. Others still have found well defined dose patterns with methylphenidate on other behavioral and learning variables in hyperactive children (Pelham Bender, Caddell, Booth, & Moorer, 1985; Rapport & Du Paul, 1986; see Werry, in press).

In our own research, we have generally favored the use of standardized doses over individualized doses for the aforementioned reasons. However, we do not wish to be polemical about this, and at present both must be regarded as valid approaches but with different advantages and drawbacks. However, this is an issue that can be clarified empirically, and a given approach for establishing dosage may be regarded as demonstrably superior for particular research questions. Therefore, in the absence of further evidence on this issue, each approach should be regarded as legitimate. On occasion, we and others have been criticized for employing standarized doses, but we hope that workers will make an effort to familiarize themselves with both sides of the issue. Finally, it should be pointed out that certain drugs (such as many of the antiepileptics) can be measured in the blood to guide their clinical use, and with time it may be possible to measure and adjust meaningfully the concentrations of many psychotropic drugs in this way (see Chapter 3).

Measures of Drug Effect

This section has been included to give the reader some grasp of the measurement techniques that are available for psychopharmacological research with developmentally disabled people. Some of the most commonly used measures have been summarized in the following sections.

Global Impressions

Ratings of overall behavior change, in terms of the rater's subjective impressions of the subject, have been and continue to be widely used in drug studies with mentally retarded persons (Wysocki & Fuqua, 1982). One of the problems with the use of global impressions as a dependent variable is that there is no objective way of knowing the criteria against which changes are judged to have occurred. For example, the importance of changes in a number of variables may be differentially rated depending on the context of the observations. Changes in learning and cognition may be rated more positively in an environment in which greater emphasis is placed on academic competence rather than compliant behavior, whereas the reverse may be true in a more custodial environment. Thus, ratings of global impressions are useful as general detectors of drug effects in that they provide a measure of change as seen by those who are responsible for the subjects. However, it is imperative that other measures also be used to provide qualitative information on the specific nature of the observed changes.

Direct Behavioral Observations

Systematic behavioral observations provide another group of measures that are less prone to bias than global impressions (Kent, O'Leary, Dietz,

& Diament, 1974; Towns, Singh, & Beale, 1984). Only recently have direct observations become widely used in psychopharmacological research, particularly with persons with developmental disabilities. For example, in reviewing studies up until 1979, Aman and Singh (1980) reported that of the 24 investigations of thioridazine in childhood disorders, only 4 used direct observations. The situation has changed dramatically over the last few years, with the use of direct observations being very common in current drug research with mentally retarded persons.

There are a number of ways in which direct observations can be used to assess the impact of drugs on behavior. It is useful to remember that the basic principles of behavioral assessment in applied behavior analysis still pertain when direct observations are used in psychopharmacology. Target behaviors can be selected on the basis of preliminary observations using the descriptive method proposed by Bijou, Peterson, and Ault (1968). This is followed by precisely defining the target behaviors with regard to objectivity, clarity, and completeness (Hawkins & Dobes, 1976). Because psychotropic drugs usually have general as well as specific effects, it is important to sample a broad range of behaviors, including both adaptive and maladaptive. Observational data on target behaviors can be collected by using one or more of the standard procedures, including frequency counts, interval recording, time sampling, and measures of response latency and duration. The procedure used will depend on a number of considerations, including the topography and rate of behaviors observed, the experience and training of the observers, and the goals of the study (Singh & Beale, 1986). These and other issues pertinent to direct observations (e.g., interobserver reliability, observation schedule) in psychopharmacological research in mental retardation are comprehensively reviewed by Aman and White (1986).

Rating Scales

Rating scales are the major source of assessment data on behavior change in pediatric psychopharmacology (Werry, 1978). However, they have not had such wide currency in drug studies with persons with developmental disabilities, and even when they have been used, more often than not investigators have tended to use ad hoc scales with unknown psychometric properties. Nevertheless, a small number of scales used in recent drug studies with mentally retarded subjects have been shown to have adequate factorial and clinical validity, including the Aberrant Behavior Checklist (Aman & Singh, 1986) and the Devereaux Child Behavior Scale (Spivack & Spotts, 1965). The Aberrant Behavior Checklist is of recent origin and is probably the most used instrument at present for assessing drugs in institutional populations. Other scales include Conners's Teacher Rating Scale (Conners, 1969), the Mental Retardation Psychiatric Rating Scale (Ruoff, Howell, Wakker, & Roberts, 1988), and the Nurses' Observation Scales for Inpatient Evaluation (NOSIE) (Honigfeld, 1974). Conners's Teacher Rating Scale has been used in only two drug studies with mentally retarded persons (see Aman & White, 1986). It was developed with children of normal IQ, and its use would appear to be questionable with children of low functional level. The Mental Retardation Psychiatric Rating Scale provides a global index of change, and while it is likely that this scale may be useful in drug research, more psychometric data on its clinical validity are needed before it can be recommended for general use. The NOSIE was devised for use with psychiatric populations, and its usefulness with developmentally disabled persons remains to be established. With the exception of one study (Heistad, Zimmermann, & Doebler, 1982), this scale has not been used for drug research with mentally retarded persons.

Although there are numerous scales designed for measuring behavior change in developmentally disabled populations (Walls, Werner, Bacon, & Zane, 1977), most have not been used in psychopharmacological investigations. It may well be the case that one or more of these scales will prove to be sensitive to drug effects, but this remains to be demonstrated. Further information and a detailed discussion of issues relating to rating scales used with mentally retarded persons can be found in Sprague and Werry (1971), Werry (1978), and Aman and White (1986). Campbell and Palij (1985) have provided an excellent summary of rating scales suitable for measuring drug effects on autistic children.

Learning Measures

Beginning with the earliest reviews of the literature, there has been a consistent call for measures of cognition and learning to be included in the assessment of drug effects in studies with developmentally disabled persons (e.g., Sprague & Werry, 1971). Given that the major problem of developmentally disabled persons is usually one of learning rather than of maladaptive behavior, it is highly desirable that drug assessment measures include indices of cognition and learning. Several such measures are now available for use in psychopharmacological investigations. These include IQ tests, achievement tests, measures relevant to classroom and vocational settings, discrimination learning tasks, and performance tests (e.g., attention tasks). It should be noted that IQ and achievement tests are not very sensitive to drug effects (Werry & Sprague, 1972) and, where possible, performance tests should be included in the test battery as they appear to be more readily influenced by medication. In addition, there is some indication in the literature that operant conditioning and discrimination learning tasks are useful indices for psychopharmacological research with developmentally disabled persons. Aman (1984) and Aman and White (1986) have reviewed a number of other tests and tasks that can be used for this purpose but, due to the rather limited data base, no conclusions can be drawn about their general utility in drug research. Suffice it to say here that the assessment of changes in learning performance is a major difficulty in this field because this is the very area in which these subjects are most deficient. It is clear from the literature, however, that few indices of cognition and learning have been employed to measure drug effects in studies with developmentally disabled people. Therefore, it is important that appropriate learning measures be developed and used much more frequently in future studies.

Other Measures

Mechanical transducers may be useful for assessing changes in physical activity, such as stereotypic behavior, movement during sleep, and hypo- or hyperactivity (see Pfadt & Tryon, 1983). Play is another important adaptive activity in this population, but it has rarely been the subject of drug research with developmentally disabled persons (Aman & White, 1986). The issue of drug effects on motor coordination and motor steadiness is certainly a relevant one, but it has similarly been neglected in this field. Finally, physiological measures comprise another group of indices that is discussed in greater detail later in this chapter. Aman and White (1986) and Werry (1978) describe a number of other measures that may be valuable for assessing pharmacological effects in this population.

Future Directions

Using the greater field of psychopharmacology as well as current social changes as a weather vane, it is possible to make some calculated guesses about future directions for research in this field. Some of our predictions are discussed in the following paragraphs.

Dual Diagnosis

One neglected aspect of psychopharmacology in this field is that of dual diagnosis (i.e., the classification of individuals with both a developmental handicap *and* a psychiatric disorder). The vast majority of past investigations have studied subjects with an amorphous collection of symptoms, which in no way could be thought to reflect a diagnosis, syndrome, or even a collection of syndromes. There is now a small but growing literature showing that some developmentally disabled people do exhibit the full spectrum of psychiatric disorders (Costello, 1982; Eaton & Menolascino, 1982; Reiss, 1982), although there is wide variability in the prevalence figures reported.

It is well established that certain classes of psychotropic drugs are effective for treating specific types of psychiatric disorders in the normal IQ population. However, a dilemma exists in the developmental disabilities field, because the expression of a given disorder may change as functional level declines. For example, it logically becomes more difficult to establish the presence of delusions, hallucinations, and so forth, or to probe about the subject's affect as verbal ability decreases. Does this mean that certain symptoms of the psychoses, for example, do not exist among severely/profoundly retarded individuals or simply that we are poorly equipped to identify them? The fact is that at this stage we do not know. The implications for the use of pharmacotherapy are profound, as the rational use of psychotropic drugs presumes an appropriate match between diagnosis and class of medication prescribed.

Two types of assessment are needed to make progress in this area. First, a valid diagnostic system is required. This may be achieved through observational procedures, the use of self-report and rating scales, and clinical assessment of signs and symptoms of psychiatric disorders. Some attempts have been made to develop diagnostic instruments, such as a modified version of the Manifest Abnormalities Scale (from the Clinical Interview Schedule, see Ballinger, Armstrong, Presly, & Reid, 1975) and the Psychopathology Instrument for Mentally Retarded Adults (Senatore, Matson, & Kazdin, 1985). Nevertheless, these systems are largely based on established patterns of psychopathology in the population of normal IQ people, and it remains to be seen whether these patterns can be applied without change across the continuum of mental handicap (Aman, 1987). At least one study suggests that this may not be appropriate (Watson, Aman, & Singh, in press).

The second form of assessment that is needed is a suitable measure of treatment effectiveness. The Aberrant Behavior Checklist (Aman & Singh, 1986), mentioned previously, is useful in drug studies with institutionalized populations. The Behavior Disturbance Scale (Leudar, Fraser, & Jeeves, 1984) may also be useful for this purpose, although it has not been used in drug studies thus far. To our knowledge, no rating scale has been developed to assess maladaptive behavior in noninstitutionalized mentally retarded children.

The pendulum has clearly swung away from the indiscriminant use of medication for suppression of isolated behavior problems not associated with a specific disorder or syndrome. At the same time, we do not have sufficient or satisfactory means of diagnosing developmentally disabled people and measuring treatment effects. Indeed, this was the sole topic at a recent workshop sponsored by the NIMH New Clinical Drug Evaluation Unit (Special Workshop, 1986). It appears, therefore, that the issue of dual diagnosis will, of necessity, be a dominant one in future work among mentally retarded populations.

Work with Noninstitutionalized Populations

Although there is a tendency for more disturbed and impaired individuals to be placed and retained within institutions, it is also true that the great majority (perhaps 90%) of mentally retarded and other developmentally disabled people do not reside in such facilities. In addition, the recent endorsement of deinstitutionalization and normalization is leading to marked reductions in the numbers of persons retained within institutions. Despite this fact, only a handful of studies with mentally retarded people have been carried out in community residential settings. As Lipman (1982) first pointed out, this is an anomaly that can no longer be ignored. If our research is to be relevant to the greatest number, then more investigators must be prepared to carry out this work with individuals who are living in the community, such as with mentally retarded children living at home or retarded adults living in group homes and foster homes. Logistically, such research is much more difficult than that conducted within large institutions, and it may demand modifications in research methodology. It is also likely that such a shift in setting will result in a new conceptualization of what is regarded as desirable change, an issue discussed next.

Quality of Care

Recently, there have been calls for the "quality of care" dimension to be taken into account in treatment evaluation (Aman, 1985; Mouchka, 1985). These workers argue that the philosophical orientation of the residential facility may determine whether a given treatment regimen is perceived as beneficial and encouraged or as an intrusion on established ward, school, or home routines and, therefore, discouraged. For example, a progressive and caring facility may perceive the use of a certain drug as beneficial if its residents are more alert and participate actively in ward programs. On the other hand, a more custodial facility may view the same drug effects as adversely affecting ward routines because the residents now demand more attention and positive social interaction. In addition to philosophical orientation, demographic and social-psychological variables have been found to influence the type of care provided to residents (Zigler, Balla, & Styfco, 1984).

Given that a large number of variables influence the behavior of both the caregiver and the subject, it could be important to measure their effects in any comprehensive evaluation of medication. Although it is difficult to see how the effects of all of these conditions can be precisely quantified, it is feasible that a global index of the quality of care provided by the residential facility can be ascertained. For example, the Child Management Scale (King, Raynes, & Tizard, 1971; McCormick, Balla, & Zigler, 1975) could be used in drug studies to describe resident care practices at the facility where the investigation is carried out. Similar evaluations of community residential facilities should perhaps be undertaken if drug studies are undertaken in these places. Such indices would enable us to appreciate treatment outcome data better, as we would then have some indication, even if only a global one, of the resident care practices of the facility.

Neuropharmacology

Current research suggests that, with time, we may be able to use blood levels of various neurochemicals as a way to classify and treat behavior disorders in developmentally disabled people. For example, one study by Greenberg and Coleman (1976) suggested that abnormalities of serotonin are related to behavioral disturbance in mentally retarded persons. A substantial body of research has suggested that serotonin levels are elevated in some mentally retarded individuals and autistic children (Coleman & Gillberg, 1985; Schain & Freedman, 1961; see Chapter 7). If serotonin exerts a causal or intermediary influence on the behavior of some of these children, then this may provide a logical avenue for modifying maladaptive behavior. This has been the rationale for a recent series of studies on a serotonin-depleting agent, fenfluramine, with autistic children (see Chapter 7; Ritvo et al., 1986). Serotonin is only one of many neurotransmitters, any one of which may be causally implicated in various developmental disabilities. The search for neurochemical imbalances and attempts to rectify these pharmacologically will undoubtedly be a major area of enquiry in future drug studies with developmentally disabled populations (see Chapters 7 and 10). However, only time will tell how productive this strategy will be for the field.

Blood Levels

It is widely accepted that patients respond differentially to many medications, even when given standardized (mg/kg) doses. Several reasons may account for this, including presence of different target disorders, variable patient compliance with the treatment regimen, and uncontrolled pharmacokinetic variables. This means that the available concentration of the drug under study, or its active metabolites, at the relevant site of action will vary between patients. The availability of blood concentration measurements opens up new strategies for drug research because such measures provide a drug index that can be related to change in clinical variables (see Chapter 3). Nevertheless, there is some disagreement in the research literature as to whether there is a clear relationship between drug concentrations in the blood and clinical response to that drug (Curry, 1978; Davis, Erickson, & Dekirmenjian, 1978). To some extent, methodological and technical problems in reliably measuring blood levels have contributed to this controversy. A number of techniques for measuring blood levels have been used (e.g., spectrophotometry, radioimmunoassay, isotope derivative dilution analysis, thin-layer chromatography, gas-liquid chromatography, mass fragmentography, and fluorimetry) (Lader, 1980; Norman & Burrows, 1981), but each has drawbacks that may limit their usefulness in drug research with developmentally disabled persons (see Lader, 1980). Recently, the radioreceptor assay has been advocated for measuring the dopamine-blocking action of neuroleptic drugs in serum or plasma (Creese & Snyder, 1977). However, there are technical problems that make the use of this procedure questionable for quantifying active drugs and metabolites in the blood (Mailman, De Haven, Halpern, & Lewis, 1984; Mailman, Pierce, et al., 1984).

An important issue insofar as the use of blood levels is concerned is the current lack of agreement on the clinically useful range of blood concentrations indicative of therapeutic change (see Chapter 3). However, measurement of blood levels may prove useful not only for research purposes but also for clinical decision making. As noted by Lewis and Mailman (Chapter 3), future research may establish "therapeutic windows" (i.e., dose response curves) for specific disorders, identify drug nonresponders, ascertain patient compliance, and assist in avoiding toxic doses. Thus, the use of drug blood levels may well help us to resolve some of the apparently conflicting results found in the literature today.

Psychophysiological Indices

Many psychiatric disorders are accompanied by physiological manifestations. For example, heart rate and blood pressure may be abnormal in mania, anxiety states, and psychotic conditions such as depression (Silverstone & Turner, 1974). Thus, psychophysiological measures may be useful in drug research for classification of initial subject status and additionally they may provide a sensitive measure of drug effects. For example, one enthusiastic group of investigators has gone so far as to claim "that every drug which has psychotropic properties produces systematic. . . effects on human brain function. . . as assessed by [computer analyzed] EGG" (p. 111) and that this particular measure can predict a given drug's "therapeutic window. . . its therapeutic potency. . . and its bioavailability in the target organ, the brain" (p. 113) (Itil et al., 1985).

Dependent measures of interest in drug research (such as learning performance) often require the subject's active cooperation, and many developmentally disabled subjects may not be able to comply with such procedures because of behavior problems or low functional levels. Physiological measures may be an attractive alternative method for assessing functional areas otherwise not amenable to measurement. A large array of psychophysiological measures is potentially available for use in pharmacological studies. Although there is not room to discuss them here, many of the available psychophysiological measures are reviewed by Katkin and Hastrup (1982), Hastings and Barkley (1978), and Silverstone and Turner (1974).

Thus far, psychophysiological indices have rarely been used in drug studies with persons with developmental disabilities, two exceptions being a study by Lobb (1968) using the Galvanic Skin Response in mentally retarded residents and an investigation by Frager, Barnet, Weiss, and Coleman (1985) in which auditory evoked potentials were assessed in autistic children. It is likely that drug researchers in the future will be attracted to psychophysiological measures to fill a noticeable void in our knowledge and to take advantage of the many technological advances that are constantly unfolding. However, it is well to remember that the clinical validity of many of these measures is far from established and, furthermore, this is a population whose clinical problems (especially among those likely to be in drug studies) make them very difficult to assess. Problems of noncompliance and lack of cooperation may pose major barriers to the use of these measures, but this is an issue that will only be resolved by serious and innovative attempts to exploit these techniques.

Conclusions

It is clear from treatment prevalence studies that psychotropic and antiepileptic drugs are prescribed frequently for mentally retarded people, although there is evidence of some reduction in recent years. Surveys have typically shown that 30% to 50% of institutionalized mentally retarded residents receive psychotropic medication. This figure drops to approximately 26% to 36% for retarded adults and to 2% to 7% of mentally retarded children living in the community. We are not aware of any drug prevalence studies among autistic children. Studies of drug patterns have suggested that age, more restrictive placement, and behavioral and sleep problems are positively associated with psychotropic drug use, whereas functional level, cerebral palsy, and epilepsy appear to be associated with fewer psychotropic drugs. There have been numerous programs to reduce the use of psychotropic medication in recent years, and these appear to result in a marked drop in drug prescription. Unfortunately, few of these programs have simultaneously monitored clinicial behavior, so that we are uncertain whether there were any behavioral/clinical costs in phasing out the medication. Studies with antiepileptic medications suggest that, after two to four seizure-free years, these drugs can be successfully withdrawn from 54% to 79% of epileptic patients (Holowach et al., 1972), although developmentally disabled people are at higher risk of relapse.

Although methodology in the field historically has been poor, there are signs of growing sophistication in recent years. The means for adjusting dosage can be a contentious issue and both individualized and standardized regimens should be acceptable in the absence of further empirical data. Traditionally, clinical global impressions have tended to be the dominant measure of drug response. Of late, however, there is a growing use of more objective measures such as direct observations of behavior and standardized rating scales. Also, workers are beginning to show far greater ingenuity in devising other suitable measures such as tests of learning. In forecasting future trends, we identify the development of more suitable diagnostic systems, specifically tailored for developmentally disabled persons, as a high priority. It also appears that the social movement toward normalization and deinstitutionalization will have profound implications for drug research and, if this work is to be relevant, more of it will have to take place in the community. This also ties in with the quality-of-care dimension, which has been almost totally ignored in the past. Specific areas in which we are likely to see greater endeavor include neurochemistry, pharmacokinetics, and the study of psychophysiological changes. It is clear that if such areas of expertise are to be integrated in a meaningful way, a much greater commitment to interdisciplinary research will need to occur than has been evident in the past.

In previous reviews, we and other writers (Aman & Singh, 1983; Lipman et al., 1978; Sprague & Werry, 1971) were forced to conclude that specific indications for the various psychotropic drugs in mental retardation were not established. This is the case despite dozens, perhaps hundreds, of studies in the field. Considerable criticism has been aimed at previous drug research, some of which was clearly inferior to parallel work occurring with other clinical populations. It is well to remember, however, that the people whom we study usually present special problems for research. Not only do they typically have cognitive dysfunction (usually in conjunction with behavioral or psychiatric disturbances), but we have been sailing uncharted waters insofar as differential diagnosis is concerned. It is clear that this field presents major challenges, even to the serious and seasoned researcher.

Acknowledgments. We wish to thank Marsha Aman for typing of the drafts leading to this manuscript. We also thank Dr. Ken Gadow (State University of New York at Stony Brook) and Professor John Werry and Dr. Rob Kydd (University of Auckland) for critical comments on the chapter. This work was supported in part by a grant from the Medical Research Council of New Zealand to Dr. M.G. Aman.

References

Ahsanuddin, K.M., Ivey, J.A., Schlotzhauer, D., Hall, K., & Prosen, H. (1983). Psychotropic medication prescription patterns in 100 hospitalized children and adolescents. *Journal of the American Academy of Child Psychiatry*, *22*, 361–364.

Aman, M.G. (1983). Psychoactive drugs in mental retardation. In J.L. Matson & F. Andrasik (Eds.), *Treatment issues and innovations in mental retardation* (pp. 455–513). New York: Plenum Press.

Aman, M.G. (1984). Drugs and learning in mentally retarded persons. In G.D. Burrows & J.S. Werry (Eds.), *Advances in human psychopharmacology* (Vol. 3, pp. 121–163). Greenwich, CT: JAI Press.

Aman, M.G. (1985). Drugs in mental retardation: Treatment or tragedy? *Australia and New Zealand Journal of Developmental Disabilities*, *10*, 215–226.

Aman, M.G. (1987). Overview of pharmacotherapy: Current status and future directions. *Journal of Mental Deficiency Research*, *31*, 215–225.

Aman, M.G., Field, C.J., & Bridgman, G.D. (1985). City-wide survey of drug patterns among non-institutionalized retarded persons. *Applied Research in Mental Retardation*, *5*, 159–171.

Aman, M.G., Richmond, G., Steward, A.W., Bell, J.C., & Kissel, R.C. (1987). The Aberrant Behavior Checklist: Factorial validity and the effect of demographic/medical variables in American and New Zealand facilities. *American Journal of Mental Deficiency*, *91*, 570–578.

Aman, M.G. & Singh, N.N. (1980). The usefulness of thioridazine for treating childhood disorders: Fact or folklore. *American Journal of Mental Deficiency*, *4*, 331–338.

Aman, M.G., & Singh, N.N. (1983). Pharmacological intervention. In J.L. Matson & J.A. Mulick (Eds.), *Handbook of mental retardation* (pp. 317–337). New York: Pergamon Press.

Aman, M.G., & Singh, N.N. (1986). *Aberrant Behavior Checklist: Manual*. East Aurora, NY: Slosson Educational.

Aman, M.G., Singh, N.N., & Fitzpatrick, J. (1987). The relationship between nurse characteristics and perceptions of psychotropic medications in residential facilities. *Journal of Autism and Developmental Disorders*, *17*, 511–523.

Aman, M.G., Singh, N.N., & White, A.J. (1987). Caregiver perceptions of psychotropic medication in residential facilities. *Research in Developmental Disabilities*, *8*, 449–465.

Aman, M.G., & White, A.J. (1986). Measures of drug change in mental retardation. In K.D. Gadow (Ed.), *Advances in learning and behavioral disabilities* (pp. 159–205). Greenwich, CT: JAI Press.

Ballinger, B.R., Armstrong, J., Presly, A.S., & Reid, A.H. (1975). Use of a standardized psychiatric interview in mentally handicapped patients. *British Journal of Psychiatry*, *127*, 540–544.

Bates, W.J., Smeltzer, D.J., & Arnoczky, S.M. (1986). Appropriate and inappropriate use of psychotherapeutic medications for institutionalized mentally retarded persons. *American Journal of Mental Deficiency*, *90*, 363–370.

Berchou, R.C. (1982). Effect of a consultant pharmacist on medication use in an institution for the mentally retarded. *American Journal of Hospital Pharmacy*, *39*, 1671–1674.

Bijou, S.W., Peterson, R.F., & Ault, M.H. (1968). A method to integrate descriptive and experimental field studies at the level of data and empirical concepts. *Journal of Applied Behavior Analysis*, *1*, 175–191.

Briggs, R., Hamad, C., Garrard, S., & Wills, F. (1985). A model for evaluating psychoactive medication use with mentally retarded persons. In J. Mulick & B. Mallany (Eds.), *Transitions in mental retardation: Advocacy, technology and science* (pp. 229–248). Norwood, NJ: Ablex.

Campbell, M., & Palij, M. (1985). Behavioral and cognitive measures used in psychopharmacological studies of infantile autism. *Psychopharmacology Bulletin*, *21*, 1047–1052.

Cohen, M.N., & Sprague, R.L. (1977, March). *Survey of drug usage in two midwestern institutions for the retarded*. Paper presented at the Gatlinburg Conference on Research in Mental Retardation, Gatlinburg, TN.

Coleman, M., & Gillberg, C. (1985). *The biology of the autistic syndromes.* New York: Praeger.

Conners, C.K. (1969). A teacher rating scale for use in drug studies with children. *American Journal of Psychiatry, 126,* 152–156.

Costello, A. (1982). Assessment and diagnosis of psychopathology. In J.L. Matson & R.P. Barrett (Eds.), *Psychopathology in the mentally retarded* (pp. 37–52). Orlando, FL: Grune & Stratton.

Craig, T.J., & Behar, R. (1980). Trends in the prescription of psychotropic drugs (1970–1977) in a state hospital. *Comprehensive Psychiatry, 21,* 336–345.

Creese, I., & Snyder, S.H. (1977). A simple and sensitive radioreceptor assay for antischizophrenic drugs in blood. *Nature, 270,* 180–182.

Curry, S.H. (1978). Pharmacokinetics and psychotropic drugs. *Psychological Medicine, 8,* 177–180.

Davis, J.M., Erickson, S., & Dekirmenjian, H. (1978). Plasma levels of antipsychotic drugs and clinical response. In M.A. Lipton, A. DiMascio, & K.F. Killam (Eds.), *Psychopharmacology: A generation of progress* (pp. 905–915). New York: Raven Press.

DiMascio, A. (1975, May). *Psychotropic drug usage in the mentally retarded: A review of 2000 cases.* Paper presented to Workshop on Psychotropic Drugs and the Mentally Retarded, Portland.

Eaton, L.F., & Menolascino, F.J. (1982). Psychiatric disorders in the mentally retarded: Types, problems, and challenges. *American Journal of Psychiatry, 139,* 1297–1303.

Ellenor, G.L., & Frisk, P.A. (1977). Pharmacist impact on drug use in an institution for the mentally retarded. *American Journal of Hospital Pharmacy, 34,* 604–608.

Emerson, R., D'Souza, B.J., Vining, E.P., Holden, K.R., Mellits, E.D., & Freeman, J.M. (1981). Stopping medication in children with epilepsy. *New England Journal of Medicine, 304,* 1125–1129.

Errickson, E., Bock, W., Young, R.C., & Silverstein, B.J. (1981). Psychotropic drug use in Title XIX (ICF-MR) facilities for the mentally retarded in Minnesota. In R. Young & J. Kroll (Eds.), *The use of medications in controlling the behavior of the mentally retarded: Proceedings* (pp. 82–88). Minneapolis, MN: University of Minnesota.

Fielding, L.T., Murphy, R.J., Reagan, M.W., & Peterson, T.L. (1980). An assessment program to reduce drug use with the mentally retarded. *Hospital and Community Psychiatry, 31,* 771–773.

Frager, J., Barnet, A., Weiss, I., & Coleman, J. (1985). A double blind study of vitamin B_6 in Down's syndrome infants: Part 2. Cortical auditory evoked potentials. *Journal of Mental Deficiency Research, 29,* 241–246.

Gadow, K.D. (1976, April). *Psychotropic and anticonvulsant drug usage in early childhood special education programs: I. Phase one: A preliminary report: Prevalence, attitude, training, and problems.* Paper presented at the annual meeting of the Council for Exceptional Children, Chicago (ERIC Document Reproduction Service No. E D 125 198).

Gadow, K.D. (1981). Prevalence of drug treatment for hyperactivity and other childhood behavior disorders. In K.D. Gadow & J. Loney (Eds.), *Psychosocial aspects of drug treatment for hyperactivity* (pp. 13–76). Boulder, CO: Westview Press.

Gadow, K.D., & Kalachnik, J. (1981). Prevalence and pattern of drug treatment for behavior and seizure disorders of TMR students. *American Journal of Mental Deficiency*, 85, 588–595.

Gerard, E., Podboy, J., & Boldt, P. (1981). A psychotropic medication monitoring system for a large developmentally disabled population. In R. Young & J. Kroll (Eds.), *The use of medications in controlling the behavior of the mentally retarded: Proceedings* (pp. 163–172). Minneapolis, MN: University of Minnesota.

Gowdey, C.W., Zarfas, D.E., & Phipps, S. (1987). Audit of psychoactive drug prescriptions in group homes. *Mental Retardation*, 25, 331–334.

Greenberg, A.S., & Coleman, M. (1976). Depressed 5-hydroxyindole levels associated with hyperactive and aggressive behavior. *Archives of General Psychiatry*, 33, 331–336.

Gualtieri, C.T., & Schroeder, S.R. (1985). *Unpublished data on children in a Class Action suit (North Carolina) for children with behavioral, developmental, and neurological handicaps*. University of North Carolina.

Hansen, P., & Keogh, B.K. (1971). Medical characteristics of children with educational handicaps. Implications for the pediatrician. *Clinical Pediatrics*, 10, 726–730.

Hastings, J.E., & Barkley, R.A. (1978). A review of psychophysiological research with hyperkinetic children. *Journal of Abnormal Child Psychology*, 6, 413–447.

Hawkins, R.P., & Dobes, R.W. (1976). Behavioral definitions in applied behavior analysis: Explicit and implicit. In B.C. Etzel, J.M. LeBlanc, & D.M. Baer (Eds.), *New developments in behavior research: Theory, methods and application* (pp. 167–188). Hillsdale, NJ: Erlbaum.

Heistad, G.T., Zimmermann, R.L., & Doebler, M.I. (1982). Long-term usefulness of thioridazine for institutionalized mentally retarded patients. *American Journal of Mental Deficiency*, 87, 243–251.

Hill, B.K., Balow, E.A., & Bruininks, R.H. (1985). A national study of prescribed drugs in institutions and community residential facilities for mentally retarded people. *Psychopharmacology Bulletin*, 21, 279–284.

Holowach, J., Thurstone, D.L., & O'Leary, J. (1972). Prognosis in childhood epilepsy: Follow-up study of 148 cases, in which therapy had been suspended after prolonged anticonvulsant control. *The New England Journal of Medicine*, 286, 169–174.

Honigfeld, G. (1974). NOSIE-30: History and current status of its use in pharmacopsychiatric research. In P. Pichot & R. Olivier-Martin (Eds.), *Modern problems in pharmacopsychiatry: Psychological measurements in psychopharmacology* (Vol. 7, pp. 238–263). Basel, Switzerland: Karger.

Hughes, P.S. (1977). Survey of medication in a subnormality hospital. *British Journal of Mental Subnormality*, 23, 88–94.

Inoue, F. (1982). A clinical pharmacy service to reduce psychotropic medication use in an institution for mentally handicapped persons. *Mental Retardation*, 20, 70–74.

Intagliata, J., & Rinck, C. (1985). Psychoactive drug use in public and community residential facilities for mentally retarded persons. *Psychopharmacology Bulletin*, 21, 268–278.

Itil, T.M., Shapiro, D.M., Eralp, E., Akman, A., Itil, K.Z., & Garbizu, C. (1985). A new brain function diagnostic unit, including the dynamic brain mapping of computer analyzed EEG, evoked potential and sleep (A new hardware/software system and its application in psychiatry and psychopharmacology). *Experimental and Clinical Psychiatry*, *1*, 107–177.

James, D.H. (1983). Monitoring drugs in hospitals for the mentally handicapped. *British Journal of Psychiatry*, *142*, 163–165.

Jonas, O. (1980). Pattern of drug prescribing in a residential centre for the intellectually handicapped. *Australian Journal of Developmental Disabilities*, *6*, 25–30.

Katkin, E.S., & Hastrup, J.L. (1982). Psychophysiological methods in clinical research. In P.C. Kendall & J.N. Butcher (Eds.), *Handbook of research methods in clinical psychology* (pp. 387–425). New York: Wiley.

Kent, R.N., O'Leary, K.D., Dietz, A., & Diament, C. (1974). Expectation biases in observational evaluation of therapeutic change. *Journal of Consulting and Clinical Psychology*, *42*, 774–780.

King, R.D., Raynes, N.V., & Tizard, J. (1971). *Patterns of residential care: Sociological studies in institutions for the handicapped*. London: Routledge & Kegan Paul.

Kirman, S.B. (1975). Drug therapy in mental handicap. *British Journal of Psychiatry*, *127*, 545–549.

Krager, J.M., Safer, D., & Earhart, J. (1979). Follow-up survey results of medication used to treat hyperactive school children. *The Journal of School Health*, *49*, 317–321.

Lader, S.R. (1980). A radioreceptor assay for neuroleptic drugs in plasma. *Journal of Immunoassay*, *1*, 57–75.

LaMendola, W., Zaharia, E.S., & Carver, M. (1980). Reducing psychotropic drug use in an institution for the retarded. *Hospital and Community Psychiatry*, *31*, 271–272.

Leudar, I., Fraser, W.I., & Jeeves, M.A. (1984). Behavioural disturbance in mental handicap: Typology and longitudinal trends. *Psychological Medicine*, *14*, 923–935.

Lipman, R.S. (1970). The use of psychopharmacological agents in residential facilities for the retarded. In F.J. Menolascino (Ed.), *Psychiatric approaches to mental retardation* (pp. 387–389). New York: Basic Books.

Lipman, R. (1982). Psychotropic drugs in mental retardation: The known and the unknown. In K.D. Gadow & I. Bialer (Eds.), *Advances in learning and behavioral disabilities* (Vol. 1, pp. 261–282). Greenwich, CT: JAI Press.

Lipman, R.S., DiMascio, A., Reatig, N., & Kirson, T. (1978). Psychotropic drugs and mentally retarded children. In M.A. Lipton, A. DiMascio, & K.F. Killam, (Eds.), *Psychopharmacology: A generation of progress* (pp. 1437–1449). New York: Raven Press.

Lobb, H. (1968). Trace GSR conditioning with benzedrine in mentally defective and normal adults. *American Journal of Mental Deficiency*, *73*, 239–246.

Mailman, R.B., De Haven, D.L., Halpern, E.A., & Lewis, M.H. (1984). Serum effects confound the neuroleptic radio receptor assay. *Life Sciences*, *34*, 1057–1064.

Mailman, R.B., Pierce, J.P., Crofton, K.M., Petitto, J., De Haven, D.L., & Lewis, M.H. (1984). Thioridazine and the neuroleptic radioreceptor assay. *Biological Psychiatry*, *19*, 833–847.

Martin, J.E., & Agran, M. (1985). Psychotropic and anticonvulsant drug use by mentally retarded adults across community residential and vocational placements. *Applied Research in Mental Retardation*, *6*, 33–49.

McCormick, M., Balla, D., & Zigler, E. (1975). Resident care practices in institutions for retarded persons: A cross-institutional cross-cultural study. *American Journal of Mental Deficiency*, *80*, 1–17.

Mouchka, S. (1985). Issues in psychopharmacology with the mentally retarded. *Psychopharmacology Bulletin*, *21*, 262–267.

Norman, T.R., & Burrows, G.D. (1981). Methods for the measurement of psychotropic drugs: Antipsychotics and antianxiety agents. In G.D. Burrows & T.R. Norman (Eds.), *Psychotropic drugs: Plasma concentration and clinical response* (pp. 83–138). New York: Marcel Dekker.

Pelham, W.E., Bender, M.E., Caddell, J., Booth, S., & Moorer, S.H. (1985). Methylphenidate and children with attention deficit disorder: Dose effects on classroom academic and social behavior. *Archives of General Psychiatry*, *42*, 948–952.

Pfadt, A., & Tryon, W.W. (1983). Issues in the selection and use of mechanical transducers to directly measure motor activity in clinical settings. *Applied Research in Mental Retardation*, *4*, 251–270.

Pulman, R.M., Pook, R.B., & Singh, N.N. (1979). Prevalence of drug therapy for institutionalized mentally retarded children. *Australian Journal of Mental Retardation*, *5*, 212–214.

Radinsky, A.M. (1984). *A descriptive study of psychotropic and antiepileptic medication use with mentally retarded persons in three residential environments.* Unpublished doctoral dissertation, University of Pittsburgh.

Rapport, M.D., & DuPaul, G.J. (1986). Methylphenidate: Rate-dependent effects on hyperactivity. *Psychopharmacology Bulletin*, *22*, 223–228.

Reiss, S. (1982). Psychopathology and mental retardation: Survey of a developmental disabilities mental health program. *Mental Retardation*, *20*, 128–132.

Ritvo, E.R., Freeman, B.J., Yuwiler, A., Geller, E., Schroth P., Yokota, A., Mason-Brothers, A., August, G.J., Klykylo, W., Leyanthal, B., Lewis, K., Piggott, L., Realmuto, G., Stubbs, E.G., & Umansky, R. (1986). Fenfluramine treatment of autism: UCLA collaborative study of 81 patients at nine medical centers. *Psychopharmacology Bulletin*, *22*, 133–140.

Ruoff, P., Howell, D.C., Wakker, E., & Roberts, B. (1988). *Development of a behavior rating scale for use in a mentally retarded population by a psychiatric consultant.* Unpublished manuscript, University of Vermont.

Schain, R.J., & Freedman, D.X. (1961). Studies on 5-hydroxyindole metabolism in autistic and other mentally retarded children. *Journal of Pediatrics*, *58*, 315–320.

Senatore, V., Matson, J.L., & Kazdin, A.E. (1985). An inventory to assess psychopathology of mentally retarded adults. *American Journal of Mental Deficiency*, *89*, 459–466.

Sewell, J., & Werry, J.S. (1976). Some studies in an institution for the mentally retarded. *New Zealand Medical Journal*, *84*, 317–319.

Silva, D.A. (1979). The use of medication in a residential institution for mentally retarded persons. *Metal Retardation*, *17*, 285–288.

Silverstone, T., & Turner, P., (Eds.). (1974). *Drug treatment in Psychiatry*. London: Routledge & Kegan Paul.

Singh, N.N., & Aman, M.G. (1981). Effects of thioridazine dosage on the behavior of severely mentally retarded persons. *American Journal of Mental Deficiency*, *85*, 580–587.

Singh, N.N., & Beale, I.L. (1986). Behavioural assessment of pharmacotherapy. *Behaviour Change*, *3*, 34–40.

Special Workshop on *Methodological problems in treatment research with mentally retarded populations who are also mentally ill*. (May, 1986). 26th Meeting of the New Clinical Drug Evaluation Unit (NIMH), Key Biscayne, FL.

Spencer, D.A. (1974). A survey of the medication in a hospital for the mentally handicapped. *British Journal of Psychiatry*, *124*, 507–508.

Spivack, G., & Spotts, J. (1965). The Devereux Child Behavior Scale: Symptom behaviors in latency age children. *American Journal of Mental Deficiency*, *69*, 839–853.

Sprague, R.L., & Sleator, E.K. (1975). What is the proper dose of stimulant drugs in children? *International Journal of Mental Health*, *4*, 75–118.

Sprague, R.L., & Sleator, E.K. (1977). Methylphenidate in hyperkinetic children: Differences in dose effects on learning and social behavior. *Science*, *198*, 1274–1276.

Sprague, R.L., & Werry, J.S. (1971). Methodology of psychopharmacological studies with the retarded. In N.R. Ellis (Ed.), *International review of research in mental retardation* (Vol. 5, pp. 147–210). New York: Academic Press.

Stores, G. (1978). Antiepileptics (anticonvulsants). In J.S. Werry (Ed.), *Pediatric psychopharmacology: The use of behavior modifying drugs in children* (pp. 274–315). New York: Brunner/Mazel.

Towns, A.J., Singh, N.N., & Beale, I.L. (1984). Reliability of observations in a double- and single-blind drug study: An experimental analysis. In K. Gadow (Ed.), *Advances in learning and behavioral disabilities* (Vol. 3, pp. 215–240). Greenwich, CT: JAI Press.

Trimble, M., & Reynolds, E. (1976). Anticonvulsant drugs and mental symptoms. *Psychological Medicine*, *6*, 169–178.

Tu, J. (1979). A survey of psychotropic medication in mental retardation facilities. *Journal of Clinical Psychiatry*, *40*, 125–128.

Tu, J., & Smith, J.T. (1979). Factors associated with psychotropic medication in mental retardation facilities. *Comprehensive Psychiatry*, *20*, 289–295.

Tu, J., & Smith, J.T. (1983). The Eastern Ontario survey: A study of drug-treated psychiatric problems in the mentally handicapped. *Canadian Journal of Psychiatry*, *28*, 270–276.

Walls, R.T., Werner, T.J., Bacon, A., & Zane, T. (1977). Behavior checklists. In J.D. Cone & R.P. Hawkins (Eds.), *Behavioral assessment: New directions in clinical psychology* (pp. 77–146). New York: Brunner/Mazel.

Watson, J.E., Aman, M.G., & Singh, N.N. (in press). The Psychopathology Instrument for Mentally Retarded Adults: Psychometric characteristics, factor structure, and relationship to subject characteristics. *Research in Developmental Disabilities*.

Werry, J.S. (1978). Measures in pediatric psychopharmacology. In J.S. Werry (Ed.), *Pediatric psychopharmacology: The use of behavior modifying drugs in children* (pp. 29–78). New York: Brunner/Mazel.

Werry, J.S. (in press). Drugs, learning, and cognitive function in children—An update. *Journal of Child Psychology and Psychiatry*.

Werry, J.S., & Aman, M.G. (1975). Methylphenidate and haloperidol in children. Effects on attention, memory, and activity. *Archives of General Psychiatry*, *32*, 790–795.

Werry, J.S., Aman, M.G., & Lampen, E. (1975). Haloperidol and methylphenidate in hyperactive children. *Acta Paedopsychiatrica*, *42*, 26–40.

Werry, J.S., & Sprague, R.L. (1972). Psychopharmacology. In J. Wortis (Ed.), *Mental retardation* (Vol. 4. pp. 63–79). New York: Grune & Stratton.

White, A.J.R. (1983). Changing patterns of psychoactive drug use with the mentally retarded. *New Zealand Medical Journal, 96,* 686–688.

Wysocki, T., & Fuqua, R.W. (1982). Methodological issues in the evaluation of drug effects. In S.E. Breuning & A.D. Poling (Eds.), *Drugs and mental retardation* (pp. 138–167). Springfield, IL: Thomas.

Zigler, E., Balla, D., & Styfco, S.J. (1984). Investigation of the effects of institutionalization on learning and other behaviors. In P. Brooks, R. Sperber, & C. McCauley (Eds.), *Learning and cognition in the mentally retarded* (pp. 129–140). Hillsdale, NJ: Erlbaum.

Zimmerman, R.L., & Heistad, G.T. (1980). Correlates of psychotropic drug treatment at Cambridge State Hospital. In R. Young & J. Kroll (Eds.), *The use of medications in controlling the behavior of the mentally retarded: Proceedings* (pp. 123–132). Minneapolis, MN: University of Minnesota.

2
Litigation and Use of Psychoactive Drugs in Developmental Disabilities

HENRY A. BEYER

Abstract

Litigation, particularly in the United States, has resulted in the establishment of a number of legal rights regarding the administration of psychoactive medication to individuals with developmental disabilities. During the last 15 years, courts have fashioned rules and standards for regulating psychoactive drug use, particularly in institutional settings. Although there is general agreement among numerous jurisdictions that high professional standards be mandated for drug use, there remain substantial differences concerning the circumstances under which such medication may be administered to refusing individuals or to persons incapable of giving an informed, competent consent. The author reviews these legal developments and suggests four general principles for regulating the administration of psychoactive drugs to people of questionable competence.

Dawn of Legal Rights

Recognition of the rights of people with developmental and other disabilities has grown enormously during the past 15 years (Beyer, 1983). Many of these newly acknowledged rights concern proper medical care and access to legal enforcement mechanisms. In 1972, for example, the General Assembly of the United Nations' "Declaration on the Rights of Mentally Retarded Persons" proclaimed that:

[t]he mentally retarded person has, to the maximum degree of feasibility, the same rights as other human beings. . . . [including] a right to proper medical care. . . (United Nations, 1972)

And in a 1975 "Declaration on the Rights of Disabled Persons," the General Assembly stated that persons with disabilities have an

inherent right to respect for their human dignity. . . . [and] the same civil . . . rights as other human beings. . . . Disabled persons shall be able to avail themselves of qualified legal aid when such aid proves indispensable for the protection of their persons. . . ." (United Nations, 1975)

Many other national and international organizations have adopted similar Bills of Rights for people with disabilities (see, e.g., International League of Societies for the Mentally Handicapped, 1968; United Cerebral Palsy Association, 1973; American Association on Mental Deficiency, 1973–75), and such provisions have achieved enforceable legal status in the legislation of several countries.[1]

In the years preceding this recognition of the rights of individuals with disabilities, there had occurred a tremendous increase in the amount of medications administered to the same population, particularly in the United States (see Chapter 1). It is not surprising, therefore, that many legal actions, particularly in the United States, have concerned the use of drugs. Although the litigation has included a wide range of different drugs, used in a variety of contexts and administered to people having significantly different disabilities, this discussion focuses principally upon the administration of psychoactive drugs, in institutions, to people with a diagnosis of mental retardation. Because some of the more important legal developments in the field have occurred in suits brought by people diagnosed as mentally ill but frequently not considered developmentally disabled,[2] several of these cases are also discussed. In part because the United States was, until recently, the only country in which people with disabilities were able to base their claims of individual rights on a written constitution (and perhaps also because of the great number of U.S. lawyers), the overwhelming majority of litigation thus far has taken place in U.S. courts. It is expected that the 1982 adoption of the Canadian Charter of Rights and Freedoms will lead to extensive judicial review in Canada in the near future.[3]

According to Gostin (1982), legal concern for the welfare and rights of the individual has traditionally stopped at the hospital door, in the belief that law should not interfere with the clinical relationship that must be established following admission. In the early 1970s, however, some courts in the United States began to take seriously the moral rights of people with disabilities that had been expounded by national and international organizations, and started to convert them into legal rights enforceable within the walls of state schools, hospitals, and developmental units (Beyer, 1983). A very important topic addressed in these new legal rights is the use of psychoactive drugs, a class of medications used extensively in psychiatric and mental retardation institutions (see Chapter 1).[4] Referring to these drugs of concern variously as "major tranquilizers," "neuroleptics," "psychotropics," or "antipsychotic drugs," courts have focused primarily upon the use and abuse of medications such as Thorazine, Mellaril, Prolixin, and Haldol that are used in treating psychoses, particularly schizophrenia.[5]

Drugs Used as Restraint

In 1971, Brakel and Rock observed that the availability of psychotropic drugs had reduced the incidence of and need for physical restraints. They also noted, however, that "[t]he line between physical restraint by mechanical device and by drugs may be a very thin one in many cases. The latter may be as open to abuse as the former" (Brakel & Rock, 1971, pp. 160–161).

As Brakel and Rock foresaw, the use and abuse of psychoactive medication for the purpose of restraint rapidly became widespread in chronically understaffed institutions for both mentally ill and mentally retarded individuals. In numerous cases, courts have found drugs being administered in institutions routinely and over extended periods, not to maximize residents' developmental potential or to prevent harm in real emergencies, but as substitutes for habilitative programs.[6] Courts have uniformly held that such use violates the residents' rights, citing state or federal statutes or the U.S. Constitution.[7] Provisions in the resulting court orders and consent decrees have typically mandated that "medication shall not be used as punishment, for the convenience of staff, as a substitute for a habilitation program, or in quantities that interfere with a resident's habilitation program."[8]

Courts have not, however, held that the use of drugs for restraint is *never* justified. The long-standing right (duty, in some cases) of staff members of state facilities to restrain individuals when necessary to prevent them from harming themselves or others was tacitly reaffirmed by the U.S. Supreme Court in 1982 in its *Youngberg v. Romeo* decision (discussed in more detail in this chapter at note 49). The Court clearly accepted the legitimate use of some restraints in a mental retardation institution by holding that a resident has a constitutional right to be free merely of "unreasonable" restraints.[9]

In determining whether psychotropic medication may be administered as a restraint in a particular situation, one must first determine whether *any* restraint may be used and, if so, whether the restraint to be used may be a drug. Restraints have been justified under either the state's policy power, used to protect society, or its *parens patriae* power (paternalistic power), used to care for individuals incapable of caring for themselves. Although the regulations authorizing the use of restraints differ significantly from state to state,[10] a clear trend is evident in the United States in the development of two legal principles governing them.

The first principle is that the use of restraints is legally justified only in an "emergency such as the occurrence of, or serious threat of, extreme violence, personal injury, or attempted suicide," not as a routine custodial convenience.[11] The second applicable principle is that of the "least restrictive alternative."[12] This principle provides guidance as to what particular action may be employed in such an emergency. It requires that the steps taken in an emergency to avoid the potential harm be those that are least intrusive, least restrictive of the individual's liberty, and yet effective under the circumstances. As one U.S. Court of Appeals explained, before administering psychotropic medication in an emergency, "an *individualized* estimation of the possibility and type of violence, the likely effects of particular drugs on a particular individual, and an appraisal of alternative, less restrictive courses of action" must be made.[13]

This formulation is similar, but somewhat narrower, than that generally followed in the British Commonwealth:

[C]ommon law emergency psychiatric treatment may be administered in two situations: (1) where the patient appears likely to injure himself or another or to damage the property of another, and where the treatment in question is the only reasonable practical mode of restraint; (2) where the treatment was necessary to preserve the patient's life or health from permanent or serious injury or to prevent grave pain and suffering (Abbott et al. 1983, p. 218; McNamara, 1981)

According to Abbott et al. (1983), this position has been codified in the U.K. Mental Health Act of 1983.

Application of the least restrictive alternative principle in this context can present difficulties. Many possible alternatives are clearly less restrictive than the use of psychoactive drugs. These would include "talking" therapies, special education and training, and many forms of behavior modification. But it is not clear whether the drugs, when used as "chemical restraints,"[14] are more or less restrictive than mechanical restraints, "timeout" (the social isolation of a client from program activities for a short period of time), involuntary commitment, or other means of restraint. Law professor David Wexler has noted that the Arizona mental health program appears to view emergency medication for control purposes as *less* restrictive than seclusion, whereas New Hampshire guidelines seem to consider chemical restraints *more* restrictive than either seclusion or physical restraints (Wexler, 1982, p. 288). Few courts have even addressed this question, much less provided an answer. In a 1981 decision entitled *Guardianship of Roe*,[15] however, a case involving an incompetent young man diagnosed as having paranoid schizophrenia, the Massachusetts Supreme Judicial Court ruled upon a similar point. It held that "in order to satisfy the least intrusive means test, the incompetent is entitled to choose by way of substituted judgment, between involuntary commitment and involuntary medication."[16] As discussed in the text below (at notes 69–76), the court indicated that, in Massachusetts, the authority to make such a substituted judgment lies with the court.

Drugs Used as Treatment

Psychotropic drugs are not used exclusively as restraints, however; they are also used as treatment. Individuals with developmental disabilities have achieved significant progress during the past 15 years in establishing their legal rights to receive treatment, training, and other habilitative services. Although the U.S. Supreme Court has declined to decide whether institutionalized individuals have a general constitutional right to treatment per se,[17] it did rule in 1982 that Nicholas Romeo, a profoundly mentally retarded man commited to a Pennsylvania state school, was constitutionally entitled to enough training to enable him to control his aggressive behavior, so that he could be permitted more freedom of movement.[18] Lower courts in many jurisdictions have gone further during the past 15 years, recognizing quite general rights to treatment or habilitation based upon state or federal constitutions[19] or on state statutes.[20] Many of these courts have also considered what role psychoactive drugs might properly play in this treatment.

Opinions differ substantially regarding the efficacy of these drugs in treating individuals with mental retardation. In 1975, the U.S. Food and Drug Administration (FDA) acknowledged that there is no evidence that phenothiazines provide any benefit to persons with "*uncomplicated* mental retardation."[21] But it approved Thorazine (chlorpromazine) and Mellaril (thioridazine) for use on persons displaying "severe behavior problems," saying that "substantial evidence" exists indicating their effectiveness in treating mentally retarded patients (Plotkin & Gill, 1979, p. 654, note 97). Plotkin and Gill (1979) have criticized the 11 studies upon which this FDA conclusion was based, arguing that many of them failed to meet basic methodological criteria required for scientific drug studies. Others have suggested that "the use of drugs in this field appears to have been established on the basis of superficial similarity of symptoms in some retarded individuals to certain psychiatric disorders" (Sprague & Baxley, 1978). They argue that the logic behind the analogy is flawed in that a specific therapeutic role for these drugs is yet to be proven. While some researchers maintain that certain maladaptive behaviors and/or psychiatric disorders of developmentally disabled persons may respond to psychotropic medications (see Chapters 6 and 7), others believe that long-term treatment with the most commonly prescribed medications, neuroleptic drugs, actually benefits only a fraction of the mentally retarded individuals now receiving them (Schatzberg & Cole, 1986; Chapter 4).

Judicial Standards for Administration of Drugs

Without attempting to resolve the question of the therapeutic value of psychoactive drugs for people with mental retardation, U.S. courts have attempted to fashion *standards* for their administration in institutions housing these individuals. Judge Frank Johnson, in his 1972 landmark ruling in a federal court in Alabama, *Wyatt v. Stickney*,[22] held that the U.S. Constitution requires, as a minimum, that:

a. No medication shall be administered unless at the written order of a physician.
b. Notation of each individual's medication shall be kept on his medical records. . . . At least weekly the attending physician shall review the drug regimen of each resident under his care. . . .
c. Residents shall have a right to be free from unnecessary or excessive medication. . . .
d. Medication shall not be used as punishment, for the convenience of staff, as a substitute for a habilitation program, or in quantities that interfere with the resident's habilitation program.
e. Pharmacy services at the institution shall be directed by a professionally competent pharmacist licensed to practice in the State of Alabama. Such pharmacist shall be a graduate of a school of pharmacy accredited by the American Council on Pharmaceutical Education. . . .[23]

Succeeding cases have emulated and elaborated upon the *Wyatt* standards. In *Halderman v. Pennhurst*, for example, a class action brought on behalf of the residents of Pennsylvania's Pennhurst State School, a federal district court ruled that "chemical restraints may be administered only upon the order of a physician,"[24] and ordered the defendant administrators to

ensure that only appropriately trained staff are allowed to administer drugs to residents . . . , to provide for at least monthly reviews by a physician of each resident's medication . . . , [and] to provide training programs to staff who administer drugs to residents. The nature of such training programs, and the qualifications to be required of staff members who administer drugs to residents shall be established in the plan. . . .[25]

Still other U.S. courts have referred to the *Wyatt* standards[26] generally, but then spelled out their own more explicit rules for drug usage. The consent decree of the federal district court for Connecticut's Mansfield Training School, for instance, requires that the state defendants "at a minimum comply with the professional staff standards set forth in *Wyatt* . . . ,"[27] and also:

. . . monitor the use of restraints and psychotropic medication and make their best efforts to reduce their utilization consistent with professional judgment.
. . . Except for emergencies, restraints and/or psychotropic medication may be employed only in conjunction with a written comprehensive behavioral treatment plan [satisfying six explicit criteria].
. . . All medication levels will be reviewed monthly by the pharmacist and team nurses and quarterly by the interdisciplinary team.
. . . Medications will be administered only by nurses or other personnel licensed under the laws of Connecticut. . . .[28]

The judiciary has generally recognized that, "without monitoring one cannot determine whether the drug has been effective and whether it should be continued."[29] But the critical importance of proper monitoring was perhaps most strongly emphasized in the 1977 consent decree in *Welsch v. Dirkswager*, a class action brought on behalf of the mentally retarded residents of Minnesota's Cambridge State Hospital.[30] The decree required that major tranquilizers for controlling behavior be used only if:

records based upon direct staff observation are consistently maintained with the frequency and according to the procedures specified in the medical record by the physician who has prescribed the major tranquilizer. . . . [They] must not be used unless the determination to prescribe or to continue the prescription of such medication and the determination of the dosage of such medication to be administered is based upon evaluation of the efficacy of the medication in controlling or modifying the specified behavior as demonstrated by the incidence of target or objectionable behaviors recorded in accordance with this paragraph. . . .[31]

Furthermore, the *Welsch* consent decree provided that the court monitor appointed to oversee implementation of the decree should retain, as consultant, a qualified physician for the purpose of periodically analyzing the files of residents receiving major tranquilizers to verify compliance with the decree's restrictions.[32]

Adverse Side Effects

The great concern U.S. courts have shown regarding the use of psychoactive drugs can be largely attributed to the evidence they have heard concerning unintended effects of such medication. Some critics claim that neuroleptic drugs of the phenothiazine class "interfere with the already limited ability of the mentally retarded individual to think, speak, ambulate, and learn" (Plotkin & Gill, 1979, p. 662). Others have strongly criticized such conclusions, saying they are based on "a highly selective review of the psychopharmacological literature and. . .emphasiz[ing] negative effects of medication in a distorted and inaccurate manner" (Gutheil & Appelbaum, 1983, p. 88).[33] One review of the literature concluded that neuroleptic drugs may well impair learning performance in mentally retarded persons, especially in those showing a poor clinical response and at high doses, but also that impairment is not an inevitable consequence of such treatment, particularly when given in low doses to people showing a favorable clinical response (Aman, 1984). A number of U.S. courts have responded sympathetically to arguments that administration of psychoactive medication without valid consent of the recipient constitutes impermissible interference with the mental process, in violation of the First Amendment.[34]

Also, although no courts are known to have yet relied upon it, the Universal Declaration of Human Rights, adopted by the United Nations General Assembly in 1948 (United Nations, 1948), may also be relevant here. That document recognizes freedom of thought, opinion, and expression, rights that may be affected, and conceivably violated, by the forced use of these drugs (Winick, 1986, pp. 7–8). In what are probably the strongest judicial sentiments expressed relative to this issue, the U.S. District Court for Massachusetts, in its 1979 decision in the *Rogers v. Okin* class action brought on behalf of state hospital patients, found it "virtually undisputed" that antipsychotic drugs are "mind altering,"[35] and that

psychotropic medication has the potential to affect and change a patient's mood, attitude and capacity to think. . . . The right to produce a thought—or refuse to do so—is as important as the right protected in *Roe v. Wade* to give birth or abort. . . . Without the capacity to think, we merely exist, not function. Realistically, the capacity to think and decide is a fundamental element of freedom.[36]

Among other side effects of psychoactive drugs noted by a number of courts are "blurred vision, constipation or diarrhea, palpitations, skin rashes, low blood pressure, faintness, and fatigue" (see Chapter 4). "Some patients experience akinesia—a state of diminished spontaneity, physical weakness, and muscle fatigue; others suffer akathesia, which is marked by . . . an inability to be still."[37]

The side effect that has received most judicial attention, however, is tardive dyskinesia. As has been noted, the legal system's handling of this issue "will probably influence to a considerable degree the day-to-day practice of psychopharmacology" (Gualtieri, Sprague, & Cole, 1986, p. 188). Tardive dyskinesia is a movement disorder manifested by involuntary, repetitive, and rhythmic movements of the tongue, lips, facial muscles, and/or the extremities, caused by chronic exposure to neuroleptics. As discussed in Chapter 9, substantial differences exist among studies regarding the prevalence of tardive dyskinesia attributable to various psychoactive drug regimens and the extent to which these symptoms are irreversible. When considering the testimony presented in a specific case, however, courts have not always recognized such differences. In the case of *Clites v. Iowa*,[38] for example, the trial court found that

[a]ll the experts agreed that [tardive dyskinesia (T.D.)] is usually permanent, disabling and interferes with coordination, personal appearance and the ability to perform as usual. Two expert witnesses interpreted differently the studies which bear on the question of whether it is proven that tardive dyskinesia causes brain damage. However, both agreed that the major tranquilizers work by affecting the transmissions of brain signals which could be affected permanently. . . . All the doctors . . . indicated that the extent of damage from T.D. depends upon the individual case.[39]

In its 1979 *Rogers v. Okin* opinion, the federal district court in Massachusetts cited various studies estimating prevalence rates of 30% to 56% among mental health patients who had received the drugs for several years.[40] A 1980 report of a task force of the American Psychiatric Association (APA) estimated that "at least 10% of patients in mental hospitals and at least 40% of elderly, chronically institutionalized or outpatients exhibit more than minimal signs of probable tardive dyskinesia attributable to or associated with neuroleptic drug treatment."[41] The situation is probably not substantially different for individuals living in mental retardation institutions (see Chapter 9).

In affirming the district court's ruling in the *Clites* case, the Iowa Court of Appeals held that

[t]he industry standard established that regular visits by a physician, tests and physical exams are necessary to properly monitor a patient under these circumstances. The State did not comply with that standard of care, as the record established Timothy was not regularly visited by a physician and physical exams had not been conducted for a three-year period.[42]

The *Clites* trial court had also addressed the practice of "polypharmacy," the administration of multiple drugs to the same patient at the same time. Although this practice has sometimes been defended on the basis that additional drugs are required to counteract side effects of the originally prescribed drug (see Ayd, 1973), it has also been criticized as complicating treatment and increasing the risk of adverse reactions due to the potentially additive effects of the prescribed medications (Sovner, 1986). In *Clites*, the district court held that the use of polypharmacy on Timothy

did not comply with the standard of care existing at that time. . . . [T]he weight of the evidence supports Plaintiffs' experts who testified that for Tim polypharmacy was unnecessary and impeded detection of side effects. Accordingly, it constituted a failure to use ordinary care. Further, the greater weight of the evidence supports the findings that the use of anti-cholinergics, along with the major tranquilizers, was improper. This also impeded the detection process and increased the likelihood that Tim's adverse reactions to the drugs would be more severe and more permanent.[43]

The dangers of impeding the detection of tardive dyskinesia and exacerbating its effects were also recognized by the Michigan Court of Appeals in 1985 in *Faigenbaum v. Oakland Medical Center*.[44] Although the defendant hospital escaped liability because of its governmental immunity and procedural errors by the plaintiff, the court found that several medical practices had fallen "below the standard of care."[45] It cited testimony that

after the onset of tardive dyskinesia, the continued prescription of neuroleptic drugs could either: (1) prevent physicians from knowing the severity of the disorder (mask it) or (2) convert a reversible case into an irreversible one. Drug therapy should be discontinued even where it is known the condition is irreversible.[46]

Deference to Professional Standards

Rather than attempting to specify acceptable dosage limits or other such technical matters regarding drug administration, courts have generally deferred to the expertise of medical professionals. For example, in *R.A.J. v. Miller*,[47] a class action brought on behalf of the mentally ill and mentally retarded residents of eight Texas state institutions, a U.S. district court approved a 1981 settlement agreement in which the state defendants agreed to "establish guidelines in the Texas formulary or elsewhere indicating professionally recognized appropriate ranges of doses for psychotropic medications. . . ."[48]

Such deference of courts to professional judgment was given substantial impetus in 1982 by the U.S. Supreme Court's decision in *Youngberg v. Romeo*.[49] The mother of Nicholas Romeo, a profoundly retarded 30-year-old man involuntarily confined in Pennsylvania's Pennhurst State School, had charged in a federal suit that he was being "improperly shackled" and was being denied adequate protection and appropriate treatment. The Supreme Court, in its most positive ruling yet concerning the rights of institutionalized persons with mental retardation, held that individuals in Mr. Romeo's situation have a constitutional right to adequate food, shelter, clothing, and medical care[50]; to safe conditions; to freedom from unreasonable restraint; and to at least "minimally adequate" training in caring for themselves.[51]

Although the *Romeo* opinion did not address drug questions directly, much of the Court's language may be highly relevant. In discussing the standard for determining the reasonableness of the use of restraints, the Court held that constitutional due process is satisfied if restraints are imposed on involuntarily confined mentally retarded individuals in accordance with the exercise of "professional judgment."[52] A decision concerning restraints,

if made by a professional, is presumptively valid; liability may be imposed only when the decision by the professional is such a substantial departure from accepted professional judgment, practice, or standards as to demonstrate that the person responsible did not base the decision on such a judgment.[53]

Furthermore, "[i]t is not appropriate for the courts to specify which of several professionally acceptable choices should have been made."[54] As for the role to be played by expert witnesses in a lawsuit concerning such issues, the Court said only that expert testimony "may be relevant to whether [institutional] decisions were a substantial departure from the requisite professional judgment."[55] The *Romeo* opinion has understandably made lower court judges considerably less prone to second guess service providers who can make a reasonable showing that their drug (or other) decisions were actually based on professional judgment.[56]

Consent to and Refusal of Drugs

The judicial actions discussed so far have focused primarily upon the conditions for administration of psychoactive medication, without devoting much attention to the wishes of the drug recipient. Yet law has traditionally accorded great weight to a person's right to control what substances enter his or her own body. It has long recognized a principle of personal autonomy, a doctrine actualized in English and U.S. common law as a right of privacy, "the right to be let alone," the "most comprehensive of rights and the right most valued by civilized men."[57]

In recent years, the U.S. Supreme Court has given the privacy right a constitutional basis in the Fourteenth Amendment's concept of personal liberty.[58] In ruling that this constitutional right to privacy extends to an institutionalized, profoundly retarded man, the Massachusetts Supreme Judicial Court described it as "an expression of the sanctity of individual free choice and self determination as fundamental constituents of life."[59] In the field of medicine, the privacy right is expressed in the doctrine of informed consent. A physician may not treat a patient until he or she has explained to the patient the expected benefits and possible risks of the proposed treatment, has outlined alternative courses of action, and has received from the patient a consent that is informed, voluntary, and competent (see Annas, 1975).

Although, as we have seen, courts have been quite active in establishing appropriate standards for the administration of psychoactive medication to institutionalized mentally retarded individuals, relatively little attention has been paid to determining how these legal privacy rights and consent requirements apply in this context. If the doctrine of informed consent applies (and there is no legal reason why at least voluntary residents should not enjoy its protection), any person to whom these drugs are to be administered for therapeutic purposes has a right, first, to receive extensive *information* concerning the significant risks, potential benefits, and possible alternatives. In the few lawsuits addressing this point, most of which have been brought by individuals diagnosed as mentally ill, courts have generally upheld this right to adequate information, even for involuntarily committed patients.[60] In a recent medical malpractice case, for example, the Texas Supreme Court ruled that a jury should have been allowed to decide the question of "whether a 'reasonable person' could have been influenced in making a decision whether to give or withhold consent to [neuroleptic drug treatment] had he known the risk [of tardive dyskinesia]."[61]

The difficulties of assuring the second requisite element, the *voluntariness* of a consent given in the institutional context, have received even less attention. In 1973, a Michigan court discussed this problem in *Kaimowitz v. Department of Mental Health*,[62] ruling that an institutionalized mental patient could not validly consent to psychosurgery. The court found that

"[t]he involuntarily detained mental patient is in an inherently coercive atmosphere even though no direct pressures may be placed upon him. He finds himself stripped of customary amenities and defenses. Free movement is restricted. He becomes a part of communal living subject to the control of institutional authorities. . . . [I]nvoluntarily confined patients tend to tell their doctor what the patient thinks these people want to hear."[63]

Members of the Mental Health Foundation of New Zealand, among others, believe that

Kaimowitz over-exaggerates the effects of institutionalization, and may operate to deprive patients of treatment by denying capacity to make treatment decisions. To the extent that institutions are potentially coercive, the best defence against such coercion is likely to be an increase, not a decrease of the opportunities given to patients for individual choice and self-determination. (Abbot, 1983, p. 216)

On the other hand, the tendency toward acquiescence is probably even more pronounced in the case of instituitionalized people who are mentally retarded (see, Bregman, 1984; Floor & Rosen, 1975; Rosen, Floor, & Zisfein, 1974; Sigelman, Budd, Spanhel, & Schoenrock, 1981). Furthermore, whether the person's institutionalization is technically classified as "voluntary" or "involuntary" is probably irrelevant in most cases. A federal court in North Dakota recognized in 1982 that the mentally retarded residents of the Grafton, North Dakota state school had not, in most cases, voluntarily consented to their confinement in any meaningful sense of the word "voluntary." The court noted that even the consent of mentally competent residents should be questioned, in light of probable pressures from family and the high cost and unavailability of alternative care.[64]

Even when the consent to drug treatment is being sought from a guardian, family member, or other representative of the disabled individual (i.e., proxy decision making, discussed below), the problem of ensuring voluntariness is not necessarily solved. Family members, keenly aware of the great power that caregivers exert over all aspects of their institutionalized loved one's life, are often reluctant to oppose any recommendation made by a service provider. A truly voluntary consent in the face of the typical disparities in bargaining positions of the parties in these situations may never be completely achievable.

The third requisite element of informed consent is the *competence* of the person consenting. Under the common law, and also by statute in some states,[65] all U.S. adults are legally competent unless they have been judged incompetent by a court. This presumption of competency applies even if they have been diagnosed as mentally retarded, and even if they live in a state school or developmental center. There are, however, many developmentally disabled individuals who have never been adjudicated incompetent but whose functional competence is very much in doubt. In such cases, some other person or group, a proxy, must be authorized to make medical and other decisions on their behalf.

Proxy Decision Making

The doctrine of informed consent, as interpreted by several U.S. courts,[66] requires that, before individuals of doubtful competence are administered psychoactive drugs (or other nonroutine medical services), a court determination be made of their competence and, if found to be not competent to make the decision at hand, a proxy decision be made on their behalf. In making the competency determination, the court is to determine whether the individual possesses the mental capacity to understand the nature and consequences of the decision to be made and can comprehend enough relevant information to come to a rational decision. If the court finds the individual to be competent for the decision, that person's choice must be respected, just as the treatment decisions of people who are not developmentally disabled are respected. If the person makes an informed, voluntary, competent decision to refuse psychoactive medication, the drugs may not legally be administered to the person as treatment.[67] It is still possible that medication might be given as a chemical restraint, but only in the event of an actual emergency, as discussed above.[68]

If, on the other hand, the court finds the person incompetent, a surrogate must make the treatment decision on the person's behalf. There is a wide variety of opinions about who this proxy decision maker should be and what standard should be used in making the decision (e.g., Kirby, 1983; President's Commission for the Study of Ethical Problems in Medicine and Biomedical and Behavioral Research, 1982). The traditional judicial solution in such situations has been for the court to appoint a legal guardian for the incompetent individual, a person then empowered to make decisions on behalf of his or her "ward." In several jurisdictions, however, courts have recently concluded that psychoactive drugs fall into a class of "extraordinary" medical treatments—treatments that are too intrusive, irreversible, or risky for even a legal guardian to consent to on behalf of another person.[69] Because there are "few legitimate medical procedures which are more intrusive than the forcible injection of antipsychotic medication . . . ,"[70] the highest court in Massachusetts, the state pioneering this approach, has ruled that the drugs may not be administered to an incompetent person, in a nonemergency situation, in either an institution or the community, without the authorization of a court.[71] Although the Massachusetts cases decided thus far have applied primarily to patients in a state psychiatric hospital who actively refused drug treatment and a noninstitutionalized mentally ill individual who also refused antipsychotic medication, the Supreme Judicial Court has explicitly noted that ,"because incompetent persons cannot meaningfully consent to medical treatment, a substituted judgment by a judge should be undertaken for the incompetent patient even if the patient accepts the medical treatment."[72] The decision thus also applies to functionally incompetent residents of mental retardation institutions who neither refuse nor meaningfully consent to drugs, and the Massachusetts Department of Mental Health is interpreting and applying the ruling in this manner.[73]

In Massachusetts, if the court finds the person incompetent to make the drug decision, the judge then makes a "substituted judgment" on the person's behalf. In making this judgment, the court tries to put itself into the shoes of the person (or, as courts sometimes say, tries to "don the mental mantle of the incompetent") and make the decision that person would make if he or she were competent, but taking into account the present and future incompetency of the individual.[74] In making a substituted judgment, the court is to consider all factors that might help it to know the actual values and preferences of the incompetent individual. Foremost among these are any preferences of the person him- or herself concerning treatment. The court also attempts to consider: the individual's religious beliefs, if known, and any effect they might have on his or her decision; the impact of the decision on the person's family, insofar as the client would have considered it in making the decision; the probability of adverse side effects; the prognosis with and without treatment; and any other relevant factors.[75] When the court determines what the individual would have decided, that decision must be respected, even if it will not achieve the restoration of the person's health, or will result in longer hospitalization. The incompetent individual "has the right to be wrong in the choice of treatment."[76]

This Massachusetts model has been criticized as being excessively legalistic, cumbersome, time consuming, and expensive. Psychiatrist Alan Stone argues that such court rulings, "by limiting use of antipsychotic drugs even in appropriate cases, create an incentive for psychiatrists to administer minor tranquilizers to their patients" (Stone, 1984, p. 155). Stone suggests that this may encourage patient dependence on these habit-forming drugs in situations where antipsychotic medication would be medically preferable (Stone, 1984). Other critics have argued that "bonded guardians" (such as family members and others whose relationship with the ward existed prior to the guardianship), when available, should have a stronger role in the decision-making process (Veatch, 1984). Still other commentators have pointed out the considerable difficulties of making a valid "substituted judgment" in actual cases (Gutheil & Appelbaum, 1985).

With some variations, however, the recognition of mental patients' qualified drug refusal rights has continued to spread through litigation in a number of other U.S. jurisdictions. Although the rationales underlying these rulings would appear equally applicable to individuals with mental retardation, the terms of most of the court judgments and decrees apply explicitly only to people in state psychiatric hospitals, and there has been little movement thus far toward extending that coverage. The Colorado Supreme Court, for example, ruled in 1985 that antipsychotic medication could be administered to an involuntarily committed, unconsenting mental patient in a nonemergency situation only after a court decides that the patient is actually incompetent to make the decision, that a "less intrusive treatment alternative is not available," and that "the patient's need for treatment by antipsychotic medication is sufficiently compelling to override any bona fide and legitimate interest in the patient refusing treatment."[77] By its terms, however, the ruling does not appear to apply to people in mental retardation institutions. A 1986 decision by the New York Court of

Appeals is quite similar in its recognition of qualified refusal rights and in limiting them to psychiatric patients.[78] And the 1983 consent decree in the California class action, *Jamison v. Farabee*,[79] which, for administration of antipsychotic medication to a nonconsenting, incompetent mental patient, requires approval by an "independent reviewer"[80] using least restrictive and best interests standards,[81] also has not been extended beyond the state mental hospital.

Effects of Newly Recognized Right to Refuse Medication

Assessments of the effects of honoring patients' refusals of medication have reached widely differing conclusions. A study by Gill (1982) of certain Massachusetts patients affected by the 1979 *Rogers v. Okin* decision[82] offered a bleak picture of these effects.[83] According to Applebaum and Hoge,

[o]f the 159 refusers [Gill] identified, 56 showed neither a worsening nor an improvement in their condition (although improvement would ordinarily have been expected following hospitalization), 89 deteriorated, and 14 who indicated that they would refuse treatment were apparently never admitted to the hospital. (Appelbaum & Hoge, 1986, p. 92)

Applebaum and Hoge caution, however, that

[t]he ways in which refusers were identified and their outcomes assessed were not specified by Gill. Nor is it clear that all refusers went without treatment entirely. Gill does note in addition, however, that the yearly use of seclusion at Boston State Hospital increased from 244 patients for 5,868 hours during the year prior to the issuance of a temporary restraining order requiring the hospital to grant patients a right to refuse, to 392 patents for 11,855 hours during the second year that the decree was in place. Similarly, referrals to the state's maximum security facility increased from an average of one per year to 6–7 per year. (Appelbaum & Hoge, 1986, p. 92).

At the other extreme is a 1980 article by Brooks of Rutgers Law School in which he analyzes the response to New Jersey's *Rennie v. Klein* suit.[84] Brooks found there was a smooth adjustment by psychiatrists and other hospital staff to *Rennie's* requirements, a reduction in the amount of medication used, and improvement in the treatment of patients (Brooks, 1980). (See also Beck, 1987).

Perhaps the most comprehensive review to date of relevant empirical knowledge on the effects of the right to refuse treatment took place in mid-1985, a little more than a decade after the right was first argued in a U.S. court (Appelbaum & Hoge, 1986). This review encompassed both published and unpublished studies of the topic, but was restricted to psychiatric patients, and focused especially on psychiatric inpatients. Among the Appelbaum-Hoge conclusions: Data suggest that when permitted to refuse drug treatment, between 20% and 50% of psychiatric patients do so at some point in their hospitalization, but that fewer than 5% refuse *consistently* and in a manner requiring outside intervention for resolution of the disagreement. Although some researchers have found refusers to be significantly more likely to be restrained and to have significantly longer lengths of stay, one study cited by Applebaum and Hoge, showed no differences between refusers and acceptors during a 1-month sample of negative behaviors. (But see Rodenhauser, Schwenkner, & Khamis, 1987). Perhaps most surprising, a study at California's Napa State Hospital found that the *Jamison* consent decree[85] had not resulted in any changes in the average dosage of medications administered, the number of successful drug refusers, the number of hours of restraint, the length of stay, or overall improvement in psychotherapy. These findings may, however, be explained by the rarity with which patient refusals have been upheld at Napa.

Appelbaum and Hoge observe that "the way in which systems respond to refusal is relatively unexplored. Those reports that exist [however] suggest that even with differing procedures and substantive criteria, most refusals are overridden and most patients treated" (Appelbaum & Hoge, 1986, p. 94). (See also Veliz & James, 1987; Hoge, Gutheil, & Kaplan, 1987). They note that varying interpretations of this phenomenon are possible: Those who are skeptical of the value of a refusal right might claim the data indicate that refusals are rarely justified. On the other hand, advocates of the right might note that "the highest rates of overriding refusals occur when the decision is in medical hands and that quite a substantial rate of upholding refusal (33 percent) was found in the single study in which that was not the case" (Appelbaum & Hoge, 1986, p. 95).

Whether conclusions of research conducted in psychiatric hospitals are applicable in other settings is, of course, problematic, and comparable studies do not yet appear to have been conducted for people with mental retardation. Attorney Steven Schwartz has, however, provided a modicum of information on this group, in discussing (also in mid-1985) the effects of the Massachusetts Supreme Judicial Court's *Rogers* decision[86] in both the mental health and mental retardation systems. According to Schwartz,

[a] large number of guardianship petitions have been filed by the Department of Mental Health with the priority on those cases involving the active refusal of treatment. As a result of internal medication reviews prior to filing petitions, a significant number of handicapped persons, particularly residents of state schools for the retarded, have had their psychotropic medication reduced or terminated altogether. Clinical observation of these persons [indicates they] have demonstrated some improvement, a marked decrease in side-effects and other damaging consequences of these drugs, and no noticeable deterioration in behavior or functioning. Data from all mental health and retardation facilities in the state indicate that there has not been any increase in accidents or injuries to institutional staff or

residents. In fact, due largely to the enactment of a separate state law that tightens restraint procedures, there has been a considerable decline in the use of all forms of restraints. (Schwartz, 1986, p. 77, footnotes omitted).

Status of U.S. Law Regarding Refusal

As mentioned above, rather few states have resolved consent questions regarding the administration of psychoactive drugs to persons of doubtful competence, even in the context of mental illness. It can be argued that the *Romeo* standard—"substantial departure from accepted professional judgment"—should be the test applied in such cases.[87] It is doubtful, however, that this rule will be extended in most jurisdictions to cover psychoactive drug therapy, a treatment that many courts and commentators consider much more intrusive than involuntary restraint (Onek, Klein, & Farr Law Firm, 1985). In the absence of definitive law, the practice of relying upon the consent of a guardian, family member, or treating physician is undoubtedly widespread, and will probably continue unless and until subject to court challenges.

When directly presented with these difficult questions, courts have found them far from easy to resolve. Consider the Third Circuit Court of Appeals' 1983 decision in New Jersey's long-running *Rennie v. Klein* suit.[88] In complying with a U.S. Supreme Court order that it reconsider the case,[89] an extremely divided appeals court attempted to apply the principles set forth in the Supreme Court's *Romeo*[90] ruling to the situation of an involuntarily confined mental patient's refusal of antipsychotic medication. Although seven of the eight judges concluded that New Jersey regulations governing the forcible administration of such drugs satisfy constitutional standards, the judges' views of precisely what those constitutional standards are differed dramatically.[91] Three judges would have ruled "only that antipsychotic drugs may be constitutionally administered to an involuntarily committed mentally ill patient whenever in the exercise of professional judgment, such an action is deemed necessary to prevent the patient from endangering himself or others."[92] One judge would have held "more explicitly. . . that the Due Process Clause at a minimum requires the authorities to administer antipsychotic drugs to an unwilling patient only when the decision is the product of the authorities' professional judgment."[93] Two judges argued, however, that

the professional judgment of a physician acting with the power of state authority requires more than comparable professional decisions in a voluntary doctor-patient relationship. In the case of the forcible use of antipsychotic drugs, a state-employed physician must, at the very least, consider the side effects of the drugs, consult with other professionals, and investigate other options available before that physician can be said to have discharged full professional judgment.[94]

And Circuit Judge Weis, joined by at least two (and probably three)[95] others, stressing the severe and potentially irreversible effects of anti-psychotic drugs,[96]

[f]eared that the latitude the majority allows in "professional judgment" jeopardizes adequate protection of a patient's constitutional rights. . . . [I]t is not enough to rely on "professional judgment" unless it includes an evaluation aimed at the least intrusive means—a cost-benefit analysis viewed from the patient's perspective.[97]

Weis insisted that "[i]ntroduction of the least intrusive means standard to these procedures does not supplant professional judgment, it merely adds an important factor to the analysis underlying that judgment."[98]

In Judge Weis's view, the hard realities of institutional conditions pose no impediment to implementation of this standard:

The realization that state institutions are understaffed, underfinanced, and overcrowded only underscores my concern that the staff may undervalue or overlook the patient's interest. . . . It surely is not asking too much of the state to require it to balance its legitimate needs with a regimen that infringes on the patient's constitutional rights to the least intrusive extent.[99]

British Commonwealth Law

It is clear that U.S. law's recognition of the autonomy rights of mentally disabled individuals with respect to drug treatment has thus far been rather uneven. The progress in a number of other countries, however, appears to have been no smoother. It has been said, for example, that courts throughout the British Commonwealth are most reluctant to support a right to refuse treatment within the mental health context. Gordon and Verdun-Jones (1983) have attributed this reluctance to "the nature of the existing mental health legislation" (p. 63). Their 1983 analysis of such legislation in Canada, Australia, New Zealand, England, and Scotland suggested that "a right to refuse treatment is virtually non-existent. Indeed, statutes tend to permit compulsory treatment to occur either explicitly or implicitly" (p. 63).

It is clear that change is underway, however. One of these researchers has since observed that the New South Wales, Australia, Mental Act of 1983 implements "to quite an amazing extent, . . . a policy of strict regulation of mental health treatments" (Verdun-Jones, 1986, p. 108). And the England and Wales Mental Health Act of 1983 is somewhat similar to California's *Jamison v. Farabee* consent decree[100] in its approach to regulation of psychoactive drugs. The Act provides that medication (and electroconvulsive therapy) may not be administered to patients who are mentally ill or have an "impairment of intelligence and social functioning" (Gostin, 1986, sections 9.02 & 9.03) in nonemergency situations except with the consent of the patient (whose competency has been verified by a medical officer) or after an independent second opinion that the treatment should be given. The independent opinion, which should assess whether the drug will alleviate or prevent a deterioration of the patient's condition,[101] may be given only by "a registered medical practitioner appointed by, or a member of, the Mental Health Act Commission who cannot be the responsible medical officer" (Gostin, 1986, section 20.21.3 [ii]). The practitioner must also consult and obtain the approval of two other persons "who have been professionally concerned with the patient's medical treatment . . ." (Gostin, 1986, section 20.21.3[ii]). These fairly stringent requirements are diluted substantially, however, by a provision stating that they apply only if three months or more have elapsed since the first occasion during the period of detention when medication was administered.[102] "The 'three month rule' was intended to give the [responsible medical officer] a period of time where he could treat a patient with medication to stabilize his condition before any statutory safeguard became applicable" (Gostin, 1982, p. 1200).

Personal Opinion

The question of whether, and how, psychoactive medication should be administered to people of questionable competence or to institutionalized individuals is one of the most difficult medicolegal issues of our day. A 1985 American Bar Association forum, which brought together leading psychiatric and legal experts from across the United States to discuss the topic, demonstrated that divisions of opinion appear as deep as ever (Rapoport & Parry, 1986). These differences can be seen in the generally negative reaction of the psychiatric community to judicial rulings restricting the use of antipsychotic medication (e.g., Stone, 1984, p. 136 et seq.; Brooks, 1987), and in the adverse reactions of *both* communities to the *Jamison v. Farabee* consent decree governing such treatment at California's Napa State Hospital.[103] Many patient advocates believe that the decree's provision that a patient's refusal can be overruled by one independent reviewer, who is a physician, eviscerates the right to refuse. They point to the rarity with which refusals are upheld as evidence of the decree's ineffectiveness (Appelbaum & Hoge, 1986, pp. 93–95). On the other hand, the American Psychiatric Association[104] and a substantial number of doctors and nursing staff at the hospital (Appelbaum & Hoge, 1986, p. 94) have expressed serious misgivings about the decree because they believe it has needlessly complicated the work of the service providers and has impaired patients' treatment.

These differences between the legal and medical views are not likely to be resolved in the near future.[105] However, it seems to me (a lawyer) that, whatever the resolution, certain principles must apply:

1. When used as a chemical restraint, psychoactive medication must be subject to controls at least as stringent as those governing the use of mechanical restraints and seclusion.[106] The strong pressures that are always present in an institutional setting to use medication for the convenience of the caregivers and as a substitute for adequate staffing and active programming, when considered in light of the undisputed evidence of the historical prevalence of such abuses, make such control indispensable.

2. Before psychoactive medications are used for therapeutic treatment of a person with development disabilities, clear, unquivocal evidence should be required that the particular drugs are likely to be effective in treating the specific problems of the individual to be treated,[107] and that the drugs' benefits are likely to outweigh their risks.[108] A number of articles in this volume make the point that a small proportion of mentally retarded individuals, having clear-cut psychiatric disorders, do benefit from appropriately selected psychotropic medication in the same way that nonretarded people do. Some experts in the field, however, continue to express concern that "only a fraction of those receiving long-term neuroleptic medication are clinically better on them than off them. . . ." (Schatzberg, & Cole, 1986, pp. 254–255; see also Chapter 4).

3. If the benefits and appropriateness of administering certain psychoactive medications to incompetent individuals for the treatment of certain problems can be demonstrated, a proper decision-making process, decision maker, and standard must be untilized.[109] Again, the lessons of history and the continuing pressures of institutional settings make clear to me that the decision maker should not be an individual responsible for, or involved in, the individual's clinical treatment. Nor does it seem adequate to entrust such a decision, with effects and risks extending beyond the medical sphere, solely to the medical profession (as is done in *Jamison*[110]). On the other hand, there seems to me considerable merit in the argument that requiring court involvement in every such decision (as in the Massachusetts *Rogers* model) is excessively cumbersome, time consuming, inefficient, and, in the long run, probably less than effective.[111] I believe further investigation is required of alternative mechanisms in which guardians or family members (where they are available) participate in an administrative decision-making process incorporating medical, legal, and social/developmental expertise (President's Commission, 1982, Vol 1, p. 188). Various models have been proposed or are now undergoing trials in several U.S. states.[122] After a few years' experience with different types, a consensus may emerge as to the best model for the purpose.

Whether the decision should be made utilizing a "best interests" or "substituted judgment" standard[113] depends, in my opinion, upon the capacities of the particular individual involved. If he or she possesses, or ever did possess, the capability of understanding and of forming an opinion regarding the proposed drug treatment, the decision maker should, I believe, utilize the substituted judgment process to attempt to determine that opinion. If, on the other hand, the individual never had the capacity to have formed a view relative to the matter, the more honest approach for the decision maker would seem to be a candid admission of the impossibility of determining what the person would do if competent, and a conscientious application of the "best interests" standard, deciding to the best of one's ability what society would consider best for the individual.

4. Finally, at any time psychoactive medications are administered to individuals with developmental disabilities, whether for restraint or for therapy, in community settings or (especially) in institutions, an effective monitoring and review mechanism must be in place to assure that the use of the drugs conforms to high professional standards such as those required by *Wyatt* and the succeeding major cases.[144]

Conclusion

It is clear that institutionalized mentally retarded individuals have enjoyed substantial progress in many jurisdictions during the past 15 years in gaining legal recognition of a number of rights regarding psychoactive drug treatment. It is equally clear that a great deal remains to be done in determining which of these legal developments best serve their interests, and in achieving universal recognition of the most salutary of these rights. These are the challenges for the next decade.

Acknowledgment. I gratefully acknowledge the research assistance of law student Douglas V. Egly.

References

Abbott, M., Dawson, J., Haines, H., Hessey, E., McBride, T., & Maule, R. (1983, December). *Towards mental health law reform: Report of the Legal Information Service/Mental Health Foundation Task Force on Revision of Mental Health Legislation*, Mental Health Foundation of New Zealand.

Aman, M.G. (1984). Drugs and learning in mentally retarded persons. In G.D. Burrows & J.S. Werry (Eds.), *Advances in human psychopharmacology* (Vol. 3, pp. 121–163). Greenwich, CT: JAI Press.

American Association on Mental Deficiency. (1973–75). *Rights of mentally retarded persons*. Washington, DC: AAMD Council.

Annas, G.J. (1975). *The rights of hospital patients*. New York: Discus/Avon.

Appelbaum, P.S., & Hoge, S.K. (1986). Empirical research on the effects of legal policy on the right to refuse treatment. In D. Rapoport & J. Parry (Eds.), *The right to refuse antipsychotic medication* (pp. 87–97). Washington, DC: American Bar Association's Commission on the Mentally Disabled.

Arkin, H.R. (1984). Forcible administration of antipsychotic medication: State laws. *Journal of the American Medical Association, 144,* 2620–2621.

Ayd, F. (1973). Rational pharmacotherapy: Once-a-day drug dosage. *Diseases of the Nervous System, 34,* 371–378.

Beck, J.C. (1987). Right to refuse antipsychotic medication: Psychiatric assessment and legal decision-making. *Mental and Physical Disability Law Reporter, 11,* 368–372.

Beyer, H.A. (1983). Litigation with the mentally retarded. In. J. Matson & J. Mulick (Eds.), *Handbook of mental retardation* (pp. 79–93). New York: Pergamon Press.

Brakel, S., & Rock, R. (Eds.). (1971). *The mentally disabled and the law.* (rev. ed.). Chicago: University of Chicago Press.

Bregman, S. (1984). Assertiveness training for mentally retarded adults. *Mental Retardation, 22,* 12–16.

Brooks, A.D. (1980). The constitutional right to refuse antipsychotic medication. *Bulletin of the American Association of Psychology and Law, 8,* 179–221.

Brooks, A.D. (1987). The right to refuse antipsychotic medication: Law and policy. *Rutgers Law Review, 39,* 339–376.

Dunphy, S.M., & Cross, J.H. (1987). Medical decision making for incompetent persons: The Massachusetts substituted judgment model. *Western New England Law Review, 9,* 153–167.

Floor, L., & Rosen, M. (1975). Investigating the phenomenon of helplessness in mentally retarded adults. *American Journal of Mental Deficiency, 79,* 565–572.

Gill, M.J. (1982). Side effects of a right to refuse treatment lawsuit: The Boston State Hospital experience. In A.F. Doudera & J.P. Swazey (Eds.), *Refusing treatment in mental health institutions: Values in conflict* (pp. 81–87). Ann Arbor, MI: AUPHA Press.

Gordon, R.M., & Verdun-Jones, S.N. (1983). The right to refuse treatment: Commonwealth developments and issues. *International Journal of Law and Psychiatry, 6,* 57–73.

Gordon, R.M., & Verdun-Jones, S.N. (1986). The impact of the Canadian Charter of Rights and Freedoms upon Canadian mental health law: The dawn of a new era or business as usual? *Law, Medicine & Health Care, 14,* 190–197.

Gostin, L. (1982). A review of the Mental Health (Amendment) Act: III. The legal position of patients while in hospital. *New Law Journal,* 1199–1202.

Gostin, L. (1986). *Mental health services—law and practice.* London: Shaw & Sons.

Gualtieri, C.T., Sprague, R.L., & Cole, J.O. (1986). Tardive dyskinesia litigation and the dilemmas of neuroleptic treatment. *Journal of Psychiatry & Law, 14,* 187–216.

Gutheil, T.G., & Appelbaum, P. (1983). "Mind control," "synthetic sanity," "artificial competence," and genuine confusion: Legally relevant effects of antipsychotic medication. *Hofstra Law Review, 12,* 77–120.

Gutheil, T.G., & Appelbaum, P.S. (1985). The substituted judgment approach: Its difficulties and paradoxes in mental health settings. *Law, Medicine & Health Care, 13,* 61–64.

Gutheil, T.G., Shapiro, R., & St. Clair, R.L. (1980). Legal guardianship in drug refusal: An illusory solution. *American Journal of Psychiatry, 137,* 347–352.

Hargreaves, W.A., Shumway, M., Knutsen, E.J., Weinstein, A., & Senter, N. (1987). Effects of the *Jamison-Farabee* consent decree: Due process protection for involuntary psychiatric patients treated with psychoactive medication. *American Journal of Psychiatry, 144*, 188–192.

Hoge, S.K., Gutheil, T.G., & Kaplan, E. (1987). The right to refuse treatment under *Rogers v. Commissioner*: Preliminary empirical findings and comparisons. *Bulletin of the American Academy of Psychiatry & Law, 15*, 163–169.

International League of Societies for the Mentally Handicapped. (1968, October). *Declaration of General and Special Rights of the Mentally Retarded.* Brussels, Belgium: ILSMH.

Kirby, M. (1983). On talking about ethics. *Australian Paediatric Journal, 19*, 208–209.

McNamara, P. (1980). Psychopharmacotherapy in South Australia. *Adelaide Law Review, 7*, 323–347.

Onek, Klein, & Farr Law Firm. (1985). *Selected legal problems in the practice of psychiatry.* Washington, DC: American Psychiatric Association.

Peay, J. (1986). The Mental Health Act 1983 (England and Wales): Legal safeguards in limbo. *Law, Medicine & Health Care 14*, 180–189.

Plotkin, R. (1977). Limiting the therapeutic orgy: Mental patients' right to refuse treatment. *Northwestern University Law Review, 72*, 461–525.

Plotkin, R., & Gill, K.R. (1979). Invisible manacles: Drugging mentally retarded people. *Stanford Law Review, 31*, 637–678.

President's Commission for the Study of Ethical Problems in Medicine and Biomedical and Behavioral Research. (1982). *Making health care decisions: A report on the ethical and legal implications of informed consent in the patient-practitioner relationship.* Washington, DC: U.S. Government Printing Office.

Rapoport, D, & Parry, J. (Eds.). (1986). *The right to refuse antipsychotic medication: A monograph including the perspectives of legal and clinical specialists based on papers presented at an ABA Presidential Showcase panel program.* Washington, DC: American Bar Association's Commission on the Mentally Disabled.

Rodenhauser, P., Schwenkner, C.E., & Khamis, H.J. (1987). Factors related to drug treatment refusal in a forensic hospital. *Hospital & Community Psychiatry, 38*, 631–637.

Rosen, M., Floor L., & Zisfein, L. (1974). Investigating the phenomenon of acquiescence in the mentally handicapped. *British Journal of Mental Subnormality, 20*, 56–68.

Schatzberg, A.F., & Cole, J.O. (1986). *Manual of clinical psychopharmacology.* Washington, DC: American Psychiatric Press.

Schwartz, S.J. (1986). Equal protection in medication decisions: Informed consent, not just the right to refuse. In D. Rapoport & J. Parry (Eds.), *The right to refuse antipsychotic medication* (pp. 74–79). Washington, DC: American Bar Association's Commission on the Mentally Disabled.

Sigelman C., Budd, E.C., Spanhel, C.L. & Schoenrock, C.J. (1981). When in doubt, say yes: Acquiescence in interviews with mentally retarded persons. *Mental Retardation, 19*, 53–58.

Sovner, R. (1986). Assessing the quality of a psychotropic drug regimen. In D. Rapoport & J. Parry (Eds.), *The right to refuse antipsychotic medication* (pp. 48–57). Washington, DC: American Bar Association's Commission on the Mentally Disabled.

Sprague, R.L., & Baxley, G.B. (1978). Drugs for behavior management, with comment of some legal aspects. In J. Wortis (Ed.), *Mental retardation and developmental disabilities* (Vol. 10, pp. 92–129). New York: Brunner/Mazel.

Stone, A.A. (1984). *Law, psychiatry, and morality: Essays and analysis*. Washington, DC: American Psychiatric Press.

Stone, A.A. (1984–85). Judges as medical decision makers: Is the cure worse than the disease? *Cleveland State Law Review, 33*, 579–592.

United Cerebral Palsy Association. (1973, May). *A Bill of Rights for the handicapped*. Washington DC: UCPA Annual conference.

United Nations. (1948). *Resolution of the General Assembly*, Dec. 10, 1948, #217, 3 GAOR (A/810).

United Nations. (1972). *Resolution of the General Assembly*, Jan. 21, 1972, Agenda Item #12 [A/Res/2856(XXVI)].

United Nations. (1975). *Resolution of the General Assembly*, Dec. 9. 1975 [A/10284/Add.1(XXX)].

Veatch, R.M. (1984). Limits of guardian treatment refusal: A reasonableness standard. *American Journal of Law and Medicine, 9*, 427–468.

Veliz, J., & James, W.S. (1987). Medicine court: *Rogers* in practice. *American Journal of Psychiatry, 144*, 62–67.

Verdun-Jones, S.N. (1986). The dawn of a "new legalism" in Australia? The New South Wales Mental Health Act, 1983 and related legislation. *International Journal of Law and Psychiatry, 8*, 95–118.

Wexler, D.B. (1982). Seclusion and restraint: Lessons from law, psychiatry, and psychology. *International Journal of Law and Psychiatry, 5*, 285–294.

Winick, B.J. (1986). The right to refuse psychotropic medication: Current state of the law and beyond. In D. Rapoport & J. Parry (Eds.), *The right to refuse antipsychotic medication* (pp. 7–31). Washington, DC: American Bar Association's Commission on the Mentally Disabled.

Notes

1. See, e.g., Canada Constitution Act 1982, § 15(1) ("Every individual is equal before and under the law and has the right to the equal protection and equal benefit of the law without discrimination and, in particular, without discrimination based on . . . mental or physical disability"); U.S. Developmental Disabilities Assistance and Bill of Rights Act, 42 U.S.C. 6010 ("The Federal Government and the States both have an obligation to assure that public funds are not provided to any . . . residential program for persons with developmental disabilities that . . . does not meet the following minimum standards: . . . Prohibition on the excessive use of chemical restraints on such persons and the use of such restraints as punishment or as a substitute for a habilitation program or in quantities that interfere with services, treatment, or habilitation for such persons . . .").

2. The U.S. Congress, for example, limits the term "developmental disability" to one which "is manifested before the person attains age twenty-two." 42 U.S.C. § 6000(7) (1978).

3. Canada Constitution Act 1982, Part I. It is clear, however, that such a dramatic change cannot occur overnight. See Gordon and Verdun-Jones (1986).

4. Many U.S. courts have cited studies indicating very widespread institutional use. See, e.g., *Wyatt v. Hardin*, Civil Action No. 3195-N (U.S.D.C., M.D. Ala., Affidavit of Dr. Robert Sprague, Sept. 8, 1977). See also Chapter 1.
5. See *Rogers v. Okin*, 634 F. 2d 650 (1st Cir. 1980), at 653 n. 1. The 1st Circuit Court of Appeals, in *Rogers*, used the term, "antipsychotic drugs," noting that "the district court used this term interchangeably with the apparently broader term 'psychotropic drugs,' which may include antidepressants and lithium, and which as far as the record shows do not have as substantial a potential for serious side effects as do the antipsychotics" (*Id*).
6. See, e.g., *Halderman v. Pennhurst*, 446 F. Supp. 1295, 1307–08 (E.D. Pa. 1977); *Gary W. v. Louisiana*, 437 F. Supp. 1209, 1229 (E.D. La. 1976); *Morales v. Turman*, 383 F. Supp. 53, 103–05 (E.D. Tex. 1974), vacated, 535 F. 2d 864 (5th Cir. 1976), reinstated, 430 U.S. 322 (1977); *Welsch v. Likins*, 373 F. Supp. 487, 503 (D. Minn 1974); *Wyatt v. Stickney*, 344 F. Supp. 387, 400 (M.D. Ala. 1972).
7. *Id.* See also *Naughton v. Bevilaqua*, 458 F. Supp. 610 (D.R.I. 1978), at 615; *Anderson v. State of Arizona*, 663 P. 2d 570 (Ariz. Ct. App. 1983).
8. *Wyatt v. Stickney*, 344 F. Supp. 387 (M.D. Ala. 1972). at 400, § 22d. Cf. *Welsch v. Dirkswager*, No. 4–72 Civil 451 (U.S.D.C., D. Minn., consent decree, Dec. 1977), at 17..
9. 475 U.S. 307, 322 (1982).
10. For example, while Utah law allows the application of restraints if "required by the needs of the patient" (Utah Code Ann., § 64-7-47), Wisconsin's statute specifies that "restraint may be used only when less restrictive measures are ineffective or not feasible and shall be used for the shortest time possible" (Wis. State Mental Health Act, § 51.61(1)(i)). See also "Seclusion and Restraint, The Psychiatric Uses: Report of the American Psychiatric Association Task Force on the Psychiatric Uses of Seclusion and Restraint" (1985), at 10: "In 23 states indications for seclusion or restraint were to prevent harm to the patient or other person. However, eight regulations included the prevention of substantial property damage and two included disruption of the treatment environment as indications."
11. *Rogers v. Commissioner*, 390 Mass. 489, at 509.
12. U.S. courts have long recognized that even when a government's action serves a legitimate societal goal, it must utilize means that curtail individual freedom no more than is necessary to secure that goal. *Lake v. Cameron*, 364 F. 2d 657, 659–660 (D.C. Cir. 1966).
13. *Rogers v. Okin*, 634 F. 2d 650 (1st. Cir. 1980), at 655–656.
14. The term "pharmacological restraints" is also used in some jurisdictions. See *Anderson v. State*, 663 P. 2d 570 (Ariz. App. 1982), at 577.
15. 421 N.E. 2d 40, 61 (Mass. 1981).
16. *Id.*, at 61.
17. *O'Connor v. Donaldson*, 422 U.S. 563 (1975), at 573; *Youngberg v. Romeo*, 457 U.S. 307 (1982), at 319.
18. *Youngberg v. Romeo*, 457 U.S. 307, 318 (1982).
19. See, e.g., *Wyatt v. Stickney*, 344 F. Supp. 387 (M.D. Ala. 1972); *New York State Association for Retarded Children v. Carey*, 393 F. Supp. 715 (E.D.N.Y. 1975).
20. See, e.g., *Association for Retarded Citizens—California v. Dept. of Developmental Services*, 696 P. 2d 150, 211 Cal. Rptr. 758 (1985).

21. Letter from A.M. Schmidt, FDA Commissioner, to D. Lehr (Nov. 11, 1975) reprinted in *Drugs in Institutions*: *Hearing Before the Subcommittee to Investigate Juvenile Delinquency of the Senate Committee on the Judiciary*, 94th Congress, 1st Session (1975), at 400, as cited by Plotkin and Gill (1979), at 653, n. 94, (emphasis added).
22. 344 F. Supp. 387 (M.D. Ala. 1972).
23. *Id.*, at 400.
24. *Pennhurst*, note 6 above, at 1328.
25. *Id.*, at 1329.
26. Or the Medicaid standards for Intermediate Care Facilities for the Mentally Retarded (ICF/MR). See 43 CFR § 442.458, 51 Fed. Reg. 7520 (Mar. 4, 1986).
27. *Conn. Association for Retarded Citizens v. Thorne*, Civil No. H-78-653 (U.S.D.C., D. Conn., consent decree, Nov. 7, 1983), at 10.
28. *Id.*, at 11–12. See also *Garrity v. Gallen*, Civil Action No. 78-116-D (U.S.D.C., D.N.H., Order for Implementation, Nov. 16, 1981).
29. See, e.g. *Halderman v. Pennhurst*, note 6, above, at 1307, quoting expert witness Dr. Robert Sprague. See also, Sovner (1986, p. 50): "Unless the prescribing physician regularly interviews the patient, it will be difficult to assess treatment-response. The physician cannot rely solely on surrogate evaluations made by nursing staff or mental health workers, although these staff do provide valuable clinical information."
30. *Welsch v. Dirkswager*, No. 4–72 Civil 451 (U.S.D.C., D. Minn., consent decree, Dec. 1977).
31. *Id.*, at 18.
32. *Id.*, at 19–20.
33. This specific criticism is directed at Plotkin, 1977.
34. See, e.g., *Rogers v. Okin*, 478 F. Supp. 1342 (D. Mass. 1979), at 1366–1367.
35. *Id.*, at 1360.
36. *Id.*, at 1366–1367. It should be noted that Alan A. Stone, professor of law and psychiatry on the Faculty of Law and the Faculty of Medicine at Harvard University, considers this decision "one of the most misguided, injudicious, juridicogenic opinions in the entire case law of law and psychiatry" (Stone, 1984–85, p. 589). "Juridicogenic" is a term coined by Dr. Stone for use in the field of law corresponding to use of the term "iatrogenic," used in medicine to refer to cures that create diseases. See also Gutheil, Shapiro, and St. Clair (1980).
37. *Rennie v. Klein*, 720 F. 2d 266 (3rd Cir. 1983), at 276.
38. *Clites v. Iowa*, Law No. 46274 (Iowa Dist. Ct. for Pottawattamie Cnty.). See also *Barclay v. Campbell*, 704 S.W. 2d 8 (Tex, 1986). But see *Frasier v. Dept. of Health and Human Resources*, 500 So. 2d 858 (La. Ct. App. 1986).
39. *Clites v. Iowa*, note 38, above, slip opinion, at 4–5.
40. *Rogers v. Okin*, 478 F. Supp. 1354 (D. Mass. 1979), at 1360.
41. American Psychiatric Association (APA) Task Force Report #18 (1980), at p. 18, as quoted by J. Kane, Chairman, Task Force on Tardive Dyskinesia, in letter to APA members (July 1985).
42. 322 N.W. 2d 917, at 920.
43. *Clites v. Iowa*, note 38, above, at 10; affirmed 322 N.W. 2d 917 (Iowa Ct. App. 1982).

44. *Faigenbaum v. Oakland Medical Center*, 373 N.W. 2d 161 (Mich. Ct. App. 1985), at 163.
45. *Id.*
46. *Id.*
47. *R.A.J. v. Miller*, No. C-A-3-74-0394-H (U.S.D.C., N.D. Tex., Settlement Agreement, Mar. 2, 1981).
48. *Id.*, at 16.
49. 457 U.S. 307 (1982).
50. *Id.*, at 315.
51. *Id.*, at 319.
52. *Id.*, at 321.
53. *Id.*, at 323 (footnotes omitted).
54. *Id.*, at 321.
55. *Id.*, at 323 n. 31.
56. See, e.g., *Society for Good Will to Retarded Children v. Cuomo*, 737 F. 2d 1239 (2nd Cir. 1984).
57. *Olmstead v. U.S.*, 277 U.S. 438, 478 (1928).
58. *Roe v. Wade*, 410 U.S. 113 (1973).
59. *Superintendent of Belchertown State School v. Saikewicz*, 370 N.E. 2d 417, 426 (Mass. 1977).
60. See, e.g., *Rennie v. Klein*, *Guardianship of Roe*, and *Rogers v. Commissioner*, discussed in text below, at notes 69–99.
61. *Barclay v. Campbell*, 704 S.W. 2d 8, 10 (Tex. 1986).
62. *Kaimowitz v. Department of Mental Health*, C.A. No. 73-19434-AW (Cir. Ct., Wayne Cty, Mich. July 10, 1973).
63. *Id.*, slip opinion at 28.
64. *ARC of N. Dakota v. Olson*, Civ. No. Al-80-141 (U.S.D.C., D.N.D., Aug. 31, 1982) (slip opinion), at 22–23.
65. See, e.g., Mass. General Laws, ch. 123 § 24.
66. See, e.g., *Rogers v. Commissioner of Mental Health*, 390 Mass. 489 (1983); *Rivers v. Katz*, 67 N.Y. 2d 485 (N.Y. Ct. App. 1986); *People v. Medina*, 705 P. 2d 961 (Colo. 1985); *In re K.K.B..*, 609 P. 2d 747 (Okla. 1980); *Wisconsin v. Gerhardstein*, 391 N.W. 2d 212 (Wis. Ct. App., 1986). See also *Henderson v. Yocum*, 11 Mental and Physical Disability Law Reporter 327 (S.D. Cir. Ct., 1st Cir., 1987); *Commmitment of M.P.*, 500 N.E. 2d 216 (Ind. App.) 1986.
67. Cf. *San Diego Dept. of Social Services v. Waltz*, 225 Cal. Rptr. 664 (Cal. Ct. App. 1986) (refusal of electroconvulsive therapy by mentally ill man with nonpsychotic periods must be respected even though his conservator consents).
68. Text, above, at note 11.
69. See *Rivers v. Katz*, 67 N.Y. 2d 485 (N.Y. Ct. App. 1986); *People v. Medina*, 705 P. 2d 961 (Colo. 1985); *Rogers v. Commissioner of Mental Health*, 390 Mass. 489 (1983); *Guardianship of Roe*, 383 Mass. 415 (1981). See also *Matter of Alleged Mental Illness of Kinzer*, 375 N.W. 2d 526 (Minn. Ct. App. 1985).
70. *Guardianship of Roe*, note 69 above, at 436.
71. *Rogers* and *Roe*, note 69 above.
72. *Rogers*, note 69, above, at 500, n. 14.
73. See Mass. Department of Mental Health Policy #84–40, Apr. 27, 1984.

74. *Rogers v. Commissioner*, note 69 above, at 500, citing the *Saikewicz* opinion, note 59 above, at 750.
75. *Rogers*, note 69 above, at 505–506.
76. *Id.*, at 501, n. 15.
77. *People v. Medina*, 705 P. 2d 961 (Colo. 1985), at 973. See also *Colorado v. Schmidt*, 720 P. 2d 629 (Colo. Ct. App. 1986).
78. *Rivers v. Katz*, 67 N.Y. 2d 485 (N.Y. Ct. App. 1986).
79. *Jamison v. Farabee*, No. C-78-0445-WHO (U.S.D.C., N.D. Cal., consent decree, Apr. 26, 1983).
80. As of March 1984, every one of the fourteen prospective appointees to the position of Independent Reviewer was a physician. Letter to H. Beyer from L. Lowden, *Jamison* Coordinator, Cal. Dept. of Mental Health (Mar. 19, 1984) (on file at the Pike Institute, Boston University School of Law). See also U.S. v. Leatherman, 580 F. Supp. 977 (D.D.C. 1983); *Opinion of the Justices*, 465 A.2d 484 (N.H. 1983).
81. The reviewer is to determine if the proposed medication is "the least restrictive form of treatment reasonably available" and is "a necessary part of the patient's treatment plan." *Id.*, Appendix A, at 1, 5, and 7.
82. Note 34, above.
83. As cited by Appelbaum & Hoge, 1986, p. 92.
84. Note 88, below.
85. See text, at note 79, above. See also Hargreaves, Shumway, Knutsen, Weinstein, and Senter (1987).
86. See text, at notes 71–76, above.
87. See text at note 53, above. See also *In re Mental Commitment of M.P.*, 500 N.E. 2d 216 (Ind. Ct. App. 1986).
88. 720 F. 2d 266 (3rd Cir. 1983).
89. The court's first decision, 653 F. 2d 836 (3rd Cir. 1983), was remanded by the U.S. Supreme Court, 458 U.S. 1119; 102 S. Ct. 3506 (1982), for reconsideration in light of *Youngberg v. Romeo*, note 49, above.
90. See text, above, at note 49.
91. Three judges joined in the opinion announcing the judgment of the court, two in one concurring opinion, three in a second concurring opinion, a lone judge wrote a third concurring opinion, and one judge wrote a dissent.
92. *Rennie v. Klein*, 720 F. 2d 266 (3rd Cir. 1983), at 269.
93. *Id.*, at 274.
94. *Id.*, at 272.
95. Judge Gibbons joined in this concurring opinion "setting forth the legal standard applicable by virtue of the fourteenth amendment. . . . [but] dissent[ed] from the judgment insofar as it modifies the preliminary injunction which was entered by the trial court" (*Id.*, at 277).
96. "The permanency of these effects is analogous to that resulting from such radical surgical procedures as a pre-frontal lobotomy" (*Id.*, at 276).
97. *Id.*, at 276.
98. *Id.*, at 277.
99. *Id.*
100. See text, above, at note 79. For a discussion of problems in implementing the act's provisions, see Peay (1986).
101. Thus, the drugs must be "*medical treatment* for mental disorder. The distinc-

tion, therefore, between 'treatment' and 'restraint' (or other measures) is important" (Gostin, 1986, at section 20.19.3).

102. England/Wales Mental Health Act 1983, § 58(1)b.

103. See text, at note 79, above.

104. "APA Decries *Jamison* Standards," 8 Mental and Physical Disability Law Reporter 496 (1984).

105. "To call [these issues] simply disputes between civil libertarians and psychiatrists following the 'medical model' is misleading. They are, instead, a manifestation of evolving societal attitudes regarding the proper balance between state interests and the liberty interests of mentally ill individuals" (Arkin, 1984, p. 2621).

106. See text, at notes 6–16, above.

107. See text, at note 21, above.

108. See text, at notes 33–46, above.

109. See text, at notes 66–81, above.

110. See text, at notes 79 and 103–104, above.

111. "Frequently, . . . it appears that the process of judicial review is merely a formality. Judges may not feel that they are able to add very much to the decisions already reached by those most intimately involved, particularly in cases that are brought simply to obtain judicial sanction for an agreed upon course of conduct" (President's Commission, 1982, Vol. 1, p. 186). See also *In re Bryant*, 10 Mental & Physical Disability Law Reporter 536 (D.C. Super. Ct., Fam. Div., 1986); Dunphy & Cross (1987).

112. New York State, e.g., has implemented a pilot project for such an administrative model, using "surrogate decision-making committees" as an alternative to requiring court orders for making certain major medical care decisions for persons with impaired decision-making capacity who do not have a guardian or family member to make such decisions (Chapter 354, N.Y. 1985 Session Laws, 7/18/85). Under a Vermont consent decree, an administrative hearing officer will conduct an adjudicatory hearing to decide medication and other medical questions for incompetent patients. *J.L. v. Miller*, 9 Mental & Physical Disability Law Reporter 261 (Vt. Super Ct., Washington Cty., 1985). A Massachusetts legislative committee has recommended institution of a trial project under which an "independent monitor," appointed by a human rights committee, would make decisions regarding antipsychotic medication for certain nonrefusing, "incapable" mental health patients as an alternative to *Rogers*-type judicial proceedings (Mass. House Bill No. 6005, 5/2/85). The District of Columbia is considering legislation to establish procedures for making health care decisions on behalf of incapacitated individuals (11 Mental and Physical Disability Law Reporter 214, 1987).

113. See text, at notes 73–76, above.

114. See text, at notes 22–32, above.

3
Psychotropic Drug Blood Levels: Measurement and Relation to Behavioral Outcome in Mentally Retarded Persons

MARK H. LEWIS AND RICHARD B. MAILMAN

Abstract

A major factor determining response to pharmacotherapy is the quantity of drug (and sometimes active metabolite) that is available to be taken up into the brain. Drug and metabolite measurements in blood are necessary to determine this bioavailability. This chapter is concerned with issues relevant to the measurement and clinical utility of blood concentrations of psychotropic drugs and their meta-bolites in mentally retarded persons. Much of the discussion addresses several confounding factors that can adversely affect the relationship between blood levels and behavioral outcome. However, despite technical and theoretical difficulties inherent in blood level measurements, such studies may improve pharmacotherapy by (a) establishing "therapeutic windows" for specific behavioral or psychiatric disorders, (b) preventing behavioral toxicity, (c) identifying non-responders or negative responders, and (d) ascertaining compliance. Relatively little research has been done quantifying drug concentrations with mentally retarded subjects as compared with other clinical populations, and many basic questions remain to be answered. The application of pharmacokinetics to drug treatment of retarded persons (who often cannot relate toxic effects or subjective indices of improvement) can only improve clinical practice and provide rational empirical criteria for treatment decisions in this field.

Despite the high prevalence of psychotropic drug use in the treatment of mentally retarded persons, basic questions concerning efficacy, specificity, dose dependency of effects, and the proportion of drug responders to non-responders or negative responders are as yet unresolved. This chapter is concerned with issues relevant to the measurement and clinical utility of determining blood concentrations of psychotropic drugs and their metabo-lites. Despite technical and theoretical difficulties inherent in such measure-ments and their correlations to clinical response, such studies should aid in establishing blood concentrations associated with changes in spe-cific behavioral disorders, preventing behavioral toxicity, and identifying nonresponders.

Much of the discussion that follows focuses on antipsychotic drug blood levels. This emphasis reflects the fact that these drugs are, by a large margin, the most frequently prescribed drugs for the treatment of behavioral disorders in retarded persons. Moreover, our work has focused on the phenothiazine antipsychotic, thioridazine. However, those factors that affect the relationship between antipsychotic drug blood levels and behavioral outcome will, to a large degree, also affect blood level and behavioral outcome relationships with other classes of drugs. Our strategy is not to review the pharmacokinetics of individual drugs, but rather to highlight issues related to the use of drug blood levels and factors that influence blood level/behavioral outcome relationships.

Many studies in the literature have failed to account for a significant portion of the variance in behavioral outcome by circulating drug concentrations. Much of the discussion that follows addresses the many factors that can adversely affect such a relationship. Careful consideration of these potential artifacts in the design of future studies should lead to increases in the magnitude of this relationship. Moreover, the available literature consists largely of studies using subjects of normal IQ with various psychiatric diagnoses. Clinical response/drug blood levels may be more strongly related in mentally retarded subjects for whom drugs such as antipsychotics are being prescribed for specific behavioral disorders. Alternatively, positive behavioral outcomes may depend upon very different plasma concentrations of a particular drug than typically expected in psychiatric populations. Finally, obtaining drug and metabolite measurements in retarded persons would seem particularly appropriate, as such persons often cannot relate adverse or toxic effects, or subjective indices of improvement.

Antipsychotic Drugs

The prevalence of antipsychotic drug use in both public and community residential facilities for mentally retarded persons has been well documented (Aman & Singh, 1983; Hill, Balow, & Bruininks, 1985; Intagliata & Rinck, 1985; Lipman, 1970; see Chapter 1). Despite the fact that up to 50% of retarded persons residing in public facilities are currently being treated with antipsychotic drugs, a number of basic questions about their use remain unanswered: (a) What is the efficacy of these drugs for specific behavioral disorders? (b) What percentage of the behaviorally disordered mentally retarded population are responders (or nonresponders) to antipsychotic drug treatment? (c) What is the relationship of dose or drug blood level to behavioral outcome? These and similar questions have received virtually no attention in this population. Adequate answers are of crucial importance because of the high prevalence of antipsychotic drug use, the paucity of controlled data evaluating efficacy, and the occurrence of serious side effects such as tardive dyskinesia. An adequate empirical response to many of these questions depends upon many factors, particularly quantification of the levels of parent drug and active metabolites (if any) in the blood. The purpose of this section is to examine issues related to the measurement of blood concentrations of antipsychotic drugs in retarded persons and the clinical utility of such information.

The clinical or behavioral effects ascribed to any psychotropic drug can be accounted for, at least in part, by its biochemical mechanisms of action (e.g., how the drug alters specific aspects of neurotransmission). Antipsychotic drugs are thought to exert their therapeutic (antipsychotic) effect by blocking dopamine receptors in specific areas of the brain (Bunney, 1984). Other biochemical and physiological effects of these drugs (e.g., adverse effects) can be accounted for by other mechanisms, including actions at other receptors, such as those for the neurotransmitters acetylcholine, norepinephrine, and histamine (see Chapter 10).

Clearly, clinical outcome (i.e., the response to a psychotropic drug) ultimately depends on the biochemical mechanisms by which drugs act, and the interaction of these mechanisms with other environmental factors. These latter pharmacodynamic factors are intimately related to pharmacokinetic events, pharmacokinetics referring to the absorption, distribution, metabolism, and elimination of drugs and their metabolites. Thus, major factors in the ultimate response of any patient include how much drug (and possibly active metabolite) gets to the brain, and the physiological changes initiated by the mechanisms of action of these drugs or their metabolites.

A basic principle of pharmacology holds that there is a direct relationship between the available concentration of drug (or its active metabolites) at the relevant site of action, and response. However, administration of a drug will initiate a cascade of biological events. Some biological responses may be due to actions occurring via several different mechanisms, with very different time courses. These factors may complicate attempts to correlate drug concentration with response. Nonetheless, knowledge of the blood levels of antipsychotic drugs may be useful in helping to adjust dose, to establish "therapeutic windows" for specific behavioral or psychiatric disorders, to confirm drug nonresponders, to assist in avoiding toxicity, and to ascertain compliance.

Historically, the value of making such blood measurements has been the subject of some controversy in clinical psychiatry. There are a number of reasons why some have argued that the measurement of antipsychotic blood levels is not clinically useful. The first is the lack of agreement on what ranges of blood concentrations may be associated with therapeutic and/or toxic effects. Thus, acceptable therapeutic windows have not been established for many of the drugs in this class (Davis, Javaid, Janicak, & Mostert, 1985). Intuitively, blood concentrations should be more highly correlated with clinical response than dose, but some studies have reported the opposite finding. This is particularly problematic as the correlation between dose and clinical outcome has often proven to be quite low.

Between-Subject Variability in Blood Levels

The often poor relationship between drug dose or blood levels and clinical response may involve a number of factors. Of particular importance is the large between-subject variability reported in blood concentrations, even in patients receiving equivalent doses of drug (Friedel, 1984). There are many factors that may cause such differences. Activity of the enzymes that metabolize antipsychotic drugs are affected by genetic, environmental, and physiological factors. Differences in the proportion of such enzymes directly affects the rate of metabolism and not only is metabolism of concern, but absorption, distribution, and elimination are also affected by these same factors. Thus, coadministration of other drugs, illness or infection, or even hormonal changes may influence markedly drug availability and action. For these reasons, it is not surprising that psychiatric patients will vary 10–20-fold or more in drug blood levels, even when a fixed-dose design is used. We (Lewis et al., 1986) and one other group (Vaisanen, Viukari, Rimon, & Raisanen, 1981) have reported large between-subject differences in mentally retarded clients receiving identical doses of antipsychotic drug. It should be noted that intramuscular administration of drug results in less variability in blood concentrations than observed following oral administration (Dahl, 1986).

Drug Metabolism

As mentioned previously, one important factor involved in the low correlations often observed between blood level and behavioral outcome is drug metabolism. Antipsychotic drugs, particularly phenothiazines, may be extensively metabolized to large numbers of compounds. This raises several clinically relevant questions, including the following: (a) Which of the metabolites have pharmacological activity and which are inactive? (b) If a metabolite is biologically active, can it cross the blood-brain barrier? (c) To what extent do the active metabolites contribute to therapeutic or adverse effects associated with the drug? Ascertaining whether the metabolites formed by antipsychotic drugs (and other psychotropic agents) have significant biological activity is quite important. If so, poor correlations between blood level and clinical response would almost certainly occur in those studies measuring only circulating concentrations of the parent compound.

Researchers in clinical psychopharmacology give at least lip service to the notion of "active" versue "inactive" metabolites. Frequently, however, the data that one uses to suggest that a metabolite may be "active" are largely dependent upon in vitro receptor binding studies. Editorially, we find this type of approach to be flawed for two reasons. First, as we discuss later in the chapter, our state of knowledge and the available technology may not always permit this technique to reflect accurately all in vivo effects. Moreover, certain drugs or their metabolites may cause important physiological effects by acting at secondary sites. Thus, for antipsychotic drugs, blockade of dopamine receptors is considered a cardinal property, yet actions at other receptors (e.g, adrenergic or histaminergic receptors) may contribute to clinical response by modulating the desired effect, or even by causing side effects. Thus, reference to "active" metabolites throughout this chapter must be taken within this editorial context.

Determining the biological significance of active metabolites can be a very complex task. For example, chlorpromazine has been hypothesized to have 168 possible metabolites. Fortunately many of the metabolic pathways required to form all of these metabolites are mutually exclusive, and only a small number of metabolites are both biologically active and occur in sufficient concentration to be considered when studying blood level/ clinical outcome relationships (Dahl, 1982). Nonetheless, many antipsychotic drugs may have one or more active metabolites that must be evaluated. The between-subject variability in the relative concentration of parent drug to metabolites may be another important factor that contributes to variability in blood level/clinical response studies.

Variability in the relative concentration of parent drug to metabolites, by necessity means a similar variability in the relative concentration of pharmacologically active compounds to inactive compounds. This latter ratio has been suggested by some to correlate significantly with clinical response (e.g., Sakalis, Traficante, Gardos, & Gershon, 1980). Recently, we examined the effect of thioridazine (Mellaril) on the stereotyped behavior of mentally retarded persons (Lewis et al., 1986). As might be expected, large between-subject differences were observed in the blood levels of thioridazine and its metabolites. We also observed large between-subject differences in the ratio of the active metabolites of thioridazine (mesoridazine and sulforidazine) to its major inactive metabolite, thioridazine-5-sulfoxide. This ratio, unlike the concentrations of the parent drug or its metabolites, did appear to be related to behavioral outcome. Subjects exhibiting a relatively high ratio of active metabolites to the major inactive metabolite exhibited increased levels of stereotyped behavior while receiving thioridazine. Those subjects whose ratio was approximately 1.0 exhibited little change in rate, whereas the client whose ratio was less than 1.0 showed some improvement on drug.

Establishing the ratio of active to inactive compounds or parent drug to metabolite(s) might well increase the predictive power of blood level determinations. Shvartsburd, Nwokeafor, and Smith (1984) observed a nonlinear relationship between thioridazine dose and plasma levels of thioridazine and metabolites in psychiatric patients. They also reported large variations in the ratio of thioridazine to mesoridazine. In drug-resistant schizophrenic patients, Sakalis et al. (1980) reported that a high mesoridazine (active metabolite) to low thioridazine-5-oxide (inactive metabolite) concentration was associated with clinical improvement. With these above exceptions, very few studies have reported attempts to examine the ratio of active to inactive compounds or parent drug to metabolite ratios.

The importance of accounting for the metabolites of antipsychotic drugs is demonstrated quite clearly with thioridazine, the most frequently prescribed psychotropic drug for mentally retarded clients exhibiting behavioral disorders (see Chapter 1). After absorption, thioridazine is metabolized into numerous compounds, although only three metabolites plus the parent compound are found in appreciable concentrations. These metabolites are mesoridazine, sulforidazine, and thioridazine-5-oxide. There are very large differences in the relative concentrations of each of the four compounds in the blood after drug administration. While one (thioridazine-5-oxide) may be devoid of antipsychotic activity, there is sufficient evidence to suggest that all can have important clinical effects in mentally retarded clients. Therefore, further understanding of the basic pharmacology of each of the metabolites becomes necessary. Studies to accomplish this goal have been ongoing in our laboratory (Kilts, Knight, Mailman, Widerlov, & Breese, 1984; Lewis, Baumeister, McCorkle, & Mailman, 1985; Lewis, Staples, McCorkle, & Mailman, 1983; Niedzwiecki, Mailman, & Cubeddu, 1984).

Our in vitro and in vivo animal studies with thioridazine support the view that various behavioral effects seen in retarded clients during both drug administration and withdrawal may depend directly on the formation and concentration of active metabolites in the individual's bloodstream. Indeed, one of our working hypotheses has been that thioridazine is a prodrug (i.e., its clinical effects are wholly dependent on the formation in the body of pharmacologically active metabolites). It then becomes logical to assume that one cannot properly predict or evaluate a retarded person's response to thioridazine without knowing how much of each metabolite (as well as thioridazine) is present in his or her blood. This hypothesis is supported by a significant body of data from preclinical experiments. Further studies in this area are possible because of the method that we developed to quantify the thioridazine metabolites (Kilts, Patrick, Breese, & Mailman, 1982).

We have been particularly interested in how metabolites of thioridazine affect pharmacological consequences ascribed to the parent compound. For example, Axelsson and co-workers (Axelesson, 1977; Axelsson & Martensson, 1977) have shown in humans that thioridazine, as well as the metabolites mesoridazine and sulforidazine, are active when given independently. In a variety of preclinical in vitro and in vivo pharmacological tests, mesoridazine and sulforidazine have been shown to be active, although the range of potencies has been shown to be between 2 and 100 times more potent than thioridazine, depending on the biochemical or pharmacological screen being used (Kilts et al., 1984; Lewis, Staples, et al., 1983; Niedzwiecki et al., 1984). It is also known that mesoridazine usually is found in higher concentrations than thioridazine in the blood of patients, and sulforidazine is found at only a slightly lower concentration (Axelsson, 1977; Axelsson & Martensson, 1977). In fact, mesoridazine is available in the United States under the trade name of Serentil, and is typically administered at half the dose prescribed for thioridazine. Another major metabolite found in plasma is thioridazine-5-sulfoxide, but this compound generally is believed to be inactive as an antipsychotic (although it may be involved in toxic side effects). Although mixed sulfoxides and sulfones may be found at trace concentrations in the circulation, these compounds are mostly urinary metabolites. Another plasma metabolite, northioridazine, has been considered, but we seldom find the latter compound in human serum, although it is one of the major metabolites in the rat.

Several groups have tried to relate the plasma concentrations of thioridazine metabolites to various clinical outcomes. Papadopoulos, Chand, Crammer, and Lader (1980) found that in schizophrenic patients, levels of mesoridazine and sulforidazine did not correlate with dose, whereas the inactive metabolite thioridazine-5-sulfoxide showed a positive correlation with dose. These workers were not able to correlate extrapyramidal side effects with thioridazine or metabolite levels, but found a positive correlation between clinical outcome and sulforidazine levels. Using the radioreceptor assay (see later discussion), Cohen, Lipinski, Pope, Harris, and Altesman (1980) studied acutely psychotic patients on a fixed dose of thioridazine and found Brief Psychiatric Rating Scale ratings to correlate highly with total antipsychotic-like activity (a sum of thioridazine plus all active metabolites). Axelsson and Aspenstrom (1982) found that Type I T-wave changes in ECG were systematically related to thioridazine concentration in blood but not to metabolite concentrations in blood. This finding is inconsistent with the earlier work of Gottschalk et al. (Gottschalk, Dinovo, Biener, & Nandi, 1978) who found thioridazine-5-sulfoxide to be related to ECG changes.

Until recently, haloperidol (Haldol, Serenace) was thought to form only inactive metabolites. This property made haloperidol a frequent choice of drug in studies attempting to relate behavioral outcome to drug blood levels. Such studies are particularly germane to the present discussion, as haloperidol is so widely used in mental retardation. While it has been argued that a therapeutic window exists for haloperidol, the evidence for such a conclusion is meager (Volavka & Cooper, 1987). Recent attention has been focused on a metabolite, reduced haloperidol, which has been characterized as either inactive or possessing little activity (e.g., Korpi & Wyatt, 1984). However, it has been reported that reduced haloperidol can be oxidized in vivo back to haloperidol (Korpi, Costakos, & Wyatt, 1985). Because reduced haloperidol is found in patient blood in high concentrations, this is an important mechanism by which this metabolite contributes to pharmacodynamics and may obscure blood level/clinical outcome relationships. We have reported a similar mechanism by which chlorpromazine-N-oxide can contribute to the clinical effects ascribed to the parent compound (Lewis, Widerlov, Knight, Kilts, & Mailman, 1983). This metabolite, found in fairly high concentrations in human blood, was previously thought to possess antidopaminergic activity. Our results demonstrated that while chlorpromazine-N-oxide had no intrinsic antidopaminergic (antipsychotic) activity, it could be converted back (reduced) to the parent compound, thereby contributing to pharmacodynamic effects. However, it has been suggested recently that our analytical methodology may have caused artifacts and the importance of this process requires further investigation (Hawes et al., 1986).

Plasma/Serum Protein Binding

Drug availability is affected by the extent to which drugs may be bound to plasma or serum proteins. Antipsychotic and tricyclic antidepressant drugs are typically highly plasma protein bound, in some cases up to 99% bound. Therefore, small changes in plasma protein binding can cause significant changes in the unbound or free pharmacologically active fraction. This may result in substantial pharmacodynamic differences. For example, thioridazine is approximately 98% plasma protein bound. Its active metabolite, mesoridazine, is 95% plasma protein bound. This difference in unbound or free drug helps to explain why clinicians prescribe mesoridazine at half or less the dose used for thioridazine.

There is another issue related to plasma protein binding. If total concentrations of the drug and metabolites are being quantified in blood, variability in plasma protein binding may confound blood level/behavioral outcome relationships. One potentially important source of such variability is alterations in the concentration of certain blood proteins secondary to physiological alterations of disease, aging, malnutrition, and so forth. Such changes may alter both distribution and clearance of many drugs. For example, α_1-acid glycoprotein is an acute phase reactant, the plasma levels of which may be elevated as a consequence of acute physiological stress, chronic inflammation, or following anticonvulsant drug administration. Increased α_1-acid glycoprotein plasma concentrations generally increase the extent of protein binding of many basic drugs. Additionally, both between- and within-subject variability in the levels of this protein may be substantial.

We should point out, however, that the assumption that only unbound or "free" drug is available to enter brain and interact with recognition sites may be too simplistic. Such an assumption does not readily account for certain important observations. For example, antipsychotics that are highly plasma protein bound may actually accumulate in higher concentrations in brain than in blood than metabolites that are less bound to plasma proteins. Thioridazine, to use a specific example, accumulates in very high concentrations in brain (> 1 μg/g tissue), yet sulforidazine (which binds less tightly to plasma proteins) achieves brain values only one-fiftieth of those obtained with thioridazine. Although there are very high concentrations of thioridazine in brain, it may be essentially unavailable at the relevant receptors.

Technical Factors in Blood Level Determinations

Any valid correlation between behavioral outcome and drug blood concentrations is highly dependent not only on the validity and reliability of the measure of clinical response, but also the accuracy and precision of the chemical analytical methodology being used. In terms of antipsychotic drugs (as well as other drugs used in psychiatry), the problems for the analytical chemist are quite imposing. For example, these drugs often are found in relatively low concentrations (one-tenth of a millionth of a gram per milliliter of blood serum [100 ng/mL] or less). Moreover, they can be extensively metabolized (i.e., biotransformed), often to other molecules with important biological activity.

Another problem is that metabolites may differ in their physicochemical properties from the parent compound. This causes problems in two ways. Extracting compounds of different chemical structures and properties from blood (a necessity prior to chemical analysis) may impose a major obstacle for the analytical chemist. Second, most commonly used analytical methods are based on gas chromatography (GC) or high performance liquid chromatography (HPLC). These methods work by separating compounds based on their chemical or physical properties, and then quantifying them. Although these methods are powerful, one always risks inadequate separation of parent drug and metabolites, and this has occurred with drugs used in this population. The consequence of inadequate separation of drug species will be invalid estimates of their concentration. In addition, sometimes more than one antipsychotic drug may be used simultaneously, or an antipsychotic may be used with other classes of drugs. This may be particularly true with mentally retarded clients, and makes this an especially important concern. Although a competent analytical chemist can minimize or avoid most of these problems, the clinician should be wary of accepting values without addressing these general concerns.

The prototypical antipsychotic drug, chlorpromazine (Thorazine) provides an excellent illustration of spurious conclusions due to technical artifacts. Although only a few of the more than 100 theoretical metabolites of this drug are of real clinical importance, even that number complicates interpretation of data. The recent widespread availability of HPLC has finally led to methods able to measure simultaneously chlorpromazine and most of its major circulating metabolites, both active and inactive. However, these assays do not quantify chlorpromazine-N-oxide, a major and pharmacologically important metabolite (Lewis, Widerlov et al., 1983) that is left behind in the schemes commonly used to extract drug or metabolites from blood.

Blood collection, prior to assay, may also involve technical factors that can lead to spurious conclusions. In the past, collection of blood into tubes containing plasticizers (chemicals that are added to plastics to give them desired physical characteristics) has yielded inaccurate estimates of the plasma concentration of some drugs. Plasticizers have been shown to alter the ratio of the concentration of drug that is free versus protein bound. Large variations in drug blood levels have been seen when certain Vacutainers were used to collect blood samples. This variability was due to contamination of the sample by tris(2-butoxyethyl)phosphate, a plasticizer used in the manufacture of the particular tube stoppers. While plasticizer-free stoppers are now available, caution should be taken to avoid tubes that may not be free of tris-butoxyethyl phosphate.

Antipsychotic Radioreceptor Assay

To circumvent these many technical problems, Creese and Snyder (1977) proposed using radioligand binding methods to monitor total antidopaminergic (i.e., antipsychotic) activity in patient blood. The idea underlying this notion was the accepted concept that both the parent antipsychotic drug and its active metabolites act by a similar mechanism, blockade of dopamine receptors. The potency of a compound is defined by its ability to block dopamine receptors. The idea is that the greater the amount of drug and active metabolites in the blood, the more the blood sample would compete for binding to dopamine receptors in animal brain tissue. The competition of a given blood sample with a radioactive antipsychotic drug for these brain receptors provides the way to make this measurement.

Although it is not intrinsically obvious to nonspecialists, the potential advantages of such a scheme are many. Most importantly, the radioreceptor assay is much faster, and requires much less laboratory expertise than commonly used analytical methods. It avoids the need for a different analytical method for every antipsychotic drug being used. These analytical methods (e.g., gas chromatography, radioimmunoassay, high performance liquid chromatography, etc.) are often technically difficult and expensive, reducing their wide clinical applicability. The radioreceptor assay can also monitor total antipsychotic-like activity in patients taking one or more antipsychotic drugs, even if they have active metabolites.

Although widely used, the radioreceptor assay has not been the powerful clinical tool originally envisioned. For example, in our clinical studies with thioridazine, the blood values we obtained from direct analytical measurements (HPLC) were about five times higher than the values as determined by the radioreceptor assay (Mailman, DeHaven, Halpern, &

Lewis, 1984; Mailman, Pierce, et al., 1984). We have shown that in the radioreceptor assay for thioridazine or its active metabolites, the presence of serum (50 μL/1 mL) significantly affects the binding of thioridazine or its metabolites to dopamine receptors, an effect not seen for chlorpromazine or haloperidol. As a consequence, when the latter drugs are used as standards, the radioreceptor assay substantially underestimates the actual neuroleptic-like activity for patients treated with thioridazine. Because of interindividual differences in the magnitude of this effect, it is not possible to control completely for it.

We have also found that sera (50 μL/1 mL) from healthy, drug-free volunteers caused marked inhibition of binding, independent of effects on the competition of a specific antipsychotic for binding sites. Although any sample of serum causes reproducible inhibition with a given preparation of bovine or rat striatal membranes, the effects of various serum samples may differ markedly when several striatal membrane preparations are compared. Moreover, samples taken from people at different times may also vary, although less than the interindividual differences. Thus, routine use of the radioreceptor assay may be limited by this nonspecific effect of serum, and this finding may offer one explanation for some of the inconsistencies found in comparing the radioreceptor assay with direct analytical methods.

Direct Analytical Methods

Attempts to correlate behavioral outcome with drug blood level using direct analytical methods like GC or HPLC also are hampered by technical issues. These issues involve specificity, sensitivity, technical difficulty, and cost. Perhaps the most commonly used assay method is gas chromatography. This method is quite sensitive, with about 1 ng/mL being the lower limit of sensitivity. Its specificity is good, although nonvolatile drugs or metabolites of the phenothiazine class of antipsychotics often require derivitization (addition of a chemical group to make the compound more volatile), which increases the time and cost associated with blood level measurement.

The use of HPLC has become an increasingly popular assay method. The cost of HPLC is probably the same as GC but, for most of these drugs, it is usually less sensitive, requiring at least 5 ng/mL of the drug or metabolite to be present in blood in order to be detected. This lower limit makes HPLC unsuitable for a number of commonly used drugs such as haloperidol. Polar metabolites of the phenothiazines are more readily assayed with HPLC than with GC, however. Gas chromatography/mass spectrometry is the most specific method available, but it requires very costly equipment and a high level of technical expertise. This method is used to validate the measurements of other assay methods such as GC or HPLC. A final method, related to the radioreceptor assay, is radioimmunoassay (RIA), which is infrequently used in measuring antipsychotic blood levels for two reasons: A specific antisera must be generated and RIAs often lack the requisite specificity.

Use of Other Medications

We have pointed out above how the use of concomitant medications can produce artifacts in the technical measurement of drug and metabolite levels. For this and other reasons, use of other medications can reduce the correlation between antipsychotic drug blood levels and behavioral response. Coadministration of two antipsychotic drugs or an antipsychotic plus other psychotropic drug(s) (antidepressants, anxiolytics, lithium, etc.) will affect the drug level/behavioral outcome relationship through pharmacokinetic and pharmacodynamic mechanisms. This is a particularly salient issue in psychopharmacology with retarded persons, as polypharmacy has been common practice.

Mentally retarded clients often suffer from seizure disorders and require anticonvulsant medication (see Chapter 1). It is widely agreed that these drugs may induce cytochrome P-450s, liver enzymes that play a major role in the metabolism of psychotropic and other drugs. One clinical consequence of coadministration of anticonvulsants with antipsychotics may be decreases in the blood levels of the antipsychotic, with a resulting need to increase the dose. As importantly, it is also possible that the patterns of metabolism may be markedly changed, and this can be of even greater importance with a drug like thioridazine. Depending upon the route or mechanism of metabolism, different antipsychotics will be differentially affected by coadministration of anticonvulsants. In a recent study, Linnoila, Viukari, Vaisanen, and Auvinen (1981) reported that in mentally retarded patients taking phenobarbital and/or diphenylhydantoin (Dilantin), significantly lower plasma levels of haloperidol and mesoridazine were found than observed in patients not receiving anticonvulsants. No difference was observed in thioridazine blood levels. However, the analytical method used to determine thioridazine and mesoridazine blood levels suffered from technical artifacts. These are described in greater detail below in the discussion of the report by Vaisanen et al. (1981).

Because of the propensity of antipsychotic drugs to induce extrapyramidal side effects, coadministration of anticholinergic (antiparkinsonian) drugs can be quite common. It is not yet clear what effect such coadministration might have on circulating concentrations, although recently several groups failed to observe an alteration in antipsychotic drug blood level (Bolvig Hansen et al., 1979; Dysken et al., 1981; Itoh, Yagi, Ohtsuka, Iwamura, & Ichikawa, 1980). However, plasma concentrations of antipsychotic drugs have been shown to be affected by lithium carbonate (Rivera-Calimlim, Kerzner, & Karch, 1978) and tricyclic antidepressants (Cooper, 1978).

Drug Blood Levels and Responders/Nonresponders/ Negative Responders

The percentage of responders or nonresponders to antipsychotic drugs in the population of mentally retarded persons receiving such drugs is currently unknown. Moreover, little systematic information is available on the proportion of patients shown to be negative responders (i.e., those exhibiting behavioral deterioration while on drugs). It is important to bear in mind that the inclusion of drug nonresponders (or negative responders) may obscure any existing relationship between behavioral outcome and drug blood levels. We know of only one study in the mental retardation literature relating the behavior of responders or nonresponders to blood level. In this study (Vaisanen et al., 1981), correlations between serum drug levels and behavioral outcome were poor for both thioridazine and haloperidol. Furthermore, drug blood levels were not found to be different between responders and nonresponders. It is difficult, however, to accept the conclusions of this study for several major reasons. First, the analytical methodology used for making thioridazine and metabolite determinations was flawed. Two flourometric assays were used, one to determine thioridazine levels and one to quantify thioridazine plus mesoridazine. The difference in assay values for any one blood sample was considered to represent mesoridazine levels. Thus, only the parent drug and mesoridazine were estimated in blood and, more importantly, the fraction thought to be thioridazine plus mesoridazine also contained other sulfones and sulfoxides, including the inactive thioridazine-5-sulfoxide. Second, the doses of haloperidol were adjusted upwards from 10 to 60 mg/day, a dose range that would be considered quite high by typical prescription practices. These high doses may have been why most of the nonresponders were negative responders. Also, despite the authors' conclusion that 21 of 30 haloperidol subjects were responders, the behavioral ratings suggested that drug treatment across all doses resulted in little or no improvement. Thus, blood level/behavioral outcome correlations would be expected to be low. Finally, it is generally accepted that HPLC, the analytical method employed to determine haloperidol blood levels, is not sufficiently sensitive for routine clinical use. Although the mean haloperidol concentration was greater than 5 ng/ml for the 20 mg/day dose in the Vaisanen et al. study, with this methodology, haloperidol would have been undetectable in a number of samples.

Despite the lack of reports relating drug blood levels to responder/ nonresponder status, the use of blood levels to aid in making this determination is of importance. For example, it has been common to observe little clinical improvement in institutionalized mentally retarded persons on what appear to be quite high doses of medication. Correct assessment of drug and metabolite blood levels may help greatly in confirming such individuals as "true" nonresponders. Also, it is difficult to evaluate adverse drug effects in this population. Measurement of drug and metabolite blood levels could be an important mechanism in avoiding "behavioral toxicity" in severely or profoundly mentally retarded people.

Measurement in Red Blood Cells Versus Plasma

Some recent research suggests that red blood cell (RBC) levels of anti-psychotic drugs might provide a better correlation with therapeutic response than plasma levels and, therefore, a better guide to dosage regulation (Casper, Garver, Dekirmenjian, Chang, & Davis, 1980; Garver, Dekirmenjian, Davis, Casper, & Ericksen, 1977; Smith et al., 1982). Other groups have found no stronger correlations with clinical response using RBC versus plasma determinations of either phenothiazines (thioridazine, fluphenazine, or chlorpromazine) or the butyrophenone, haloperidol (Alfredsson & Sedvall, 1976; Mavroidis, Kanter, Hirschowitz, & Garver, 1984; Neborsky, Janowsky, & Perel, 1982; Neborsky, Janowsky, Perel, Munson, & Depry, 1984; Smith et al., 1984). Conversely, with the neuroleptic, butaperazine, RBC levels do appear to be more strongly related to clinical outcome than do plasma concentrations (Garver et al., 1976). Interestingly, Shvartsburd et al. (1984) found large interpatient variability in the ratios of RBC to plasma for both thioridazine and meso-ridazine.

Diagnosis and Objective Evaluation of Clinical Change

Two other factors that contribute substantially to low correlations between blood levels and behavioral outcome are subject or diagnostic heterogeneity and the methodology used to evaluate clinical change. This latter consideration is an often neglected, albeit critically important, factor in establishing blood level/clinical outcome relationships. Many studies in the psychiatric literature have not paid sufficient attention to the validity and reliability of various behavioral assessment instruments. Other methodological short-comings include insufficient statistical power, an insufficient observation period, carry-over effects from other medications, inconsistent timing of blood samples relative to time of drug administration, and use of a heterogeneous subject population (Dahl, 1986).

The measurement of behavioral change in drug studies with mentally retarded clients has been the subject of several previous reviews (e.g., Sprague, 1977; Sprague & Werry, 1971). Much of the earlier literature is methodologically flawed to the point of being uninterpretable. More recent studies have used direct observations of behavior, often within a single-subject design. While this is a powerful methodology, it may not allow a large enough number of subjects to be evaluated to generate behavioral outcome/blood level correlations between subjects. Furthermore, progress in this field has been hampered by the lack of behavioral assessment instruments that have been demonstrated to have the requisite validity, reliability, and sensitivity to drug effects. In this regard, the recent development of the Aberrant Behavior Checklist by Aman and his colleagues (Aman, Singh, Stewart, & Field, 1985a, b) is quite promising, as this instrument has the potential to be both psychometrically sound and sensitive to drug effects. However, its ultimate utility must await further testing by other groups.

The use of flexible-dose regimens, where dose is titrated according to clinical judgement, may also lead to spurious conclusions regarding the nature of the relationship between blood levels and behavioral outcome. This is due, in part, to the often high blood levels of drug seen in nonresponders. Adjusting dose during the course of a study may well result in a restriction of range, and, hence, a lower correlation (Nunnally, 1967). For that reason, attempts to correlate blood level and clinical response should include use of a fixed-dose design.

In future attempts to enhance pharmacotherapy in mentally retarded patients by measuring blood levels of drug and metabolites, care should also be given to the issue of psychiatric diagnosis. Emotional disturbance has been demonstrated to occur in mentally retarded persons with much greater frequency than in nonretarded persons (Lewis & MacLean, 1982). This raises the important issue of subject homogeneity. Care should be taken to ensure diagnostic homogeneity as far as possible and to separate drug effects on dually diagnosed clients from those without demonstrable emotional disturbance.

Blood Levels and Behavioral Outcome in Mentally Retarded Clients

There are very few data available on drug blood levels in retarded clients. This is unfortunate as conclusions regarding therapeutic and adverse effects on responders and nonresponders should not be made in the absence of blood level determinations. To our knowledge, only our own work (Lewis et al., 1986) and the work of Vaisanen et al. (1981) have attempted to correlate blood level to clinical response. The latter group has also examined the effect of anticonvulsants on antipsychotic blood levels in retarded clients (Linnoila et al., 1980) and the relationship of antipsychotic blood levels to prolactin secretion (Linnoila, Viukara, Vaisanen & Auvinen, 1981). Our initial work cited above suggested that increases in stereotyped responding following thioridazine administration were related to relatively high ratios of the active metabolites (mesoridazine plus sulforidazine) to the inactive metabolite, thioridazine-5-sulfoxide. Recently, we have begun to study the effect of gradual withdrawal of thioridazine on such behavioral disorders as aggression, disruption, and self-injury. We have preliminary evidence to suggest that thioridazine is effective in suppressing clinically important problem behaviors in this population, that withdrawal from thioridazine will result in rapid behavioral deterioration, and that such deterioration is correlated with a dose-dependent reduction in drug and metabolite blood levels. Finally, the analysis of drug and metabolite blood concentrations suggests that the clinical dose equivalence of thioridazine to mesoridazine may be 3:1 or 4:1 rather than the 2:1 ratio typically quoted.

Blood Levels and Tardive Dyskinesia

A major risk factor associated with the long-term use of antipsychotic drug administration is tardive dyskinesia (TD). TD is a sometimes irreversible neurological syndrome typically consisting of buccal-lingual-masticatory movements often observed in conjunction with other choreoathetotic and/ or dystonic movements (see Chapter 9). The pathophysiology of TD is still unclear although alterations in dopamine receptor sensitivity may be involved. Effective treatments are not yet available (Baldessarini et al. 1980).

Although the prevalence of TD in retarded persons has been estimated to be approximately 30% (Gualtieri, Breuning, Schroeder, & Quade, 1982; Richardson, Haugland, Pass, & Craig, 1986; see Chapter 9), the high rate of abnormal spontaneous motor movements in developmentally disabled people makes reliable determinations difficult. The results of several studies in psychiatric patients by one group have suggested that monitoring antipsychotic drug blood levels might reduce the risk of TD, presumably by ensuring lower blood concentrations (Jeste et al., 1981; Jeste, Rosenblatt, Wagner, & Wyatt, 1979). Should this prove to be the case, it would provide more than sufficient rationale for routine antipsychotic blood level determinations in clinical practice. However, our group (Widerlov et al., 1982), also studying schizophrenic adults, was not able to replicate the results that Jeste et al. (1979) obtained. Furthermore, a number of other groups have not been able to establish a positive correlation between incidence of tardive dyskinesia and antipsychotic blood level (Cseransky, Kaplan, Holman, & Hollister, 1983; Fairbairn et al., 1983; Itoh et al., 1984; Rowell, Rich, Hall, Fairbairn, & Hassanyeh, 1983; Smith et al., 1980).

Antidepressant and Antianxiety Drugs

Lithium Carbonate

The study of lithium carbonate (Eskalith, Lithobid) in mentally retarded persons has been limited largely to case studies of its effect on aggressive (e.g., Dale, 1980) or self-injurious behavior (e.g., Cooper & Fowlie, 1973), or manic-depressive illness (e.g., Rivinus & Harmatz, 1979). A recent double-blind, crossover design that included 25 aggressive patients has been a notable exception (Tyrer, Walsh, Edwards, Berney, & Stephens, 1984). While reported findings suggest the efficacy of lithium, the lack of well-controlled studies using larger numbers of subjects makes it difficult to draw conclusions about the utility of this drug in the pharmacotherapy of retarded persons (see also Chapter 6). Despite the growing appreciation of the increased prevalence of psychiatric disorders, particularly affective disorders, among retarded persons (Lewis & MacLean, 1982), fewer than 1% of the retarded persons recently surveyed were receiving lithium (Hill et al., 1985; Intagliata & Rinck, 1985). Use of this medication is likely to increase as treatment programs for "dually diagnosed" clients become more common. However, drug trials of lithium should be undertaken with caution because of the problem of lithium toxicity, the inability of mentally retarded clients to verbalize untoward side effects, potential alterations in renal or thyroid function, and maintenance of adequate fluid and electrolyte balance. As with nonretarded psychiatric patients, the therapeutic dosage of lithium will probably be close to the toxic range.

Lithium is quite unlike antipsychotic and antidepressant drugs in that blood levels correlate highly with clinical end points. For example, lithium blood concentrations of approximately 0.9–1.4 mEq/L have been correlated with positive clinical response, while concentrations greater than 1.5 mEq/L or less than 0.9 mEq/L result in side effects or the lack of clinical response, respectively. If blood values exceed 2.0 mEq/L, lithium toxicity is generally the result, manifested as anorexia, slurred speech, decreased motor behavior, drowsiness, vomiting, and, at higher blood levels, frequently coma. The blood concentrations necessary for prophylaxis in bipolar disorder have been demonstrated to be in the range of approximately 0.5–0.8 mEq/L.

Lithium blood levels generally take about 5 days to reach steady state, and blood samples are typically taken 12 hours after the last dose, the so-called "12-hour standardized serum lithium concentration" (12hstSLi). Lithium is absorbed rapidly and reaches peak blood concentrations in approximately 2 hours and has a half-life of 12–30 hours or more (Lydiard & Gelenberg, 1982). Blood determinations of lithium are technically quite simple to perform and are routinely done by flame photometry or atomic absorption.

Tricyclic Antidepressant Drugs

Like the antipsychotic drugs previously described, tricyclic antidepressants, which have been the mainstay of biological treatments for depression, are extensively metabolized by hepatic enzymes, undergo a large "first pass" effect, and are highly plasma protein bound. Also like the antipsychotic drugs, large variations in steady state blood levels are observed in patients on a fixed dose. Blood levels of the prototypical tricyclic antidepressant, imipramine (Tofranil), and its active demethylated metabolite, desipramine, have been shown to correlate positively with clinical response. Favorable clinical outcome increases as blood levels increase to 200–250 ng/ml (Task Force on the Use of Laboratory Tasks in Psychiatry, 1985). Higher concentrations do not seem to increase the antidepressant effect and untoward effects are observed with greater frequency. Using imipramine in the treatment of childhood depression, Preskorn and co-workers (Preskorn, Weller Hughes, & Weller, 1986) reported optimal plasma concentrations to be in the range of 125–250 ng/ml. Below this range, clinical effects were not different from placebo, whereas above this range, toxic effects could be observed.

For reasons that are not clear, a "therapeutic window" exists for nortriptyline (Aventyl, Pamelor) blood levels, such that concentrations either less than 50 ng/ml or greater than 150 ng/ml are associated with unfavorable antidepressant response. Any systematic relationship between amitriptyline (Tryptanol) blood levels and clinical outcome has yet to be adequately demonstrated (Task Force Report, 1985). Little information is available on more recently introduced antidepressants that exert their clinical effect by mechanisms different from those of the tricyclic antidepressants.

Many of the same issues that have been raised when considering antipsychotic drug blood levels and behavioral outcome (e.g., responders versus nonresponders, active metabolites, technical problems in quantification, etc.) apply equally well when considering antidepressant drugs. Despite these potential artifacts, the Task Force on the Use of Laboratory Tasks in Psychiatry (1985) has judged plasma level measurements of tricyclic antidepressants to be "unequivocally useful."

The use of antidepressants in both community and public residential facilities for mentally retarded persons is limited. By recent estimates only slightly more than 1% of the residents of such facilities are being treated with antidepressant medication. This can be contrasted with antipsychotic drug use, which has been estimated to involve 30–40% of the clients surveyed. To the best of our knowledge no attempt has been made to quantify antidepressant blood levels and their relationship to behavioral outcome in retarded persons.

Antianxiety Agents

The principal group of antianxiety drugs currently in use is the benzodiazepines, which include such well-known drugs as diazepam (Valium), chlordiazepoxide (Librium), and triazolam (Halcion). Differences in the clinical effects exerted by various benzodiazepines are due in large measure to their pharmacokinetics, particularly to the elimination half-life and the formation of active metabolites (Shader & Greenblatt, 1977). The pharmacokinetics of benzodiazepines have been reviewed extensively (e.g., Greenblatt, Divoll, Abernethy, Ochs, & Shader, 1984) and so will not be discussed here. As with other drug classes already reviewed, large between-subject variations are seen even after chronic dosing. Furthermore, benzodiazepines are highly plasma protein bound and so small changes in protein binding can have clinically important effects, and active metabolites (e.g., desmethyldiazepam) play an important role in clinical outcome. While the importance of pharmacokinetic differences in clinical outcome is undisputed, the predictive utility of benzodiazepine blood concentrations is in doubt. In fact, little support can be found in the literature for any systematic relationship between benzodiazepine blood levels and clinical outcome (Norman & Burrows, 1984).

Summary

Davis, Erickson, and Dekirmenjian (1978) have outlined several conditions under which blood level determinations may improve clinical practice. These include a long interval between initiation of drug and clinical response, "clinically silent" toxicity, a narrow therapeutic index (therapeutic doses are close to toxic doses), large between-patient differences in blood levels, and drug-drug interactions. These conditions are quite relevant to the pharmacological treatment of retarded persons and argue for the utility of drug blood level determinations. Relatively little progress has been made in the psychopharmacology of mentally retarded persons, as compared with other clinical populations, and many basic questions remain to be answered. It is our belief that an adequate response to these questions requires carefully controlled pharmacological investigations that include a pharmacokinetic component. Moreover, in the case of drugs that are extensively metabolized, there may be a need for sound basic data about the neuropharmacology of the metabolites. Often, such experiments have led to surprising conclusions (Lewis, Widerlov et al., 1983). The application of clinical pharmacokinetics to drug treatment of retarded persons can only improve clinical practice and provide rational, empirical criteria for clinical treatment decisions.

Referenecs

Alfredsson, G., & Sedvall, G. (1976). Mass fragmentographic analysis of chlorpromazine in human plasma. In G. Sedvall, B. Uvnas, & Y. Zotterman (Eds.), *Antipsychotic drugs: Pharmacokinetics.* (pp. 367–372) Oxford: Pergamon Press.

Aman, M.G., & Singh, N.N. (1980). The usefulness of thioridazine for treating childhood disorders—fact or folklore? *American Journal of Mental Deficiency, 84,* 331–338.

Aman, M.G., & Singh, N.N. (1983). Pharmacological intervention. In J.L. Matson & J.A. Mulick (Eds.), *Handbook of mental retardation.* (pp. 317–337). Elmsford, NY: Pergamon.

Aman, M.G., Singh, N.N., Stewart, A.W., & Field, C.J. (1985a). The Aberrant

Behavior Checklist: A behavior rating scale for the assessment of treatment effects. *American Journal of Mental Deficiency*, *89*, 485–491.

Aman, M.G., Singh, N.N., Stewart, A.W., & Field, C.J. (1985b). Psychometric characteristics of the Aberrant Behavior Checklist. *American Journal of Mental Deficiency*, *89*, 492–502.

Axelsson, R. (1977). On the serum concentrations and antipsychotic effects of thioridazine, thioridazine side-chain sulfoxide and thioridazine side-chain sulfone in chronic psychotic patients. *Current Therapeutic Research*, *21*, 588–589.

Axelsson, R., & Aspenstrom, G. (1982). Electrocardiographic changes and serum concentrations in thioridazine-treated patients. *Journal of Clinical Psychiatry*, *43*, 332–335.

Axelsson, R., & Martensson, E. (1977). The concentration pattern of nonconjugated thioridazine metabolites in serum by thioridazine treatment and its relationship to physiological and clinical variables. *Current Therapeutic Research*, *21*, 561–586.

Baldessarini, R.J., Cole, J.O., Davis, J.M., Gardos, G., Preskorn, S.H., Simpson, G.M., & Tarsy, D. (1980). Tardive dyskinesia: Task Force Report. Washington DC: American Psychiatric Association.

Bolvig Hansen, L., Elley, J., Christensen, T.R., Larsen, N-E., Naestoft, J., & Hvidberg, E.J. (1979). Plasma levels of perphenazine and its major metabolites during simultaneous treatment with anticholinergic drugs. *British Journal of Clinical Pharmacology*, *7*, 75–80.

Bunney, B.S. (1984). Antipsychotic drug effects on the electrical activity of dopaminergic neurons. *Trends in Neurosciences*, *7*, 212–215.

Casper, R., Garver, D.L., Dekirmenjian, H., Chang, S., & Davis, J. (1980). Phenothiazine levels in plasma and red blood cells. *Archives of General Psychiatry*, *37*, 301–305.

Cohen, B.M., Lipinski, J.F., Pope, H.G., Harris, P.Q., & Altesman, R.I. (1980). Neuroleptic blood levels and therapeutic effect. *Psychopharmacology*, *70*, 191–193.

Cooper, T.B. (1978). Plasma level monitoring of antipsychotic drugs. *Clinical Pharmacokinetics*, *3*, 14–38.

Cooper. A.F., & Fowlie, H.C. (1973). Control of gross self-mutilation with lithium carbonate. *British Journal of Psychiatry*, *122*, 370–371.

Creese, I., & Snyder, S.H. (1977). A simple and sensitive radioreceptor assay for antischizophrenic drugs in blood. *Nature*, *270*, 180–182.

Cseransky, J.G., Kaplan, J., Holman, C.A., & Hollister, L.E. (1983). Serum neuroleptic activity, prolactin, and tardive dyskinesia in schizophrenic outpatients. *Psychopharmacology*, *81*, 115–118.

Dahl, S.G. (1982). Active metabolites of neuroleptic drugs: Possible contribution to therapeutic and toxic effects. *Therapeutic Drug Monitoring*, *4*, 33–40.

Dahl, S.G. (1986). Plasma level monitoring of antipsychotic drugs: Clinical utility. *Clinical Pharmacokinetics*, *11*, 36–61.

Dale, P.G. (1980). Lithium therapy in aggressive mentally subnormal patients. *British Journal of Psychiatry*, *137*, 469–474.

Davis, J.M., Erickson, S., & Dekirmenjian, H. (1978). Plasma levels of antipsychotic drugs and clinical response. In M.A. Lipton, A. DiMascio, & K.F. Killam (Eds.), *Psychopharmacology: A generation of progress.* (pp. 905–916). New York: Raven Press.

Davis, J.M., Javaid, J.I., Janicak, P.G., & Mostert, M. (1985). Antipsychotics: Plasma levels and clinical response. In G.D. Burrows, T.R. Norman, & B. Davies (Eds.), *Drugs in psychiatry: Vol. 3. Antipsychotics.* (pp. 57–70). Amsterdam: Elsevier.

Dysken, M.W., Javaid, J.I., Chang, S.S., Schaffer, C., Shahid, A., & Davis, J.M. (1981). Fluphenazine pharmacokinetics and therapeutic response. *Psychopharmacology*, *73*, 205–210.

Fairbairn, A.F., Rowell, F.J., Hui, S.M., Hassanyeh, F., Robinson, A.J., & Eccleston, D. (1983). Serum concentrations of depot neuroleptics in tardive dyskinesia. *British Journal of Psychiatry*, *142*, 579–583.

Friedel, R.O. (1984). An overview of neuroleptic plasma levels: Pharmacokinetics and assay methodology. *Journal of Clinical Psychiatry Monograph*, *2*, 7–12.

Garver, D.L., Davis, J.M., Dekirmenjian, H., Jones, F.D., Casper, R., & Haraszti, J. (1976). Pharmacokinetics of red blood cell phenothiazine and clinical effects. *Archives of General Psychiatry*, *33*, 862–866.

Garver, D.L., Dekirmenjian, H., Davis, J.M., Casper, R., & Ericksen, S. (1977). Neuroleptic drug levels and therapeutic response: Preliminary observations with red blood cell-bound butaperazine. *American Journal of Psychiatry*, *134*, 304–307.

Gottschalk, L.A., Dinovo, E., Biener, R., & Nandi, B.R. (1978). Plasma concentrations of thioridazine metabolites and ECG abnormalities. *Journal of Pharmaceutical Sciences*, *67*, 155–157.

Greenblatt, D.J., Divoll, M., Abernethy, D.R., Ochs, H.R., & Shader, R.I. (1984). Benzodiazepine pharmacokinetics: An overview. In G.D. Burrows, T.R. Norman, & B. Davies (Eds.), *Drugs in psychiatry: Vol. 2. Antianxiety agents*, (pp. 79–92). Amsterdam: Elsevier.

Gualtieri, C.T., Breuning, S.E., Schroeder, S.R., & Quade, D. (1982). Tardive dyskinesia in mentally retarded children, adolescents and young adults: North Carolina and Michigan studies. *Psychopharmacology Bulletin*, *18*, 62–65

Hawes, E.M., Hubbard, J.W., Martin, M., McKay, G., Yeung, P.K.F., & Midha. K.K. (1986). Therapeutic monitoring of chlorpromazine: III. Minimal interconversion between chlorpromazine and metabolites in human blood. *Therapeutic Drug Monitoring*, *8*, 37–41.

Hill, B.K., Balow, E.A., & Bruininks, R.H. (1985). A national study of prescribed drugs in institutions and community residential facilities for mentally retarded people. *Psychopharmacology Bulletin*, *21*, 279–284.

Intagliata, J., & Rinck, C. (1985). Psychoactive drug use in public and community residential facilities for mentally retarded persons. *Psychopharmacology Bulletin*, *21*, 268–278.

Itoh, H., Yagi, G., Ohtsuka, N., Iwamura, K., & Ichikawa, K. (1980). Serum level of haloperidol and its clinical significance. *Progress in Neuropsychopharmacology and Biological Psychiatry*, *4*, 171–183.

Itoh, H., Yagi, G., Tateyama, M., Fuji, Y. Iwamura, K., & Ichikawa, K. (1984). Monitoring of haloperidol serum levels and its clinical significance. *Progress in Neuropsychopharmacology and Biological Psychiatry*, *8*, 51–62.

Jeste, D.V., DeLisi, L.E., Zalcman, S., Wise, C.D., Phelps, B.H., Rosenblatt, J.E., Potkin, S.G., Bridge, T.P., & Wyatt, R.J. (1981). A biochemical study of tardive dyskinesia in young male patients. *Psychiatry Research*, *4*, 327–331.

Jeste, D.V., Rosenblatt, J.E., Wagner, R.L., & Wyatt, R.L. (1979). High serum neuroleptic levels in tardive dyskinesia? *New England Journal of Medicine, 301,* 1184.

Kilts, C.D., Knight, D., Mailman, R.B., Widerlov, E., & Breese, G.R. (1984). Effects of thioridazine and its metabolites on dopaminergic function: Drug metabolism as a determinant of the antidopaminergic actions of thioridazine. *Journal of Pharmacology and Experimental Therapeutics, 231,* 334–342.

Kilts, C.D., Patrick, K.S., Breese, G.R., & Mailman, R.B. (1982). Simultaneous determination of thioridazine and its S-oxidized and N-demethylated metabolites using HPLC on radially compressed silica. *Journal of Chromatography, 232,* 377–391.

Korpi, E.R., Costakos, D.T., & Wyatt, J.R. (1985). Interconversions of haloperidol and reduced haloperidol in guinea pig and rat liver microsomes. *Biochemical Pharmacology, 34,* 2923–2927.

Korpi, E.R., & Wyatt, R.J. (1984). Reduced haloperidol effects on striatal dopamine metabolism and conversion to haloperidol in the rat. *Psychopharmacology, 83,* 34–337.

Lewis, M.H., Baumeister, A.A., McCorkle, D., & Mailman, R.B. (1985). A computer-supported method for analyzing behavioral observations: Studies with stereotypy. *Psychopharmacology, 85,* 204–209.

Lewis, M.H., & MacLean, W.E., Jr. (1982). Issues in treating emotional disorders. In J.L. Matson & R.P. Barrett (Eds.), *Psychopathology in the mentally retarded.* (pp. 1–36). New York: Grune & Stratton.

Lewis, M.H., Staples, L., McCorkle, D., & Mailman, R.B. (1983). Thioridazine pharmacodynamics: In vitro correlations and dependence on drug metabolism. *Society for Neuroscience Abstracts, 9* : 432.

Lewis, M.H., Steer, R.A., Favell, J.E., McGimsey, J., Clontz, L., Trivette, C., Jodry, W., Schroeder, S., Kanoy, R. & Mailman, R.B. (1986). Thioridazine metabolism and effects on stereotyped behavior in mentally retarded patients. *Psychopharmacology Bulletin, 22,* 1040–1044.

Lewis, M.H., Widerlov, E., Knight, D.L., Kilts, C.D., & Mailman, R.B. (1983). N-oxides of phenothiazine antipsychotics: Effects on in vivo and in vitro dopaminergic function. *Journal of Pharmacology and Experimental Therapeutics, 225,* 539–545, 1983.

Linnoila, M., Viukari, M., Vaisanen, K., & Auvinen, J. (1980). Effect of anticonvulsants on plasma haloperidol and thioridazine levels. *American Journal of Psychiatry, 137,* 819–821.

Linnoila, M., Viukari, M., Vaisanen, K., & Auvinen, J. (1981). Plasma neuroleptic and prolactin levels in mentally retarded patients. *Acta Pharmacologica et Toxicologica, 46,* 159.

Lipman, R.S. (1970). The use of psychopharmacological agents in residential facilities for the retarded. In F.J. Menolascino (Ed.), *Psychiatric approaches to mental retardation.* (pp. 387–398). New York: Basic Books.

Lydiard, R.B., & Gelenberg, A.J. (1982). Hazards and adverse effects of lithium. *Annual Review of Medicine, 33,* 327–344.

Mailman, R.B., DeHaven, D.L., Halpern, E., & Lewis, M.H. (1984). Serum effects confound the neuroleptic radioreceptor assay. *Life Sciences, 34,* 1057–1064.

Mailman, R.B., Pierce, J.P., Crofton, K.M., Petitto, J., DeHaven, D.L., & Lewis, M.H. (1984). Thioridazine and the neuroleptic radioreceptor assay. *Biological Psychiatry*, *19*, 833–847.

Mavroidis, M.L., Kanter, D.R., Hirschowitz, J., & Garver, D.L. (1984). Therapeutic blood levels of fluphenazine: Plasma or RBC determinations? *Psychopharmacology Bulletin*, *20*, 168–170.

Neborsky, R.J., Janowsky, D.S., & Perel, J.M. (1982). Red blood cell/plasma haloperidol ratios and antipsychotic efficacy. *Psychiatry Research*, *6*, 123–124.

Neborsky, R.J., Janowsky, D.S., Perel, J.M., Munson, E., & Depry, D. (1984). Plasma/RBC haloperidol ratios and improvement in acute psychotic symptoms. *Journal of Clinical Psychiatry*, *45*, 10–13.

Niedzwiecki, D.M., Mailman, R.B., & Cubeddu, L.X. (1984). Greater potency of mesoridazine and sulforidazine than thioridazine on striatal dopamine autoreceptors *Journal of Pharmacology and Experimental Therapeutics*, *228*, 686–689.

Norman, T.R. & Burrows, G.D. (1984). Benzodiazepine plasma concentrations and anxiolytic response. In G.D. Burrows, T.R. Norman, & B. Davies (Eds.), *Drugs in psychiatry: Vol. 2. Antianxiety drugs.* (pp. 93–106). Amsterdam: Elsevier. Nunnally, J. (1967). *Psychometric theory.* New York: McGraw-Hill.

Papadopoulos, A.S., Chand, T.G., Crammer, J.L., & Lader, S. (1980). A pilot study of plasma thioridazine and metabolites in chronically treated patients. *British Journal of Psychiatry*, *136*, 591–596.

Preskorn, S.H., Weller, E., Hughes, C., & Weller, R. (1986). Plasma monitoring of tricyclic antidepressants: Defining the therapeutic range for imipramine in depressed children. *Clinical Neuropharmacology*, *9* (suppl. 4), 265–267.

Richardson, M.A., Haugland, G., Pass, R., & Craig, T.J. (1986). The prevalence of tardive dyskinesia in a mentally retarded population. *Psychopharmacology Bulletin*, *22*, 243–249.

Rivera-Calimlim, L., Kerzner, B., & Karch, F.E. (1979). Effect of lithium on plasma chlorpromazine levels. *Clinical Pharmacology and Therapeutics*, *23*, 451–455.

Rivinus, T.M., & Harmatz, J.S. (1979). Diagnosis and lithium treatment of affective disorder in the retarded: Five case studies. *American Journal of Psychiatry*, *136*, 551–554.

Rowell, F.J., Rich, C.G., Hall, G., Fairbairn, A.F., & Hassanyeh, F. (1983). Serum chlorpromazine levels in tardive dyskinesia. *British Journal of Clinical Pharmacology*, *15*, 141–142.

Sakalis, G., Traficante, L.J., Gardos, G., & Gershon, S. (1980). Treatment of drug-resistant schizophrenics with mesoridazine. In E. Usdin, H. Eckert, & I.S. Forrest (Eds.), *Phenothiazines and structurally related drugs: Basic and clinical studies.* (pp. 207–214). New York: Elsevier/North Holland.

Shader, R.I., & Greenblatt, D.J. (1977). Clinical implications of benzodiazepine pharmacokinetics. *American Journal of Psychiatry*, *134*, 652–655.

Shvartsburd, A., Nwokeafor, V., & Smith, R.C. (1984). Red blood cell and plasma levels of thioridazine and mesoridazine in schizophrenic patients. *Psychopharmacology*, *82*, 55–61.

Smith, R.C., Baumgartner, R., Ravichandran, G.K., Shvartsburd, A., Schoolar, J.C., Allen, P., & Johnson, R. (1984). Plasma and red cell levels of thioridazine and clinical response in schizophrenia. *Psychiatry Research*, *12*, 287–296.

Smith, R.C., Vroulis, G., Shvartsburd, A., Allen, R., Lewis N., Schoolar, J.C., Chojnacki, M., & Johnson, R. (1982). RBC and plasma levels of haloperidol and clinical response in schizophrenia. *American Journal of Psychiatry, 139*, 1054–1056.

Smith, R.C., Vroulis, G., Misra, C.H., Schoolar, J.C., DeJohn, C., Korivi, P., Leelavathi, D.E., & Arzu, D. (1980). Receptor techniques in the study of plasma levels of neuroleptics and antidepressant drugs. *Communications in Psychopharmacology, 4*, 451–465.

Sprague, R.L. (1977). Overview of psychopharmacology for the retarded in the United States. In P. Mittler (Ed.), *Research to practice in mental retardation: Vol. 3. Biomedical aspect.* (pp. 199–202). Baltimore: University Park Press.

Sprague, R.L., & Werry, J.S. (1971). Methodology of psychopharmacological studies with the retarded. In N.R. Ellis (Ed.), *International review of research in mental retardation* (Vol. 5, pp. 147–210). New York: Academic Press.

Task Force on the Use of Laboratory Tests in Psychiatry. (1985). Tricyclic antidepressants-blood level measurements and clinical outcome: An APA task force report. *American Journal of Psychiatry, 142*, 155–162.

Tyrer, S.P., Walsh, A., Edwards, D.E., Berney, T.P., & Stephens, D.A. (1984). Factors associated with a good response to lithium in aggressive mentally handicapped subjects. *Progress in Neuropsychopharmacology and Biological Psychiatry, 8*, 751–755.

Vaisanen, K., Viukari, M., Rimon R., & Raisanen, P. (1981). Haloperidol, thioridazine and placebo in mentally subnormal patients: Serum levels and clinical effects. *Acta Psychiatrica Scandanavica, 63*, 262–271.

Volavka, J., & Cooper, T.B. (1987). Review of haloperidol blood level and clinical response: Looking through the window. *Journal of Clinical Psychopharmacology, 7*, 25–30.

Widerlov, E., Haggstrom, J.-E., Kilts, C.D., Andersson, U., Breese, G., & Mailman, R.B. (1982). Serum concentrations of thioridazine, its major metabolites and serum neuroleptic-like activities in schizophrenics with and without tardive dyskinesia. *Acta Psychiatrica Scandanavica, 66*, 294–305.

4
Neuroleptic Medications for Persons with Developmental Disabilities

STEPHEN R. SCHROEDER

Abstract

Since the many methodological reviews of the early 1980s, there have been a number of neuroleptic studies with persons who have developmental disabilities. Generally these recent studies are better designed, with multimodal assessment packages and double-blind placebo controls. Prospective studies tend to support the view that low doses of neuroleptics may inhibit inappropriate behaviors, especially stereotypy, to a modest degree and may promote learning in some cases, whereas high doses tend to produce untoward effects. However, the results so far present a very incomplete mosaic of findings, and much more systematic research is required before firm conclusions can be reached.

In the United States the main issues in the psychopharmacology of high prevalence, low severity developmental disorders revolve around the use of stimulants like methylphenidate among school-aged children living in community settings (Gadow, 1985). The main issues in low prevalence/high severity developmental disorders still center around neuroleptic drugs (Gualtieri & Keppel, 1985) in both public and community residential facilities (Hill, Balow, & Bruininks, 1985).

More recently there has been a substantial decrease in the use of neuroleptics for behavioral control in public residential facilities (PRFs): Hill, et al., 1985), but not in community residential facilities (CRFs), largely because quality assurance standards have been applied much more loosely in CRF programs (Mouchka, 1985). This dramatic shift in trend is likely a result of several important developments within the past decade. The purpose of this paper is to review these developments and to discuss recent studies within the past 5–10 years that flow from them. We will only touch lightly on those topics that are discussed more fully in other chapters in this book.

Preliminary Considerations

Prevalence Studies on Use of Neuroleptics in Developmental Disabilities

Early prevalence studies (e.g., Lipman, 1970) called attention to widespread use of neuroleptic drugs in public residential mental retardation facilities. Cross-cultural studies (see Chapter 1) suggested that neuroleptics are used much more sparingly in Europe, Scandinavia, Australia, and New Zealand than in the United States. Indeed within the United States there is tremendous variability in use from one institution to the next, which is unlikely to be related to heterogeneity among the populations, size, location, or a number of other factors (Jonas, 1980; LaMendola, Zaharia, & Carver, 1980; Lipman, 1970; Silva, 1979; Tu, 1979). These studies suggested that neuroleptics were often being used excessively or unnecessarily. Since 1980 the rate of use of neuroleptics in PRFs in the United States has been reduced by more than 50% (Hill et al., 1985).

Monitoring Medication Programs

As in many areas of clinical behavior analysis, the best approach to behavioral pharmacological management is to obtain good data. Until 10 years ago most facilities lacked an organized centralized system for tracking the use or the effects of neuroleptic medication. The result was a proliferation of polypharmacy, long regimens with no drug holidays, and increased doses when drug tolerance appeared. In studies where a well-designed drug evaluation technology was used in mental retardation facilities (Fielding, Murphy, Reagan, & Peterson, 1980; James, 1983; Kalachnik, Miller, Jamison, & Harder, 1983; LaMendola et al., 1980), the overwhelming result was a reduction in number of neuroleptic prescriptions, polypharmacy, lower average doses, and removal of unnecessary medications (see also Chapter 1). The involvement of an interdisciplinary team in making decisions about medications is an essential element that is now a familiar process to professionals in this field. The development of better measurement and monitoring instruments (Kalachnik, Larum, & Swanson, 1983) is an important new area of research in behavioral pharmacotherapy.

Critical Reviews of Previous Neuroleptic Treatment Research

Concerning reviews of the clinical research literature on neuroleptic treatment among developmentally disabled persons, it can be said that never was there written so much, by so many, about so little. Of the many good reviews available covering different aspects of the topic, the following are particularly recommended: (a) general (Aman, 1983); (b) effects of neuroleptics on learning (Aman, 1984); (c) dose effects (Cole, 1982);

(d) behavioral measurement techniques (Aman & White, 1986; Johnston et al., 1983; Poling, Picker, & Hall-Johnson, 1983); (e) methodology (Sprague & Werry, 1971); and (f) drug-behavior interactions (Schroeder, Lewis, & Lipton, 1983). These reviews tend to agree that: (a) with a few notable exceptions (e.g., Alexandris & Lundell, 1968; Davis, 1971; Davis, Sprague, & Werry, 1969; Marholin, Touchette, & Stewart, 1979), most of the research on neuroleptics in developmental disabilities before 1980 can be safely ignored because of faulty methodology; (b) higher doses of neuroleptics rarely improved behavior control more than lower doses in this population. The minimum effective dosage is probably much lower than is commonly believed.

Methodological Considerations

The state-of-the-art methodological review of psychopharmacological research in developmental disabilities is still that by Sprague and Werry (1971), which listed six minimum design requirements: (a) placebo control; (b) random assignment of treatments and/or subjects; (c) double-blind evaluation, (d) multiple standardized doses, so that dose response can be evaluated; (e) standardized (reliable and valid) evaluations; and (f) appropriate statistical analyses. These are stiff requirements for neuroleptic studies with severely handicapped clients who are often treated for violent aggression, destructiveness, self-injurious behavior, tantrums, and screaming, the main behaviors for which neuroleptics are used for control (Jonas, 1980; Tu & Smith, 1983). In such clinical populations one can anticipate the following methodological problems: (a) lack of adequate sample size; (b) extreme heterogeneity of subjects; (c) subject attrition; (d) idiosyncratic all-or-none response by some subjects; (e) lack of specificity of treatment effects for individual subjects; (f) ethical difficulties in using placebo groups or wait lists (e.g., with severely self-injurious subjects); and (g) difficulty of maintaining double-blind conditions (e.g., if serious side effects such as extrapyramidal symptoms emerge) (Chassan, 1979). It is a rare study that does not have to compromise on at least some of these issues. Single-subject designs come much closer to the clinically accepted methods of titrating the clinically effective dose of the drug. They take longer and are usually more arduous than group studies. Their external validity comes from replication across subjects. Treatment orders can be randomized or counterbalanced, so that statistical analyses can be performed. Group studies are more useful in detecting smaller effects, because of the power of group statistics. However, they trade off internal validity for external validity in that, with neuroleptic studies of the type in question, one is usually hard pressed to find a subject who is typical of the population. It is difficult to generalize about a group or to predict a priori who will respond to a neuroleptic drug and who will not.

A number of additional methodological concerns have emerged from recent studies, such as drug × behavior × setting interactions, confounding due to side effects, staff reactivity, attribution bias, failure to replicate effects across repeated treatment conditions, acute versus chronic dose effects, and rate dependency. These are discussed when more recent studies are reviewed in a subsequent section.

Diagnostic Issues

Persons with behavioral disturbances and developmental disabilities have often been the victims of neglect and avoidance of both the mental health and developmental disabilities bureaucracies. Thus, as a group they are underdiagnosed, and a poor prognosis is frequently unjustifiably attributed to them (Reiss, Levitan, & Szyszko, 1982). If schizophrenia (Eaton & Menolascino, 1982), depression (Sovner & Hurley, 1983), and other biologically based mental illnesses (Breese, Mueller, & Schroeder, 1986) precipitate maladaptive behaviors, then a differential diagnosis and prescriptive pharmacological treatment might be indicated. For instance, we have recently outlined and reviewed three neurochemical hypotheses that might be setting factors for self-injurious behavior (Schroeder, Bickel, & Richmond, 1986): (a) the neonatal dopamine depletion hypothesis, (b) the opioid peptide model, and (c) the altered physiological state model. Each of these models is designed to account for the interactions of certain physiologically determined susceptibilities and environmental setting events that act to select a specific behavioral phenotype (e.g., self-biting, head-banging, etc). If any of them prove to be correct, then a theory-guided basis for prescribing specific neuroleptics for specific behaviors would be available for the first time. At present, selection of the specific neuroleptic for treatment is still done largely by trial and error (Gualtieri & Keppel, 1985).

Toxic Side Effects

The term *neuroleptic* comes from the Greek phrase, "seize the neuron." It is believed that neuroleptics exert their antipsychotic effects by modulating dopamine receptors in the basal ganglia. Some toxic effects are thought to occur as a result of "supersensitivity" related to chronic blockade of dopamine neurons. Although the evidence from humans is mainly epidemiological, there is a substantial animal literature demonstrating this phenomenon experimentally.

A number of *short-term* side effects may be confounded with desirable treatment outcomes, so that their effects must also be assessed when evaluating a main drug effect. The first class of such effects are apathy, drowsiness, and lethargy, which can usually be attenuated by titrating the dosage or by waiting for the client to develop a tolerance for the drug. A second class includes somatic complaints such as dry mouth, blurred vision, urinary retention, or abdominal pain.

A third class of short-term side effects involves acute extrapyramidal side effects (EPS), such as akathisia, dystonia, and pseudoparkinsonism. Akathisia is characterized by restlessness, an inability to sit still, foot tapping, leg bouncing, constant pacing, and shifting of weight while standing. Dystonia is defined as sustained contraction of a skeletal muscle group with simultaneous relaxation of the opposing group. Dystonia may be observed in spasms of the neck (torticollis, retrocollis), eyes (oculogyric crisis), and face (grimacing face, locked jaw). Pseudoparkinsonism is characterized by lack of spontaneous movement, cogwheel rigidity, resting tremor, pill rolling and loss of postural reflexes, masklike or expressionless face, drooling, infrequent blinking, and shuffling gait. Each of these three side effects has a critical relationship to the initiation of treatment. Akathisia is most likely to occur within the first 5 to 60 days of neuroleptic use; dystonia within the first 1 to 5 days of neuroleptic use; and pseudoparkinsonism within 5 to 30 days after neuroleptic use.

The main *long-term* side effect, tardive dyskinesia, is also an extrapyramidal side effect, although not always listed as such, that occurs much later in the course of drug treatment or upon drug withdrawal and "is characterized by a variable mix of involuntary movements of the face, mouth, tongue, upper limbs and lower limbs" (Kalachnik, Harder, & Kidd-Nielsen, 1984). The diagnostic criteria for tardive dyskinesia require a minimum of several months of drug treatment before consideration of diagnosis (Schooler & Kane, 1982). We will not treat this topic further, as there is a separate chapter devoted to it in this book (see Chapter 9).

"Withdrawal symptoms" after reduction or discontinuation of neuroleptic treatment include nausea, anorexia, vomiting, diaphoresis, hyperactivity, or insomnia. These have been found both in developmentally disabled children (Gualtieri, Quade, Hicks, Mayo, & Schroeder, 1984) and adults (Gualtieri, Hicks, Quade, & Schroeder, 1986). Clients may or may not have dyskinesia. On rare occasions, seizures occur (see James, 1983, for review). For this reason gradual rather than abrupt withdrawal is indicated, particularly for those who have been on high doses for long periods of time. Withdrawal symptoms usually appear shortly after drug changes and dissipate within a few weeks.

Some workers believe that the presence of withdrawal symptoms and dyskinesias is often paralleled by a "behavioral supersensitivity" related to behavioral disturbances (Schroeder & Gualtieri, 1985). Gualtieri et al. (1986) have referred to these as "a behavioral analog of tardive dyskinesia." This phenomenon may be similar to "supersensitivity psychosis" observed in the rapid relapse in some schizophrenic patients after neurolepic withdrawal (Chouinard, & Jones, 1980).

"Cholinergic rebound supersensitivity" may also be a side effect of those neuroleptic drugs that possess a relatively strong anticholinergcic activity, although this is usually weaker than their antidopaminergic activity (Snyder, Benerjee, Yamamura, & Greenberg, 1974). Anticholinergic drugs (e.g., benztropine) are often used to treat extrapyramidal symptoms resulting from neuroleptic treatment. However, chronic treatment with anti-cholingeric drugs can create a "cholinergic supersensitivity" of cholinergic receptors in the basal ganglia (similar to dopaminergic supersensitivity resulting from neuroleptic treatment) such that a rebound in EPS may be seen upon withdrawal or reduction of these antiparkinsonian drugs (Carter, 1983; Inoue, 1982). The control of EPS apparently is mediated by influencing the dopaminergic-cholinergic balance in the basal ganglia.

Another sometimes overlooked side effect that may occur upon treatment with dopamine blockers such as neuroleptics or upon withdrawal of dopaminergic drugs such as the antiparkinsonian drugs is the "neuroleptic malignant syndrome" (Caroff, 1980; Levenson, 1985; Mueller, 1985; Varia & Taska, 1985). Neuroleptic malignant syndrome is characterized by unexplained hyperpyrexia (fever), muscular rigidity, altered consciousness (i.e., stupor, coma, and eventually death [if untreated] and autonomic dysfunctions such as diaphoresis [profuse sweating], dyspnea [irregular breathing], urinary incontinence, labile blood pressure, and tachycardia). About 50 cases have been reported in the literature. Incidence is estimated at less than 1% of those receiving neuroleptics. Mortality from neuroleptic malignant syndrome is calculated at 14% for oral dosage and 38% for intramuscular administration. All ages and both sexes may be affected. Onset may occur within minutes of the first dose or after prolonged treatment. The etiology and pathogenesis are unknown, but the first symptom is usually a high fever. If discovered, it must be treated immediately, by stopping all neuroleptics, administering dantroline sodium (Dantrium), a muscle relaxant, and/or dopamine agonists such as amantadine and bromo-criptine, and treatment for shock. Persons who have had a neuroleptic malignant syndrome attack are prone to have more attacks. It is believed that neuroleptic malignant syndrome occurs more with high-potency neuroleptics such as haloperidol and fluphenazine, although it has also been reported with low-potency neuroleptics such as thioridazine.

Such devastating side effects of neuroleptic treatment call for a more refined definition of toxicity, a term that contains many surplus meanings. For instance, a commonly used definition is that of DiMascio, Soltys, and Shader (1970):

Behavioral toxicity is a phrase used to describe those pharmacological actions, that, when administered within the dosage range in which a drug has been found to possess clinical utility, produce—through mechanisms not immediately specifiable—alternations in perceptual and cognitive functions, psychomotor performance, motivation, mood, interpersonal relationships, or intrapsychic processes of an individual to the degree that they interfere with or limit the capacity of the individual to function within his setting or constitute a hazard to his physical well-being. (p. 127)

Such a definition covers all negative side effects, while remaining neutral with respect to theoretical substrates. In the light of recent research on neuroleptic side effects, it would seem to be time to update this definition, in order to explore new models for different types of toxic responses. Neurotoxicity-based postsynaptic receptor supersensitivity or other models based upon behavioral models (e.g., symptom substitution or covariation, reinforcement schedule-induced effects, state dependency, addiction, etc.) are heuristic concepts that need to be exploited more than they have been. As neuroleptics are ever more widely prescribed, our knowledge of side effects needs to increase.

Recent Neuroleptic Studies

The modern era of pharmacotherapy was ushered in by Aman and Singh's (1980) critical review of the effectiveness of thioridazine, the most frequently used neuroleptic in mental retardation. Since that time there have been a number of withdrawal and prospective studies using double-blind crossover designs and multimodal assessment strategies of the type recommended by Sprague and Werry (1971).

Coldwater Studies

Breuning and his colleagues have published a number of very influential neuroleptic withdrawal and prospective studies based on data collected at the Coldwater Regional Center for Developmental Disabilities (Breuning, 1982; Breuning & Davidson, 1981; Breuning, Davis, Matson, & Ferguson, 1982; Breuning, Davis, & Poling, 1982; Breuning, Ferguson, Davidson, & Poling, 1983; Breuning, O'Neill, & Ferguson, 1980; Wysocki, Fuqua, Davis, & Breuning, 1981). As a group, these studies stand somewhat alone in the literature as showing uniformly negative effects of neuroleptics on learning, adaptive behavior, and habilitation in mental retardation. Aman and Singh (1986) have reviewed these studies in the light of the controversy they have created, and have suggested that their results were likely related to the high doses of neuroleptics used and the fact that subjects were selected based upon their failure to respond to behavioral intervention. The latter has been a common practice in other studies, however, and is often explicit in accreditation guidelines. Furthermore, single fixed-dose studies of neuroleptics in normal humans (Janke, 1980) suggest a generally negative influence on mental activity and an increase in activity at low doses (e.g., chlorpromazine, 50 mg; haloperidol, 2 mg; perphenazine, 8 mg; pimozide, 2 mg; promethazine, 50 mg; promazine, 50 mg; reserpine, 5 mg). On the other hand, some studies have suggested enhanced learning (Anderson et al., 1984; Werry & Aman, 1975). So many pieces of this puzzle still remain to be found before a conclusion is possible.

Recently, there have been allegations of scientific fraud insofar as the Coldwater studies are concerned (Holden, 1986, 1987; see also Ferguson,

Cullari, & Gadow, 1987; Gadow, 1987; Gualtieri, 1987; Sprague, 1987; see also Preface) and they have been the subject of a review panel by the National Institute of Mental Health. Recently the panel's report was released, and it alleged that Breuning

knowingly, willfully, and repeatedly engaged in misleading and deceptive practices in reporting results of research . . . that he did not carry out the described research; and that only a few of the experimental subjects described in publications and progress reports were ever studied; and that the complex designs and rigorous methodologies reported were not employed (Holden, 1987, p. 1566; see also Hostetler, 1987).

It is obvious that the Coldwater studies cannot be accepted at face value and, indeed, replication studies, which attempt to duplicate the procedures reported by Breuning, would provide a great service for the field.

Other Recent Neuroleptic Withdrawal Studies

Neuroleptic withdrawal studies need to be considered separately from prospective studies because: (a) it is rare that current or cumulative dose was under the control of the experimenter; (b) control for the passage of time or effects of the behavioral intervention since the client was first put on the drug is rarely possible; and (c) confounding due to withdrawal symptoms, tardive dyskinesia, and short-term side effects must be dealt with when assessing behavioral effects.

Heistad, Zimmerman, and Doebler (1982) took advantage of a court-ordered drug holiday for all the residents of Cambridge State School, a PRF in Minnesota, to conduct a 4- to 5-week double-blind, placebo-controlled, crossover study of thioridazine in 106 patients (54% male, mean age 28.5). Subjects were randomly assigned to either one of two orders, drug-placebo or placebo-drug. More than 50% were diagnosed as profoundly retarded, but their mean level of retardation was less severe as compared with the total hospital population. The data collection package consisted of the following: (a) a 31-category observation system patterned after Jones, Reid, and Patterson (1975) (performed daily); (b) the Nurses Observation Scale for Inpatient Evaluation (Honigfeld, 1973) (completed once per treatment); (c) the Abnormal Involuntary Movement Scale (AIMS) (filled in once per subject); (d) global impressions by a physician, nurse, and resident staff members on 64 of the patients; and (e) daily behavior reports of resident maladaptive behavior from resident care staff. Statistical results generally favored thioridazine for a moderate suppression of inappropriate behaviors, with a nonsignificant tendency for increased positive behaviors to occur more frequently while on thioridazine. The most consistent effect was on self-stimulation, which increased by 18% on placebo. AIMS scores showed no suggestion of increased involuntary movements on placebo compared to drug. Heistad et al. (1982) attribute this latter result to inexperience of the raters. Indeed, recent studies by Kalachnik et al. (1984), using the Dyskinesia Identification System–Coldwater (DISCO) (Sprague et al., 1984), found tardive dyskinesia in nearly half of the subjects in a study conducted at the same hospital. This is a key point since we now know that short-term side effects occur precisely within the first 4 to 8 weeks upon neuroleptic withdrawal and usually recede later (Gualtieri et al. 1984, 1986). The brief drug holiday effects in this study are not surprising, but they may not tell us much about the long-term efficacy of chronically administered thioridazine, because of the apparent failure of these investigators to detect relevant withdrawal effects.

Schroeder and Gualtieri (1985) reported on a double-blind, crossover, placebo-controlled withdrawal study of 23 profoundly retarded residents, two of whom had been receiving haloperidol and 21 thioridazine, for at least 6 months, in two PRFs in North Carolina. They were assigned randomly to a 2-, 3-, 4- or 5-week baseline period and then to either abrupt or gradual withdrawal of at least 8 weeks, in order to keep the staff blind for as long as possible. The data base consisted of: (a) weekly ratings of tardive dyskinesia using the AIMS by the attending physician and a trained research assistant; (b) daily modified frequency observations by the teacher for ½ hour, time-locked to drug or placebo administration; (c) weekly observations of the client on the ward with a 26-category modified frequency observational instrument by a trained research assistant; and (d) twice daily ratings of the client by direct care staff on the morning and afternoon shifts using the Resident Behavior Rating Scale (Sprague, 1978). The main results were that there was a small but statistically significant increase in staff ratings of inappropriate behavior upon drug withdrawal that appeared to be tied to the occurrence of tardive dyskinesia. This effect was not apparent in directly observed behavioral data recorded by teachers and research assistants. There were complex interactive effects on behavior depending on the setting (dayroom verse classroom), presence of tardive dyskinesia, and staff reactions to the clients upon drug withdrawal. Inspection of the data of individuals revealed a wide array of results ranging from improvement to serious deterioration of target behaviors. Neuroleptic withdrawal studies should take into account these interactions by the use of appropriate statistical models (e.g., covariance analyses or multiple regression analyses).

Lewis et al. (1986) performed a double-blind, placebo-controlled, crossover BABA design intensively studying the effects of withdrawal of chronically administered thioridazine in three profoundly retarded adults. Subjects had been selected for their high rates of stereotyped behavior (between 30% and 70% of all sessions). Continuous recording of selected behavioral topographies was carried out for either three or four 30-minute sessions each day. Two observers recorded simultaneously on 20% of the sessions. The AIMS was completed by the attending psychiatrist and a trained research assistant. Time series analysis was used to assess the single-subject data statistically. Change from drug to placebo was statistically reliable but inconsistent across subjects. Blood levels were also taken in this study. Metabolism of the drug was related to behavioral response in a very complex manner (see Chapter 3). No dyskinesia was observed in these clients, although one client exhibited withdrawal symptoms of screaming, pacing, and irritability.

Recent Prospective Neuroleptic Studies Involving Thioridazine

Prospective studies have the advantage that they do not have to deal with a preexisting history of neuroleptics if a sufficient washout period is used. Therefore, there is less concern for long-term side effects. Short-term side effects can often be handled by titrating the dose.

Only a few recent prospective studies of thioridazine have been reported. The Lewis et al. (1986) study previously discussed also had a cohort of three subjects run in a prospective ABAB study, with essentially the same inconsistent results as those reported in the withdrawal study. Dose had been started at 100 mg of thioridazine per day and adjusted to be equal to approximately 1,000 ng of "thioridazine equivalents" per ml from blood samples drawn on Days 3 and 5.

Singh and Aman (1981) performed a dose response prospective study of thioridazine on 19 severely or profoundly retarded adolescent residents of a PRF in New Zealand. All subjects were first withdrawn from their chronic regimen of thioridazine (mean = 5.23 mg/kg; range = 1.28–17.54 mg/kg) for a 4-week washout period. Then they received their previous titrated dosage, or a standard dosage (2.5 mg/kg), or placebo in a double-blind crossover design. There were 4 weeks per treatment condition and a 1-week transition period in which the dosage was set midway between the previous and forthcoming dosage levels. Conditions were counterbalanced and assessments were conducted within the last 5 days of each period. It was found that both active drug conditions were significantly related to a reduction in hyperactivity, bizarre behavior, and stereotyped behavior, while not affecting cognitive behaviors (i.e., instruction-following and attention as measured by the continuous performance test). There were no significant therapeutic differences between the lower standard dose and the substantially higher titrated doses.

Jakab (1984) conducted a study of the short-term effect of thioridazine tablets versus thioridazine in suspension on emotionally disturbed mentally retarded children. Behavioral observations were conducted by blind observers before and after medication in a classroom during structured activity and during free play. On short-term observation both forms of thioridazine (mean = 3.44 mg/kg; range = 2.14–5.71 mg/kg) were effective in reducing aggression, disruptive tantrumming, self-abuse, stereotyped self-stimulation, and pica. Average symptom reduction was 27.4% within 35 minutes following medication intake. This study was not really an efficacy study comparing thioridazine with placebo. Instead it compared pre- and postmedication intervals. There were substantial changes over the course of the assessment periods, suggesting that time since administration is an important variable to be controlled when evaluating the drug's effect.

Menolascino, Ruedrich, Golden, and Wilson (1985) compared the effects of thiothixene to thioridazine in a rater-blind study on 61 randomly assigned retarded and nonretarded schizophrenics in an inpatient psychiatric hospital setting. There were equal numbers of males and females and the subjects ranged in age from 18 to 60 years. Patients received no psychotropic medication for a month, and then were given a titrated dose of thioridazine (mean = 264 mg; range = up to 800 mg) or of thiothixene (mean = 34.5 mg; range = up to 80 mg) for a maximun of 3 months. Ratings were performed at baseline and at Weeks 1, 2, 3, 4, 8, and 12 on the Global Evaluation Scale, Katz Rating Scale, Brief Psychiatric Rating Scale (BPRS), the Nurse's Observation Scale for Inpatient Evaluation, and a Motor Steadiness Battery. Apparently, no placebo condition, double-blind precaution, ratings scales for side effects, or interrater reliability sessions were used. Nevertheless, both drugs were found to produce considerable improvement on the BPRS but not the other rating scales. Time of onset of effect was reported to be faster for thiothixene than thioridazine in the retarded group, although thiothixene also produced more extrapyramidal side effects. There are a number of methodological problems, as noted above, which make the interpretation of this study difficult.

Recent Prospective Studies Involving Haloperidol and Other Neuroleptics

Aman, White, and Field (1984) examined the effects of chlorpromazine (2.0–3.5 mg/kg) on the suppression of stereotyped behavior and adaptive behavior in six profoundly retarded residents of a PRF in New Zealand who had been preselected for the presence or absence of stereotypic behavior in a well-conducted placebo-controlled, crossover study. Chlorpromazine caused noticeable drowsiness in all subjects over the 2-week drug period. Body rocking was significantly suppressed in the wards, but other clinical behaviors were not influenced by the drug. Performance on an operant lever-pulling task was significantly impaired in most subjects. Body rocking, which was also assessed during operant responding, was unrelated to presence or absence of clinical stereotypy observed on the wards. Aman et al. (1984) suggested that chlorpromazine may have a selective effect on stereotyped behavior.

To the best of our knowledge, the best placebo-controlled, double-blind study of drug-behavior therapy interactions was a study with autistic children by Campbell et al., (1978). In this study, they examined the effects of clinically titrated doses of haloperidol or placebo in combination with contingent or noncontingent reinforcement of language training according to the program designed by Lovaas (1977). The subjects were autistic inpatient children ranging in age from 2.6 to 7.2 years and in severity from profound to mild impairment from the nursery of Bellevue Psychiatric Hospital. Language training consisted of 30 minutes of individualized training a day involving attending to the therapist, vocalizing, word imitation, object identification, responsive speech, and so forth. Subjects were assigned randomly to each of the four groups: each factorial combination of drug or placebo, and contingent or noncontingent language training (i.e., reinforcement, dependent or not, on correct responding). In addition to the language measures, other measures taken were five ward rating scales and a battery of cognitive tests compiled by the Child Psychopharmacology Branch of the National Institute of Mental Health (EDCEU, 1976). Dosage of haloperidol was titrated for each individual in weekly increments until an optimal dose was found. The mean dose for children below 4.5 years was 0.07 mg/kg per day; above 4.5 years it was 0.15 mg/kg per day.

The main results were: (a) Haloperidol was significantly related to decreases in stereotyped behaviors and withdrawal behaviors of older but not younger children. This may have been a dose effect. (b) Contingent reinforcement was significantly related to improvement of ward behaviors. (c) Contingent reinforcement was related to more compliance and imitation during language training. (d) Haloperidol plus the Lovaas (1977) language program was more effective than either alone in promoting language performance, especially imitative speech. When either treatment was presented alone, contingent reinforcement, but not haloperidol, significantly affected language performance. (e) Results from the cognitive battery revealed no effect on performance of either treatment. (f) The most frequent side effect of haloperidol was sedation. This well-conducted experiment is an excellent example of the multiple interactions that can occur (but usually go unnoticed) in a study on pharmacotherpay, unless an integrated drug-behavior therapy design is used. Drug placebos do not necessarily ensure an inert treatment unless a behavioral baseline placebo (in this case noncontingent reinforcement) is also used for comparing behavioral treatments.

The Campbell et al. (1978) study has been updated several times, as fuller data analyses have been completed (Campbell et al., 1982; Cohen et al., 1980). The most recent update (Anderson et al., 1984) reversed an earlier result, in that it was found that haloperidol at low doses (0.019–0.217 mg/kg per day) produced greater facilitation and retention of discrimination learning in the laboratory with no adverse side effects. Untoward effects were noted only above the optimum titrated dose or during the dosage regulation period. They found that this was not true in a more severely disturbed population of aggressive children hospitalized for conduct disorders. With such clients, Anderson et al. noted that the higher doses of haloperidol required to suppress these symptoms (0.04–0.21 mg/kg per day; mean = 0.096) also suppressed performance on laboratory tests of cognition (Platt, Campbell, Green, & Grega, 1984).

Durand (1982) performed a single-subject drug-behavior interaction design on a 17-year-old profoundly retarded institutionalized young man, using haloperidol (4 mg per day) alone or in combination with punishment (hand squeeze contingent on SIB). The two together were more effective than either alone. Caution must be used when interpreting this study, which was nonblind and not placebo controlled. The animal literature suggests that neuroleptics tend to disrupt rather than facilitate avoidance learning and to have very little effect on punished responding (Cook & Davidson, 1973), and hence the present results are counterintuitive.

Aman, Teehan, White, Turbott, and Vaithianathan (in press), performed the best study to date on haloperidol in the mental retardation population. Twenty residents, ages 13 to 35 years, from a PRF in New Zealand (most of whom had previously received neuroleptic maintenance therapy) were assessed in a double-blind, placebo-controlled crossover study. Haloperidol was administered in standardized doses of 0.025 and 0.05 mg/kg per day, for 3 weeks each in a counterbalanced Latin Square Design. Behavior ratings were collected on the Aberrant Behavior Checklist (Aman, Singh, Stewart, & Field, 1985) and the Fairview Problem Behavior Checklist (Barron & Sandman, 1983). In addition, direct observations were collected (using an interval recording technique) on movement, stereotypic behavior, inactivity, appropriate isolated behavior, appropriate social behavior, and inappropriate behavior. Instruction-following, heart rate, and seizure frequency were also recorded. There was a significant reduction in stereotypic behavior and an increase in gross motor activity at the high dose of the drug. There was a tendency for reinforced instruction-following to improve on the drug. Aman et al. also divided the group into high and low stereotypy subgroups. There were a number of significant drug-by-subgroup interactions, suggesting that individuals with high levels of stereotypy may show a more favorable response to neuroleptic medication than those with low levels of stereotypy.

White and Aman (1985) subjected eight severely retarded residents to a double-blind placebo-controlled trial of pimozide. The drug did not alter behavioral adjustment as assessed by behavior observations. However, ratings on the Aberrant Behavior Checklist showed significant drug-induced improvements on two dimensions (irritability and hyperactivity/noncompliance). Learning on a discrimination learning task was not affected by the drug.

Lynch, Eliatamby, and Anderson (1985) performed a double-blind, placebo-controlled, crossover study of intramuscular pipothiazine palmitate (50 mg) on 30 aggressive mentally handicapped patients. Target symptoms and global impressions were rated at monthly intervals. Patients showed marked improvement on pipothiazine palmitate. Extrapyramidal side effects occurred in seven patients.

Finally, a study by Goldstein, Anderson, Reuben, and Dancis (1985) involved a double-blind placebo-controlled trial of fluphenazine (1.5 mg twice daily) on a 20-month-old Lesch-Nyhan syndrome child, which resulted in a dramatic elimination of self-biting. A subsequent open trial (5 mg per day) with a 15-year-old boy who had been stable for years did not show a dramatic effect, perhaps because of years of practicing self-mutilation. These results are particularly interesting in that the Lesch-Nyhan syndrome has been notoriously refractory to neuroleptic therapy (Breese, Mueller, & Schroeder, 1986). Perhaps this is due to the fact that Lesch-Nyhan syndrome self-mutilatory behavior is due to dopamine supersensitivity at the D1 rather than the D2 receptor site. Fluphenazine, a D1 and D2 receptor blocker, may therefore have advantages over other neuroleptics like haloperidol or thioridazine, which are largely D2 blockers. Unfortunately, there is not a pure D1 blocker approved for clinical use in the United States at this time. If Goldstein's theory is correct, this will be the first neuroleptic with such a selected effect on a specific behavioral phenotype. It could be a breakthrough and could force a reconceptualization of the role of specific neuroleptics on specific behaviors in different subpopulations of persons with developmental disabilities. However, it is also clear that these preliminary encouraging results require replications to determine their robustness.

Summary and Conclusions

Since 1980 there has been a welcome increase in sophistication of neuroleptic studies. With this upgrading of technology, it is likely that in future years we will learn more about dose response functions of selected drugs (e.g. haloperidol versus fluphenazine) on specific behaviors (e.g., stereotyped versus self-injurious behaviors) and in specific populations (e.g., autistic versus mentally retarded versus Lesch-Nyhan syndrome). It appears that specific neuropharmacological theories will be available to guide our choice of drugs rather than the hit-or-miss strategy of pharmacotherapy to which we are currently condemned. However, we are only on the threshold of this era. For us, each new client will still constitute a single-subject experiment until we have filled in many more pieces of the mosaic that constitutes the fascinating puzzle of pharmacotherapy with persons who have developmental disabilities.

Acknowledgment. I wish to acknowledge Grants HD 03110, HD *20980*, and MCH Project 916 for support during the writing of this paper.

References

Alexandris, A., & Lundell, F.W. (1986), Effect of thioridazine, amphetamine, and placebo on the hyperkinetic syndrome and cognitive area in mentally deficient children. *Canadian Medical Association Journal*, 98, 92–96.

Aman, M.G. (1983). Psychoactive drugs in mental retardation. In J.L. Matson & F. Andrasik (Eds.), *Treatment issues and innovations in mental retardation* (pp. 455–513). New York: Plenum Press.

Aman, M.G. (1984). Drugs and learning in mentally retarded persons. In G.D. Burrows & J.S. Werry (Eds.), *Advances in human psychopharmacology* (Vol. 3, pp. 121–163). Greenwich, CT: JAI Press.

Aman, M.G., & Singh, N.N (1986). A critical appraisal of recent drug research in mental retardation: The Coldwater studies. *Journal of Mental Dificiency Research*, *30*, 203–216.

Aman, M.G., & Singh, N.N. (1980). The usefulness of thioridazine for treating childhood disorders—Fact or folklore? *American Journal of Mental Deficiency*, *84*, 331–338.

Aman, M.G., Singh, N.N., Stewart, A.W., & Field, C.J. (1985). The Aberrant Behavior Checklist: A behavior rating scale for measurement of treatment effects. *American Journal of Mental Deficiency*, *89*, 485–491.

Aman, M.G., Teehan, C.J., White, A.J., Turbott, S.H., & Vaithianathan, C. (in press). Haloperidol treatment with chronically medicated residents: Dose effects on clinical behavior and reinforcement contingencies. *American Journal of Mental Retardation*.

Aman, M.G., & White, A.J. (1986). Measures of drug change in mental retardation. In K.D. Gadow (Ed.), *Advances in learning and behavioral disabilities* (Vol. 5). Greenwich, CT: JAI Press, pp. 157–202.

Aman, M.G., White, A.J., & Field, C.J. (1984). Chlorpromazine effects on stereotypic and conditioned behavior—A pilot study. *Journal of Mental Deficiency Research*, *28*, 253–260.

Anderson, L.T., Campbell, M., Grega, D.M., Perry, R., Small, A.M., & Green, W.H. (1984). Haloperidol in the treatment of infantile autism: Effects on learning and behavioral symptoms. *American Journal of Psychiatry*, *141*, 1195–1202.

Barron, J., & Sandman, C.A. (1983). Relationship of sedative-hypnotic response to self-injurious behavior and stereotypy by mentally retarded clients. *American Journal of Mental Deficiency*, *88*, 177–186.

Breese, G.R., Mueller, R.A., & Schroeder, S.R. (1986). The neurochemical basis of symptoms in the Lesch-Nyhan syndrome: Relationship to control symptoms in other developmental disorders. In E. Schopler (Ed.), *Current neurobiological issues in autism*. New York: Academic Press. pp. 145–156.

Breuning, S.E. (1982). An applied dose-response curve of thioridazine with the mentally retarded: Aggressive, self-stimulatory, intellectual and workshop behaviors—A preliminary report. *Psychopharmacology Bulletin*, *18*, 57–59.

Breuning, S.E., & Davidson, N.A. (1981). Effects of psychotropic drugs on intelligence test performance of institutionalized mentally retarded adults. *American Journal of Mental Deficiency*, *85*, 575–579.

Breuning, S.E., Davis, V.J. Matson, J.L., & Ferguson, D.G. (1982). Effects of thioridazine and withdrawal dyskinesias on workshop performance of mentally retarded young adults. *American Journal of Psychiatry*, *139*, 1447–1454.

Breuning, S.E., Davis, V.J., & Poling, A.D. (1982). Pharmacotherapy with the mentally retarded: Implications for clinical psychologists. *Clinical Psychology Review*, *2*, 79–114.

Breuning, S.E., Ferguson, D.G., Davidson, N.A., & Poling, A.D. (1983). Effects of thioridazine on the intellectual performance of mentally retarded drug responders and nonresponders. *Archives of General Psychiatry*, *40*, 309–313.

Breuning, S.E., O'Neill, J., & Ferguson, D.G. (1980). Comparison of psychotropic drug, response cost, and psychotropic drug plus response cost procedures for controlling institutionalized retarded persons. *Applied Research in Mental Retardation*, *1*, 253–168.

Campbell, M., Anderson, L.T., Meier, M., Cohen, I.L., Small, A.M., Samit, C., & Sachar, E.J. (1978). A comparison of haloperidol and behavior therapy and their interaction in autistic children. *Journal of the American Academy of Child Psychiatry*, *17*, 640–655.

Campbell, M., Anderson, L.T., Small, A.M., Perry, R., Green, W.H., & Caplan, R. (1982). The effects of haloperidol on learning and behavior in autistic children. *Journal of Autism and Developmental Disorders*, *12*, 167–176.

Caroff, S.N. (1982). The neuroleptic malignant syndrome. *Journal of Clinical Psychiatry*, *41*, 79–83.

Carter, G. (1983). The abrupt withdrawal of antiparkinsonian drugs in mentally handicapped patients. *British Journal of Psychiatry*, *142*, 166–168.

Chassan, J.B. (1979). *Research design in clinical psychology and psychiatry*. New York: Halstead Press.

Chouinard, G., & Jones, B.D. (1980). Neuroleptic-induced supersensitivity psychosis: Clinical and pharmacological characteristics. *American Journal of Psychiatry*, *137*, 16–21

Cohen, I.L., Campbell, M., Posner, D., Small, A.M., Trickel, D., & Anderson, L.T. (1980). Behavioral effects of haloperidol in young autistic children. *Journal of the American Academy of Child Psychiatry*, *19*, 665–677.

Cole, J.O. (1982). Psychopharmacology update: Antipsychotic drugs: Is more better? *McLean Hospital Journal*, *VII*, 61–87.

Cook, L., & Davidson, A.B. (1973). Effects of behaviorally active drugs in a conflict-punishment procedure in rats. In S. Garattini, E. Massini, & L.O. Randall (Eds.), *The benzodiazepines*. New York: Raven Press.

Davis, K.V. (1971). The effect of drugs on stereotyped and nonstereotyped operant behaviors in retardates. *Psychopharmacologia*, *22*, 195–213.

Davis, K.V., Sprague, R.L., & Werry, J.S. (1969). Stereotyped behavior and activity level in severe retardates: The effect of drugs. *American Journal of Mental Deficiency*, *73*, 721–727.

DiMascio, A., Soltys, J.J., & Shader, R.I. (1970). Psychotropic drug side effects in children. In R.I. Shader & A. DiMascio (Eds.), *Psychotropic drug side effects* (pp. 235–260). Baltimore: Williams & Wilkins.

Durand, V.M. (1982). A behavioral/pharmacological intervention for the treatment of severe self-injurious behavior. *Journal of Autism and Developmental Disorders*, *12*, 243–251.

Eaton, L.F., & Menolascino, F.H. (1982). Psychiatric disorders in the mentally retarded: Types, problems, and challenges. *American Journal of Psychiatry*, *139*, 1297–1303.

EDCEU. (1976). *Assessment manual*. Rockville, MD: National Institute of Mental Health.

Ferguson, D.G., Cullari, S., & Gadow, K.D. (1987). Comment on the "Coldwater" studies. *Journal of Mental Deficiency Research*, *31*, 219–220.

Fielding, L.T., Murphy, R.J., Reagan, M.W., & Peterson, T.L. (1980). An assessment program to reduce drug use with the mentally retarded. *Hospital and Community Psychiatry*, *31*, 771–773.

Gadow, K.D. (1985). Prevalence and efficacy of stimulant drug use with mentally retarded children and youth. *Psychopharmacology Bulletin, 21*, 291–303.

Gadow, K.D. (1987). Comments on the community drug treatment prevalence survey by Davis et al. (1981). *Journal of Mental Deficiency Research, 31*, 215–219.

Goldstein, M., Anderson, L.T., Reuben, R., & Dancis, J. (1985). Self-mutilation in Lesch-Nyhan disease is caused by dopaminergic denervation. *The Lancet, February 9*, 338–339.

Gualtieri, C.T. (1987). Letter to the editor. *Journal of Mental Deficiency Research, 31*, 222–223.

Gualtieri, C.T., Hicks, R.E., Quade, D., & Schroeder, S.R. (1986). Tardive dyskinesia in young mentally retarded adults. *Archives of General Psychiatry, 43*, 335–340.

Gualtieri, C.T., & Keppel, J.M. (1985). Psychopharmacology in the mentally retarded and a few related issues. *Psychopharmacology Bulletin, 21*, 304–309.

Gualtieri, C.T., Quade, D., Hicks, R., Mayo, J.R., & Schroéder, S.R. (1984). Tardive dyskinesia and other clinical consequences of neuroleptic treatment in children and adolescents. *American Journal of Psychiatry, 141*, 20–23.

Heistad, G.T., Zimmerman, R.L., & Doebler, M.I. (1982). Long-term usefulness of thioridazine for institutionalized mentally retarded patients. *American Journal of Mental Deficienty, 87*, 243–254.

Hill, B.K., Balow, E.A., & Bruininks, R.H. (1985). A national study of prescribed drugs in institutions and community residential facilities for mentally retarded people. *Psychopharmacology Bulletin, 21*, 279–284.

Holden, C. (1986). NIMH review of fraud charge moves slowly. *Science, 234*, 1488–1489

Holden, C. (1987). NIMH finds a case of "serious misconduct." *Science, 235*, 1566–1567.

Honigfeld, G. (1973). NOSIE-30: History and current status of its use in pharmacopsychiatric research. In P. Pichot & R. Olivier-Martin (Eds.), *Modern problems in pharmacopsychiatry: Vol. 7 Psychological measurement* (pp. 238–263). Basel: Karger.

Hostetler, A.J. (1987, July) NIMH sends fraud case to Justice. *The APA Monitor, 18*, 18.

Inoue, F. (1982). Neuroleptic withdrawal behavior-cases of cholinergic rebound supersensitivity. *Clinical Pharmacy, 1*, 567–569.

Jakab, I. (1984). Short-term effect of thioridazine tablets versus suspension on emotionally disturbed/retarded children. *Journal of Clinicial Psychopharmacology, 4*, 210–215.

James, D.H. (1983). Monitoring drugs in hospitals for the mentally handicapped. *British Journal of Psychiatry, 142*, 163–165.

Janke, W. (1980). Psychometric and psychophysiological actions of antipsychotics in men . In F. Hoffmeister & G. Stille (Eds.), *Handbook of Experimental Pharmacology* (Vol. 55, pp. 305–336). Berlin: Springer-Verlag.

Johnston, J.M., Wallen, A., Partin, J., Neu, E., Cade, R.F., Stein, G.H., Goldstein, M.K., Pennypacker, H.S., & Gfeller, E. (1983). Human operant laboratory measurement of the effects of chemical variables. *The Psychological Record, 33*, 457–472.

Jonas, O. (1980). Pattern of drug prescribing in a residential center for the intellectually handicapped. *Australian Journal of Developmental Disabilities, 6–7*, 25–29.

Jones, R.R., Reid, J.B., & Patterson, G.R. (1975). Naturalistic observation in clinical assessment. In P. McReynolds (Ed.), *Advances in psychological assessment* (Vol. 3, pp. 42–95). San Francisco: Jossey-Bass.

Kalachnik, J.E., Harder, S.R., & Kidd-Nielsen, P. (1984). Persistent tardive dyskinesia in randomly assigned neuroleptic reduction, neuroleptic nonreduction, and no-neuroleptic history groups: Preliminary results. *Psychopharmacology Bulletin, 20*, 27–32.

Kalachnik, J.E., Larum, J.G., & Swanson, A. (1983). A tardive dyskinesia monitoring policy for applied facilities. *Psychopharmacology Bulletin, 19*, 277–282.

Kalachnik, J.E., Miller, R.F., Jamison, A.G., & Harder, S. (1983). Results of a system to monitor effects of psychotropic medication in an applied setting. *Psychopharmacology Bulletin, 19*, 12–15.

LaMendola, W., Zaharia, E.S., & Carver, M. (1980). Reducing psychotropic drug use in an institution for the retarded. *Hospital and Community Psychiatry, 31*, 271–272.

Levenson, J.L. (1985). Neuroleptic malignant syndrome. *American Journal of Psychiatry, 142*, 1137–1145.

Lewis, M.H., Steer, R.A. Favell, J., McGimsey, J., Clontz, L., Trivette, C., Jodry, W., Schroeder, S.R., Kanoy, R.C., & Mailman, R.B. (1986). Thioridazine and metabolite blood levels and effects on human stereotyped behavior. *Psychopharmacology Bulletin, 22*, 1040–1044.

Lipman, R.S. (1970). The use of psychopharmacological agents in residential facilities for the retarded. In F.J. Menolascino (Ed.), *Psychiatric approaches to mental retardation* (pp. 387–398). New York: Basic Books.

Lovaas, O.I. (1977). *Language development through behavior modification.* New York: Wiley.

Lynch, D.M., Eliatamby, C.L.S., & Anderson, A.A. (1985). Pipothiazine palmitate in the management of aggressive mentally handicapped patients. *British Journal of Psychiatry, 146*, 525–529.

Marholin, D., Touchette, P., & Stewart, R.M. (1979). Withdrawal of chronic chlorpromazine medication: An experimental analysis. *Journal of Applied Behavior Analysis, 12*, 159–171.

Menolascino, F.J., Reudrich, S.L., Golden, C.J., & Wilson, J.E. (1985). Diagnosis and pharmacotherapy of schizophrenia in the retarded. *Psychopharmacology Bulletin, 21*, 316–322.

Mouchka, S. (1985). Issues in pharmacology with the mentally retarded. *Psychopharmacology Bulletin, 21*, 262–267.

Mueller, P.S. (1985). Neuroleptic malignant syndrome. *Psychosomatics, 26*, 654–662.

Platt, J.E., Campbell, M., Green, W.H., & Grega, D.M. (1984). Cognitive effects of lithium carbonate and haloperidol in treatment-resistant aggressive children. *Archives of General Psychiatry, 41*, 657–662.

Poling, A., Picker, M., & Hall-Johnson, E. (1983). Human behavioral pharmacology. *The Psychological Record, 33*, 473–493.

Reiss, S., Levitan, G.W., & Szyszko, J. (1982). Emotional disturbance and mental retardation: Diagnostic overshadowing. *American Journal of Mental Deficiency, 86*, 567–574.

Schooler, N., & Kane, J. (1982) Research diagnoses for tardive dyskinesia. *Archives of General Psychiatry, 39*, 486–487.

Schroeder, S.R. Bickel, W., & Richmond, G. (1986). Primary and secondary prevention of self-injurious behavior. In K. Gadow (Ed.), *Advances in learning and behavioral disabilities* (Vol. 5, pp. 65–87). Greenwich, CT: JAI Press.

Schroeder, S.R., & Gualtieri, C.T. (1985). Behavioral interactions induced by chronic neuroleptic therapy with persons with mental retardation. *Psychopharmacology Bulletin, 21*, 323–326.

Schroeder, S.R., Lewis, M.H., & Lipton, M.A. (1983). Interactions of pharmacotherapy and behavior therapy among children with learning and behavioral disorders. In K. Gadow & I. Bialer (Eds.), *Advances in learning and behavioral disabilities* (Vol. 2, pp. 179–225). Greenwich, CT: JAI Press.

Silva, D.A. (1979). The use of medication in a residential institution for mentally retarded persons. *Mental Retardation, 17*, 285–288.

Singh, N.N., & Aman, M.G. (1981). Effects of thioridazine dosage on the behavior of severely retarded persons. *American Journal of Mental Deficiency, 85*, 580–587.

Snyder, S.H., Benerjee, S.P., Yamamura, H., & Greenberg, D. (1974). Drugs, neurotransmitters and schizophrenia. *Science, 184*, 1243–1253.

Sovner, R., & Hurley, A.D. (1983). Do the mentally retarded suffer from affective illness? *Archives of General Psychiatry, 40*, 61–67.

Sprague, R.L. (1978). *The Resident Behavior Rating Scale.* Unpublished instrument, available from the author, Institute for Child Behavior and Development, University of Illinois, Champaign.

Sprague, R.L. (1987). Letter to the editor. *Journal of Mental Deficiency Research, 31*, 223–225.

Sprague, R.L., Kalachnik, J.E., Breuning, S.E., Davis, V.K., Ullman, R.K., Cullari, S., Davidson, N.A., Ferguson, D.G., & Hoffner, B.A. (1984). The Dyskinesia Identification System–Coldwater (DISCO): A tardive dyskinesia rating scale for the developmentally disabled. *Psychopharmacology Bulletin, 30*, 328–338.

Sprague, R.L., & Werry, J.S. (1971). Methodology of psychopharmacological studies with the retarded. In N.R. Ellis (Ed.), *International review of research in mental retardation* (Vol. 5, pp. 147–219). New York: Academic Press.

Tu, J. (1979). A survey of psychotropic medication in mental retardation facilities. *Journal of Clinical Psychiatry, 40*, 125–128.

Tu, J., & Smith, J.T. (1983). The eastern Ontario Survey: A study of drug-treated psychiatric problems in the mentally handicapped. *Canadian Journal of Psychiatry, 28*, 270–276.

Varia, I.M., & Taska, R.J. (1985). The neuroleptic malignant syndrome. *Resident and Staff Physician, 31*, 83–85.

Werry, J.S., & Aman, M.G. (1975). Methylphenidate and haloperidol in children. Effects on attention, memory, and activity. *Archives of General Psychiatry, 32*, 790–795.

White, T.J., & Aman, M.G. (1985). Pimozide treatment in disruptive severely retarded patients. *Australian and New Zealand Journal of Psychiatry, 19*, 92–94.

Wysocki, T., Fuqua, W., Davis, V., & Breuning, S.E. (1981). Effects of thioridazine (Mellaril) on titrating delayed matching-to-sample performance of mentally retarded adults. *American Journal of Mental Deficiency, 85*, 539–547.

5
Antiepileptic Drugs

GREGORY STORES

Abstract

Antiepileptic drug (AED) treatment is an important part of the care of developmentally disabled people, but modern treatment principles are often overlooked in this group. Special assessment and treatment difficulties may well be encountered in such patients. The study of the psychological effects of AED treatment is complicated by special methodological problems in the epilepsies. Psychological measures of clinical value have been employed to only a limit extent. Assessment of seizure severity and frequency, also of obvious relevance to the patient's psychological well-being, may be difficult to achieve. Ideally a distinction would be made between side effects, intoxication, idiosyncrasy, and withdrawal effects. Claims have been made that many AEDs can have beneficial effects on behavior independent of their antiepileptic action. Research provides limited support for such claims. Adverse effects are commonly reported, especially with the older AEDs such as phenobarbitone and phenytoin, although benzodiazepines can also cause problems in this respect. Combinations of drugs are best avoided. There is a need to incorporate modern treatment principles into the care of persons with developmental disabilities and to investigate more systematically the effects of AEDs in such patients by means of appropriately well-designed studies.

Epilepsy commonly complicates the management of mental retardation and autism. In this chapter, *antiepileptic* drugs is used rather than *anticonvulsant* drugs on the grounds that many forms of epileptic attack for which drug treatment is used are not convulsive in type. *Seizure* implies an attack that is epileptic in nature.

The likelihood of recurrent seizures in retarded people is greatest in those severely affected and in need of institutional care. Corbett, Harris, and Robinson (1975) found that 50% of such patients had a history of epilepsy. Richardson, Katz, Koller, and McLaren (1979) quoted an even higher figure. About 25% of autistic patients develop epilepsy (Deykin & MacMahon, 1979; Rutter, 1970), curiously at about the time of adolescence in most cases.

Not surprisingly, therefore, antiepileptic drug (AED) treatment features prominently in the care of these patients. Aman (1984) presents evidence to suggest that this type of treatment is extremely common in both institutionalized and nonstitutionalized retarded patients (see also Chapter 1). It is, then, unfortunate that standards in the use of such drugs in these patients have been repeatedly shown to be low. O'Neill, Ladon, Harris, Riley, and Dreifuss (1977), for example, reported the unsatisfactory nature of AED treatment in a long-term center for mentally retarded persons and how improvements could often be readily achieved by basic readjustments in prescribing practices. A similar account was given by Wilkinson, Murphy, Georgeson, and D'Souza (1982). Particularly alarming was the report by Kaufman and Katz-Garris (1979) that in another group of institutionalized patients, AEDs were being administered to many patients without adequate evidence that they had ever had epilepsy. Further disquieting results come more recently from surveys by Aman, Paxton, Field, and Foote (1986) and Iivanainen, Viukari, Seppalainen, and Helle (1978) in which evidence of intoxication was commonly found in retarded patients taking AEDs, particularly with phenytoin.

Recent Advances in AED Treatment

This type of evidence suggests that the considerable advances that have taken place elsewhere in the last 15 years or so in the use of AEDs may not have been incorporated into the care of retarded patients. It is not easily judged how prevalent such shortcomings have been, but they may well be commonplace.

What are these recent advances? In pediatric practice, there has been a change in the drugs preferred. Sodium valproate and carbamazepine are now used more often (at least in the United Kingdom) than the older drugs such as phenobarbitone and phenytoin. Good practice dictates that an attempt be made to match choice of drug to type of seizure. Simple drug regimes are now preferred, with emphasis on treatment with a single drug wherever possible, administered as few times a day as necessary. Ideally, patient care includes systematic evaluation of compliance, the drug's effectiveness in reducing seizure occurrence, and the possible adverse effect of both physical and psychological types. Welcome though these changes are, there still exists an imbalance between the generally sophisticated clinical pharmacology of AEDs and the relatively crude assessments of drug efficacy and possible complications.

Special Treatment Problems in Patients with Developmental Disabilities

These modern treatment principles should be encouraged in the field of developmental disabilities, but special difficulties are likely to be encountered in trying to implement them. The epilepsies associated with mental retardation (especially as functional level declines) are complex and usually difficult to treat. Whether this is true of the epilepsies that develop in autistic patients is uncertain because of a lack of data. There is a clear need for studies of epilepsy and autism in which the high diagnostic standards now expected in relation to autism are matched by a comparable degree of accuracy in identifying the clinical and electrographic types of coexisting epilepsy.

However, as far as epilepsy in mentally retarded people is concerned, special problems also exist in the recognition and precise classification of seizures and the introduction of rational, simple, and effective treatment, including the evaluation of its effects and the detection of complications. In fact, problems of recognition seem to exist on a large scale even in non-retarded patients. There are many types of attack at all ages. Some are physical and others psychological in type; some are transient, others persist and need special treatment. In many cases these various types are confused with each other. A report by Jeavons (1983) illustrates the point. Of both children and adults referred to his epilepsy clinic, 25% were shown on review to have been mistakenly diagnosed as having epilepsy. Nonepileptic attacks misdiagnosed in this way included syncope, behavioral problems, and sleep disorders. How often is epilepsy misdiagnosed in retarded patients who may exhibit a particularly wide range of nonepileptic episodic changes of behavior? Conversely, how often are nonconvulsive epileptic seizures (perhaps at least as common as convulsive seizures) not recognized as epileptic and attributed to psychological causes?

Pedley (1983) provides a good account of the various types of attack and emphasizes that the means to correct diagnosis is essentially clinical assessment of the precise nature of the episodes. Where diagnostic doubt persists, intensive EEG monitoring, including the comparatively recently developed ambulatory cassette monitoring, can be very helpful (Stores, 1985a). Although the value of this sort of procedure has now gained widespread recognition, there seems to be a reluctance to use such investigations with retarded patients on the unjustified assumption that they will not tolerate the procedure.

Even where epilepsy is correctly diagnosed in the retarded individual, standards of care may be particularly unsatisfactory, with insufficient attention to correct dosage or to the attainment of satisfactory blood levels. These shortcomings can readily be corrected for many patients but, as it is often difficult to treat the epilepsies associated with retardation, basic modern principles of prescribing (notably, treatment with a single drug) may have to be modified. In addition, it may be necessary to resort to second-line treatments or combinations of drugs with the attendant increased risk of adverse effects.

Overall, those who care for developmentally disabled persons need to have a sound knowledge of the epilepsies and their treatment because of their common occurrence in retarded and autistic patients. Modern standards of diagnosis and treatment are required, but special difficulties are likely to be met because of the relatively complicated nature of the seizure disorders and general problems of patient assessment.

Psychological Effects of AEDs

Reports about AEDs on mental state and overt behavior are by no means new. However, in the last 15 years or so the subject has become increasingly popular, although the outcome of the various studies has not provided very much precise information.

Methodological Problems

There are various reasons for this lack of conclusive information. In the first place, there is often a conflict between using the ideal research design and good patient care. For example, the use of placebo controls (almost a standard procedure in psychopharmacological research) is not ethically defensible in patients having seizures. Additionally, it is generally impossible to control fully for all the physical, psychological, and social factors that might influence the psychological outcome in the treated patient. A recent review by Trimble and Reynolds (1984) illustrates how the published reports form a rather confused miscellany. Most studies have been conducted on adult patients and others on normal adult volunteers. The relevance of these findings to children with epilepsy is uncertain. Many studies involve mixed age groups or subjects with a wide range of intelligence, or patients who have been taking several drugs at once. Frequently the type of seizure disorder, and its cause and severity, are not indicated and treatment details may well be lacking. Furthermore, it may be difficult to disentangle the *antiepileptic* properties of a given drug (i.e., it may be more or less successful in suppressing seizures) from its *behavioral* effect.

A further limitation on the value of many reported accounts is the relatively crude form of psychological assessment used. Even where pharmacological sophistication has been displayed in treatment, the measures of outcome are often judged impressionistically and without attention to specific aspects of behavior or cognition.

Psychological Assessment

Methods of assessment have varied widely. The theoretical ideal would be directly to observe behavior continuously. This is clearly impossible for most practical purposes. Performance in the formal, one-to-one testing situation with a psychologist may be poorly related to the patient's everyday behavior and circumstances and, therefore, may lack external validity. The same is possibly true of automated testing used in several recent studies. Likewise, laboratory performance tests need to be compared with naturalistic measures to ascertain their predictive value for real-life behavior. Naturalistic measures, such as standardized questionnaires of cognitive dysfunction, have begun to interest psychologists in recent times (Bennett-Levy & Stores, 1984; Broadbent, Cooper, Fitzgerald, & Parkes, 1982).

Some attempts have been made to establish characteristic profiles of adverse AED effects, but the relative lack of sophistication in the psychological methods characteristically used so far do not easily permit this degree of precision. It may be naive to expect circumscribed cognitive deficits in the face of day-to-day alterations in motivation, feeling, or well-being and other nonspecific variables likely to be experienced by patients with epilepsy. For a long time it has been thought that measures of intelligence, for example, are characteristically labile in such patients, making it difficult to compare the results of repeated assessments. The after-effects of overt seizures may well cause these variations. In addition, there is increasing interest in the subtle influence of "subclinical" seizure discharge (Stores, in press), including very brief discharges traditionally considered insignificant yet apparently capable in some patients of causing "transient cognitive impairment" (Aarts, Binnie, Smit, & Wilkins, 1984). In this complex situation, circumscribed effects on cognitive function of AEDs may well be difficult to discern.

Seizure Frequency and Severity

One further consideration that is very basic to the claim that certain AEDs might have a direct beneficial effect on people with epilepsy is the need to establish seizure frequency and severity accurately in relation to treatment. Clearly, improvements in psychological well-being may result from fewer or less serious seizures. This possibility needs to be excluded before claims for a direct psychotropic action can be made convincingly. Assessment of seizure variables can be very difficult, especially in the case of nonconvulsive seizures or other types of attack in which the clinical changes are subtle.

The usual way of judging seizure variables is by means of interviews with patients or relatives. There are many sources of error in this form of assessment that may well be increased with retarded individuals where communication problems exist so commonly. Patients may not be aware of all their seizures or they may confuse epileptic and nonepileptic attacks, which commonly coexist. Some patients or their relatives may be motivated to underestimate or overestimate the seizure frequency.

In an attempt to provide more objective accounts, prolonged video recordings and ambulatory cassette monitoring can be used to provide a more accurate assessment of seizure accounts than ordinary clinical reporting. While it is not a practical possibility to employ these means on a wide scale, consideration should be given to their use in systematic investigations of AED effects where change in seizure frequency is a crucial variable.

Types of Adverse Drug Effects

Adverse psychological effects of treatment may occur as side effects, intoxication, idiosyncratic response, or as a withdrawal symptom. The distinctions between these conditions require exact information on dosage or plasma levels that may not be provided, especially in earlier reports. The most common complication of treatment takes the form of *side effects* that occur within the supposed "optimal" or "therapeutic" range of plasma concentrations for seizure control. This range simply represents plasma levels at which control is likely to be achieved in most patients without the development of gross adverse effects. Side effects are usually unpredictable because of marked individual differences in response to treatment.

Intoxication is more predictable above clearly specified plasma levels for most AEDs, although even here individual differences are seen. Children may present a different picture of intoxication from adults. For example, Vallarta, Bell, and Reichert (1974) described cases of phenytoin intoxication in children without the classical cerebellar-vestibular signs. As discussed later, some drug combinations carry a special risk of intoxication. Surveys of intoxication with AEDs suggest that it may be quite common in some mentally retarded groups (Aman, Paxton, Field, & Foote, 1986; Iivanainen et al., 1978). The reason for this is not entirely clear, although Aman et al. suggested that some caregivers may be confusing symptoms of toxicity with nonspecific correlates of the developmental disabilities (e.g., clumsiness, slurred speech). *Idiosyncratic responses* are unusual. Finally, although rarely discussed in relation to AED treatment, *withdrawal effects* are also possible, especially with barbiturates and benzodiazepines.

Beneficial Psychological Effects

Drugs now used mainly in the treatment of epilepsy have for many years also been prescribed for their supposed beneficial effects on behavior in nonepileptic patients, including people with mental retardation. The details of this use (and the limited justification for the practice) were discussed by Stores (1978). A more positive account (at least for carbamazepine) was recently provided by Post and Uhde (1986). For some time *carbamazepine* has been used in Europe quite widely in psychiatry but generally without justification, although recent reports more convincingly suggest that it has some psychotropic properties. Remschmidt (1976) reviewed the claims made in the early 1970s that carbamazepine could be an effective psychotropic agent. At best there were hints that overactivity and aggressive behavior might be helped by carbamazepine, but the picture was very confused, largely because of the poor quality of the reports. Recently, more promising accounts of its use with adult psychiatric patients have been published. These reports have been reviewed by Post and Uhde (1986), who also discussed the possible place of other AEDs in general psychiatry.

Their review does not distinguish between retarded and nonretarded psychiatric patients, but there is no reason in principle why a psychotropic effect should be confined to one or other of these groups. The authors conclude that carbamazepine has already been established as a useful treatment for lithium-resistant manic-depressive illness. It might also be effective in schizoaffective illness and some forms of aggression in adults. However, at least one review suggests that the place of carbamazepine in child psychiatry remains very uncertain (Evans, Clay, & Gualtieri, 1987).

There seem to have been few attempts to evaluate the psychotropic properties of carbamazepine specifically in retarded patients. However, the study by Reid, Naylor, and Kay (1981) suggested that the drug reduces overactivity associated with elevation of mood in severely retarded young adults, and the individual case report of a very disturbed retarded patient by Rapport, Sonis, Fialkov, Matson, and Kazdin (1983) raises the possibility that this drug might enhance the effects of behavior modification. However, Gay (1984) has demonstrated how seizure type might interact with AED treatment to affect operant conditioning adversely in mentally retarded patients.

Since the 1940s *phenytoin* has been used in the United States for various psychological disorders in both adults and children. Little justification can be found for this practice and it is significant that the drug has been given FDA approval only for use in the treatment of epilepsy. Nevertheless, there have been a few interesting experimental reports that small doses of phenytoin can have selectively beneficial effects on cognitive function, and some claims that similarly small amounts of the drug can bring about various cognitive and behavioral improvements in retarded children (Goldberg & Kurland, 1970). However, only a small minority of variables showed improvement in the Goldberg and Kurland study, and there was the suggestion of worsening on other measures.

The claim that *sodium valproate* has a psychotropic action is of particular relevance to developmentally disabled persons because this drug, compared with other AEDs, has had some impact on the difficult epilepsies associated with retardation and is, therefore, quite often used. The reviews by Stores (1978) and Post and Uhde (1986) illustrate the inconsistent results obtained, although again the latter authors are rather more positive about its possible value in general psychiatry. Trimble and Thompson (1984) reviewed the reported effects of valproate on cognitive function in normal volunteers and the results were found to be contradictory. Since then Ko, Korpi, Freed, Zaleman, and Bigelow (1985) and Harding, Pullen, and Drasdo (1980) have failed to demonstrate any cognitive effects of this drug used with schizophrenic and normal adults, respectively.

Some of the *benzodiazepines* (notably nitrazepam, clonazepam, and clobazam) have also found a place in the treatment of the otherwise drug-resistant seizures (such as myoclonic and atonic attacks) often associated with retardation. Aman and Field (1985), in discussing the use of diazepam and chlordiazepoxide as anxiolytics and hypnotics in retarded patients, point out the unconvincing evidence that these drugs have a beneficial effect on behavior. Indeed, the better designed studies suggest behavioral deterioration as a consequence of their use (see also Chapter 6).

At one time *sulthiame* was marketed as being especially useful in the control of not only seizures but also behavior disturbance. For the most part, neither claim withstood close scrutiny and the drug is now little used. It is interesting, however, that some well-designed studies did raise the possibility that it was helpful in reducing excitement and aggression even in nonepileptic retarded patients (Al-Kaisi & McGuire, 1974; Moffatt, Siddiqui, & Mackay, 1970).

One other drug for which beneficial psychological effects have been claimed when used in nonepileptic patients is *ethosuximide*. This drug is sometimes used in combination with sodium valproate for the control of otherwise drug-resistant seizures, especially atypical absences, and therefore its possible psychological effects are relevant to some developmentally disabled patients (see Stores, 1978).

So far this section has been concerned with the possible beneficial effects on behavior and cognitive processes of AEDs used in nonepileptic patients. In fact, most of the claims for their psychotropic action come from studies in which the drug has been used primarily for the treatment of seizures. Evaluation of these claims is particularly difficult.

It is indisputable that some patients with epilepsy improve psychologically with the introduction of some of the drugs mentioned, but there are two explanations (other than direct psychotropic action of the drugs) which may apply in most instances. The first is that the treatment is effective in controlling the seizures themselves and it is this control that improves behavior. The second is that new drugs have replaced other forms of AED treatment that were affecting behavior adversely. For example, it comes as no surprise that behavior improved when sodium valproate was substituted for clonazepam (Lance & Anthony, 1977), in view of the consistent tendency for the latter drug to cause behavioral problems. These alternative explanations for improvement when AEDs are changed may explain most of the putative "psychotropic" properties of AEDs, but carbamazepine does seem a likely exception in view of its effect on the mental state of some nonepileptic patients, especially those with affective disorders. This claim should not be overstated, as there is clearly a need to improve on the relatively limited information currently available.

Adverse Psychological Effects

Information on adverse effects is derived almost exclusively from reports on people with epilepsy, most of whom, presumably, have not been retarded. As in other sections of this chapter, the aim is not to present a detailed coverage of the literature. Comprehensive reviews are available elsewhere (Hirtz & Nelson, 1985; Reynolds, 1983; Stores, 1978). In few reports are treatment effects discussed in retarded and nonretarded patients separately. It is necessary, therefore, to draw on the published accounts as a whole, including studies of both adults and children, to estimate the likelihood of psychological harm occurring when AEDs are given to developmentally disabled persons. Any of the common AEDs are likely to be prescribed for such patients with a tendency towards the use of older drugs and towards drug combinations.

The shortcomings discussed at the start of this chapter of most studies in this field need to be remembered. All studies concerned with the psychological consequences of epilepsy are difficult to interpret in that it is rarely possible to ascribe outcome to one factor alone out of the many variables that operate in the epilepsies. Adequately controlled investigations are virtually impossible to achieve because of the methodological and ethical constraints to which reference has already been made. Add to this individual differences in response to treatment, and it is not surprising that detailed information is not available. Indeed, it is difficult to see how, in principle, anything more than broad generalizations will ever be possible in this area of enquiry.

Given these provisos, the overall picture concerning the risk of adverse psychological effects is as follows. As far as possible, a distinction is made between the various types of adverse effects described earlier, and between effects on cognitive function and general behavior. Only AEDs in common use are considered. The interested reader is referred to Rivinus (1982), who has catalogued both positive and negative effects of a very wide range of antiepileptic treatments, including those not often used.

BARBITURATES

Phenobarbitone and related drugs (including primidone) carry a considerable risk of side effects. It is largely for this reason that, especially in pediatric practice, other AEDs (particularly carbamazepine and valproate) are preferred nowadays. Side effects take the form of behavioral disturbance, especially excitement, irritability, tearfulness, aggression, and possibly sleep disorder. In children, these problems may be so distressing that some parents discontinue the treatment without the doctor being told (Wolfe & Forsythe, 1978), which, in itself, can be a serious risk. A few studies have shown that, in the cognitive sphere, phenobarbitone selectively impairs sustained attention, although the results of various clinical studies suggest that this drug is not as harmful as would be expected from experimental findings.

The clinical picture of intoxication in adults (with ataxia, dysarthia, nystagmus, and intellectual deterioration) is well known, but overdosage in children, particularly if they are mentally retarded, may well be missed, especially as these physical signs do not necessarily accompany intoxication.

An idiosyncratic response to primidone is well recognized, but not to phenobarbitone, unless the extreme degree of gross motor overactivity shown by some children on this drug is an example. Discontinuation of barbiturates needs to be performed with caution to avoid withdrawal effects, including seizures.

PHENYTOIN

The main psychological risk with phenytoin usually is not the direct behavioral side effects, but embarrassment or distress because of the drug's tendency to cause cosmetic problems. These are principally gum hypertrophy, hirsutism, acneiform rashes, and coarsening of the facial features. These are the reasons for the reluctance of many pediatricians to use this drug, especially for female patients.

Various cognitive and behavioral side effects have been reported in patients taking phenytoin, including intellectual deterioration, impairment of motor skills, poor reading, and personality change (Dodrill, 1975a; Reynolds & Travers, 1974; Stores & Hart, 1976). There is a suggestion that such problems are more likely to occur in the higher plasma concentrations optimal for seizure control. A recent comparison of phenytoin and carbamazepine, used singly in newly diagnosed cases, tended to confirm previous reports of the development of cognitive deficits (especially memory) in patients taking phenytoin (Andrewes, Bullen, Tomlinson, Elwes, & Reynolds, 1986)

Individual differences in response to this drug appear to be particularly prominent not only in the development of side effects but also in the type of clinical picture seen when plasma levels reach the toxic range. Intoxication is a particular risk because of the drug's unusual pharmacokinetics. Changes of dosage should be made only by small degrees. Apart from the usual textbook picture of intoxication, with prominent cerebellar-vestibular signs, other phenytoin intoxication syndromes have been described, some of which are purely behavioral or extrapyramidal in type. It is mainly in retarded patients that chronic phenytoin intoxication has been mistaken for neurodegenerative disorder (Logan & Freeman, 1969; Vallarta et al., 1974). In some of these cases, reduction or discontinuation of treatment has not been followed by recovery to the preintoxication state. Idiosyncrasy or withdrawal effects of a primarily psychological type are not described.

CARBAMAZEPINE AND SODIUM VALPROATE

Both carbamazepine and sodium valproate have acquired the reputation of being effective in a wide range of epilepsies without carrying such high risk, as the barbiturates or phenytoin, of physical or psychological complications. Some patients react adversely to even modest doses of these drugs, but in general side effects appear to be unusual. This opinion is based mainly on collective clinical impressions, but also on the results of a series of studies, most of which are subject to the difficulties of interpretation discussed earlier. The results of current investigations of these drugs taken singly are, therefore, awaited with interest.

In the meantime there have been various reports, mentioned by Trimble and Reynolds (1984), that suggest that carbamazepine is generally less psychologically harmful than most other AEDs. This seems to be true not only in adults but also in children (Schain, Ward, & Guthrie, 1977). Direct psychotropic properties are impossible to judge from such reports. More recently, it was observed that epileptic children, when tested under different concentrations of carbamazepine, showed improved performance on a test of attention span and less seat activity shortly after taking medication when drug concentrations were higher (Aman, Werry, Paxton, & Turbott, 1988).

As for valproate, the evidence suggests that its independent effect on mental state is neutral. Trimble and Thompson's (1984) review points to the inconsistent findings on the psychological changes seen in epileptic patients on this drug, but in most studies no convincing changes attributable to the drug itself were seen. Aman, Werry, Paxton, and Turbott (1987) suggest that higher serum levels of valproate are associated with impaired performance in children with epilepsy, although in this study severity of the seizures may have been a confounding variable. In some patients, valproate indirectly causes psychological or social upset by inducing excessive weight gain.

Intoxication with carbamazepine produces obvious disorder with drowsiness, ataxia, and diplopia. There is a less well-defined upper plasma concentration with valproate above which toxicity is seen, but very high plasma levels are associated principally with drowsiness or stupor. Idiosyncratic reactions and withdrawal effects of carbamazepine and valproate have not been convincingly described.

OTHER AEDs

Benzodiazepines are probably second only to barbiturates as far as the risk of psychological complications is concerned. As mentioned earlier, some members of this group have been found more effective than other AEDs in controlling seizures associated with retardation. There is often a need, however, to balance the advantage of improved seizure control against the behavioral upset caused by the medication (see Chapter 6).

Clonazepam appears to be the most troublesome in this respect. Few studies of this drug have been performed, but clinical experience has shown restlessness, irritability, and disinhibition to be common side effects (see Trimble, 1983). Intoxication with benzodiazepines causes a nonspecific picture of drowsiness, confusion, and ataxia. Dennis and Hunt (1985) have described a high rate of such problems in children with tuberose sclerosis who take nitrazepam. Psychiatrists have become increasingly aware of the occurrence of insomnia, dysphoria, and other psychological disorders following the cessation of long-term treatment with benzodiazepines (Anon, 1985). Although little discussed, withdrawal of such drugs used to treat epilepsy can be expected to have the same effects.

Ethosuximide (of limited use in retarded patients) sometimes causes lethargy and dysphoria as side effects, but the frequency with which this happens is uncertain. More dramatic, psychotic states have also been reported (Wolf, 1980). Certainly, drowsiness occurs at high plasma concentrations without distinctive features.

Although little used now, *sulthiame* is worth further mention because of its popularity in the past as a treatment for epilepsy associated with behavioral disturbance, perhaps especially in mentally retarded individuals. There was little convincing justification for its use. Indeed, systematic evaluation suggested that it commonly caused a variety of unpleasant physical and psychological side effects (Dodrill, 1975b).

The ketogenic diet and corticosteroids (or adrenocorticotropic hormone) are other unusual forms of antiepileptic treatments used in particularly difficult seizure disorders in mentally retarded persons, usually when other treatments have failed. It seems that no reliable accounts exist of psychological complications of their use in this context, although it is easy to see how difficulties might arise from the dietary restrictions imposed with a ketogenic diet.

Drug Combinations

Because of the difficulty often encountered in controlling seizures in persons with mental retardation, these patients are at special risk of multiple drug treatments, even when the modern drugs have replaced more traditional treatments (Sheppard, Ballinger, & Fenton, 1987). Some combinations readily lead to intoxication. Sulthiame often raises previously therapeutic phenytoin plasma concentrations to toxic levels. Stupor or coma can result from combinations of valproate and barbiturates or benzodiazepines (perhaps especially clonazepam), and the plasma concentration of ethosuximide can also be raised to toxic levels by valproate. Some patients on multiple treatments (including combined preparations) may be taking several doses of the same drug (usually phenobarbitone), which produces a state of chronic intoxication. A different type of drug interaction with possible psychological consequences is that between certain AEDs and other treatments including antidepressants, the serum levels of which may be reduced by barbiturates, phenytoin, and carbamazepine.

Recommendations

Modern Treatment Principles

The most basic clinical need appears to be the extension of modern principles of prescribing to retarded patients, who seem to have been bypassed by many of the recent advances in the use of AEDs. The effect of appropriate choice of drugs, preferably used singly, and avoidance of overdosage, with systematic checks for possible physical and psychological complications, should not only produce better seizure control than multiple therapy with outmoded drugs, but also promote the patient's general well-being. Where combined or otherwise complicated treatment is necessary, extra caution to avoid harmful effects is required. Compliance with treatment guidelines cannot be assumed and should be checked. Some findings suggest that there is a special need for this in retarded patients (Gibbons, Frewin, Hallpike, & Chryssidis, 1983).

Measurement of plasma levels can still be helpful in certain circumstances—especially when phenytoin is used because of the difficulty of assessing this drug's plasma levels clinically. Again, individual differences in these respects are prominent. A few patients will benefit from plasma levels below the optimal range; others will tolerate levels above this range. Being within the optimal range does not preclude side effects, some of which may be subtle yet significant. Several studies (Aman et al., 1987; Reynolds & Travers, 1974; Thompson & Trimble, 1983) have suggested that higher plasma levels within the optimal range increase the risk of adverse effects.

In general, the minimal dose of treatment that will achieve effective control should be used. Because of difficulties of seizure control in mentally retarded persons, it is often necessary to explore such drugs to their limits and the risk of exceeding an acceptable dose exists, more so than in other patients. Similarly, the general principle of discontinuing treatment after 2 to 4 years of freedom from seizures applies less commonly with this population, with the result that retarded patients are often exposed to very long periods (perhaps a lifetime) of treatment. It is unfortunate that the logistic difficulties of studying very long-term effects of AED treatment have meant that there is very little information on this potentially important point, although Corbett, Trimble, and Nichol (1985) found that long-term treatment with phenytoin and phenobarbitone was associated with cognitive deterioration. Lesser, Luders, Wyllie, Dinner, and Morris (1986) have discussed the difficulties of attributing mental deterioration of people with epilepsy to any one cause. For example, progressive neurological deterioration may be a more basic and largely independent factor leading to such deterioration.

Research Design

As stated earlier, research design in even basic aspects of the epilepsies is particularly difficult, and this is probably more so where psychological effects are concerned. It is for this reason that so many investigations of the psychological consequences of AEDs are unsatisfactory. Although some recent studies have shown or suggested that certain AEDs have psychological effects, and that these effects are often dose related, the impact of these studies themselves (compared with clinical impressions) on prescribing practice has been limited partly because of inconsistent or marginal results, or confounding of drug variables with clinical variables. In principle at least, how might research be improved in the hope of providing results of more definite clinical value? The following are some of the relevant considerations that have been discussed more fully elsewhere (Stores, 1985b).

It seems reasonable that the difficulties of interpreting results would be reduced if studies involved newly diagnosed cases about to undergo treatment with a single drug. Pretreatment assessment could be carried out with further assessments at intervals in order to detect possible short- and long-term effects. In this way each patient would act as his or her own control, and the problem of comparisons between groups (usually impossible to match accurately) could be avoided. In research with children, a comparison group needs to be assessed, mainly to measure changes associated with development, practice, and other time-related variables. It seems desirable that, as far as possible, groups studied should be relatively homogeneous for age and overall intellectual level. Heterogeneity in these respects complicates the type of psychological assessment that is appropriate and the statistical analysis required. The measures used are crucial, of course, and ideally would include a combination of well-defined aspects of cognitive function and other real-life measures of behavior, the results of which can be readily incorporated into the patient's clinical care. Even clinical measures need to be based on sufficiently refined concepts rather than terms that, although hallowed by long use, may represent a complex of different behaviors. The term *inattentiveness* is an obvious example (Stores, Hart, & Piran, 1978).

Needless to say, compliance with the prescribed treatment regimen should be demonstrated rather than assumed, and changes in seizure frequency should also be documented accurately because of their potentially confounding influence on the interpretation of results. In the mentally retarded population, the possibility of subtle seizures, including nonconvulsive status (Stores, 1986), to which such patients are particularly prone, should be borne in mind and appropriate monitoring carried out.

The final issue is that of individual differences. The challenge here is to identify patients who are particularly predisposed to develop psychological or other complications of treatment. This is a surprisingly underresearched area of enquiry. At a commonsense level, it might be expected that if a patient's behavior is already disordered in some way, drugs such as phenobarbitone or clonazepam, which carry a high risk of inducing such behavior, would make that behavior worse. Apart from pretreatment behavior, other possibly significant subject variables are type and extent of brain damage, age, and sex. Additionally, the patient's social environment may well act as a modifying influence. The difficulties of research into the psychological effects of AEDs in developmentally disabled persons should not be underestimated, nor should they act as a deterrent to the investigation of this important and interesting aspect of clinical care.

Conclusion

It appears that modern principles of antiepileptic treatment for some reason have not been used as extensively in the management of mentally retarded individuals as they have been in many intellectually normal epileptic patients. In addition, there are a number of reasons why special precautions should be observed with the developmentally disabled population so that toxic and side effects are not overlooked. Finally, an approach to research design is recommended, including the use of monotherapy, newly diagnosed cases, appropriate comparison groups, well-defined cognitive and clinical measures, and close monitoring of seizure control. It is hoped that if modern principles are adopted more widely, clinical management of persons with developmental disabilities will be improved immediately. Furthermore, the use of more satisfactory research designs should enhance our knowledge so that future treatment of this group of patients can be advanced still further.

References

Aarts, J.H.P., Binnie, C.D., Smit, A.M., & Wilkins, A.J. (1984). Selective cognitive impairment during focal and generalised epileptiform EEG activity. *Brain*, *107*, 293–308.

Al-Kaisi, A., & McGuire, R. (1974). The effect of sulthiame on disturbed behaviour in mentally subnormal patients. *British Journal of Psychiatry*, *124*, 45–49.

Aman, M.G. (1984). Drugs and learning in mentally retarded persons. In G.D. Burrows & J.S. Werry (Eds.), *Advances in human psychopharmacology*, Vol. 3, pp. 121–163. Greenwich, CT: Jai Press.

Aman, M.C., & Field, C.J. (1985). Pharmacological management. In N.N. Singh & K.M. Wilton (Eds.), *Mental retardation in New Zealand: Provisions, services and research* (pp. 223–249). Christchurch: Whitcoulls.

Aman, M.G., Paxton, J.W., Field, C.J., & Foote, S.E. (1986). Prevalence of toxic anticonvulsant drug concentrations in mentally retarded persons with epilepsy. *American Journal of Mental Deficiency*, *90*, 643–650.

Aman, M.G., Werry, J.S., Paxton, J.W., & Turbott, S.H. (1987). Effect of sodium valproate on psychomotor performance in children as a function of dose, fluctuations in concentration, and diagnosis. *Epilepsia*, *28*, 115–124.

Aman, M.G., Werry, J.S., Paxton, J.W., & Turbott, S.H. (1988) *Effects of carbamazepine on psychomotor performance in children as a function of dose, fluctuations in concentrations, and diagnosis.* Unpublished manuscript in preparation, Ohio State University.

Andrewes, D.G., Bullen, J.G., Tomlinson, L., Elwes, R.D.C., & Reynolds, E.H. (1986). A comparative study of the cognitive effects of phenytoin and carbamazepine in new referrals with epilepsy. *Epilepsia, 27*, 128–134.

Anon. (1985). Some problems with benzodiazepines. *Drug and Therapeutics Bulletin, 23*, 21–23.

Bennett-Levy, J., & Stores, G. (1984). The nature of cognitive dysfunction in schoolchildren with epilepsy. *Acta Neurologica Scandinavica, 69*, (Suppl. 99) 79–82.

Broadbent, D.E., Cooper, P.F., Fitzgerald, P., & Parkes, K.R. (1982). The cognitive failures questionnaire (CFQ) and its correlates. *British Journal of Clinical Psychology, 21*, 1–16.

Corbett, J.A., Harris, R., & Robinson, R. (1975). Epilepsy. In J. Wortis (Ed.), *Mental retardation and developmental disabilities* (Vol. VII, pp. 79–111). New York: Brunner/Mazel.

Corbett, J.A., Trimble, M.R., & Nichol, T.C. (1985). Behavioural and cognitive impairments in children with epilepsy: the long-term effects of anticonvulsant therapy. *Journal of the American Academy of Child Psychiatry, 24*, 17–23.

Dennis, J., & Hunt, A. (1985). Prolonged use of nitrazepam for epilepsy in children with tuberous sclerosis. *British Medical Journal, 291*, 692–693.

Deykin, E.Y., & MacMahon, B. (1979). The incidence of seizures among children with autistic symptoms. *American Journal of Psychiatry, 136*, 1310–1312.

Dodrill, C.B. (1975a). Diphenylhydantoin serum levels, toxicity and neuropsychological performance in patients with epilepsy. *Epilepsia, 16*, 593–600.

Dodrill, C. (1975b). Effects of sulthiame upon intellectual, neuropsychological and social functioning abilities among adult epileptics: Comparison with diphenylhantoin. *Epilepsia, 16*, 617–625.

Evans, R.W., Clay, T.H., & Gualtieri, C.T. (1987). Carbamazepine in pediatric psychiatry. *Journal of the American Academy of Child and Adolescent Psychiatry, 26*, 2–8.

Gay, P.E. (1984). Effects of antiepileptic drugs and seizure type on operant responding in mentally retarded persons. *Epilepsia, 25*, 377–386.

Gibbons, K.S., Frewin, D.B., Hallpike, J.F., & Chryssidis, E. (1983). Compliance with anticonvulsant drug therapy in retarded and non-retarded epileptics. *Australian Journal of Hospital Pharmacy, 13*, 58–60.

Goldberg, J.R., & Kurland, A.A. (1970). Dilantin treatment of hospitalised cultural-familial retardates. *The Journal of Nervous and Mental Disease, 150*, 133–137.

Harding, G.F.A., Pullen, J.J., & Drasdo, N. (1980). The effect of sodium valproate and other anticonvulsants on performance of children and adolescents. In M.J. Parsonage & A.D.A. Caldwell (Eds.), *The place of sodium valproate in the treatment of epilepsy* (pp. 61–71). London: Academic Press.

Hirtz, D.G., & Nelson, K.B. (1985). Cognitive effects of antiepileptic drugs. In T.A. Pedley & B.S. Meldrum (Eds.), *Recent advances in epilepsy* (Vol. 2, pp. 161–181). Edinburgh: Churchill Livingstone.

Iivanainen, M., Viukari, M., Seppalainen, A., & Helle, E. (1978). Electroencephalography and phenytoin toxicity in mentally retarded epileptic patients. *Journal of Neurology, Neurosurgery and Psychiatry, 41*, 272–277.

Jeavons, P.M. (1983). Non-epileptic attacks in childhood. In F.C. Rose (Ed.), *Research progress in epilepsy* (pp. 224–230). London: Pitman.

Kaufman, K.R., & Katz-Garris, L. (1979). Epilepsy, mental retardation, and anti-convulsant therapy. *American Journal of Mental Deficiency*, *84*, 256–259.

Ko, G.N., Korpi, E.R., Freed, W.J., Zaleman, S.J., & Bigelow, L. (1985). Effect of valproic acid on behavior and plasma amino acid concentrations in chronic schizophrenic patients. *Biological Psychiatry*, *20*, 199–228.

Lance, J.W., & Anthony, M. (1977). Sodium valproate and clonazepam in the treatment of intractable epilepsy. *Archives of Neurology*, *34*, 14–17.

Lesser, R.P., Luders, H., Wyllie, E., Dinner, D.S., & Morris, H.H. (1986). Mental deterioration in epilepsy. *Epilepsia*, *27*, (Suppl. 2) S105–S123.

Logan, W., & Freeman, J. (1969). Pseudodegenerative disease due to diphenylhydantoin intoxication. *Archives of Neurology*, *21*, 631–637.

Moffat, W., Siddiqui, A., & Mackay, D. (1970). The use of sulthiame with disturbed mentally subnormal patients. *British Journal of Psychiatry*, *117*, 673–678.

O'Neill, B.P., Ladon, B., Harris, L.M., Riley, H.L., & Dreifuss, F.E. (1977). A comprehensive, interdisciplinary approach to the care of the institutionalised person with epilepsy. *Epilepsia*, *18*, 243–250.

Pedley, T.A. (1983). Differential diagnosis of episodic symptoms. *Epilepsia*, *24* (Suppl. 1), S31–S44.

Post, M., & Uhde, T.W. (1986). Anticonvulsants in non-epileptic psychosis. In M.R. Trimble & T.G. Bolweg (Eds.), *Aspects of epilepsy and psychiatry* (pp. 177–212). Chichester: Wiley.

Rapport, M.D., Sonis, W.A., Fialkov, M.J., Matson, J.L., & Kazdin, A.E. (1983). Carbamazepine and behaviour therapy for aggressive behaviour. *Behaviour Modification*, *7*, 255–265.

Reid, A.H., Naylor, G.J., & Kay, D.S.G. (1981). A double-blind placebo-controlled, crossover trial of carbamazepine in overactive severely mentally handicapped patients. *Psychological Medicine*, *11*, 109–113.

Remschmidt, H. (1976). The psychotropic effect of carbamazepine in non-epileptic patients, with particular reference to problems posed by clinical studies in children with behavioural disorders. In W. Birkmeyer (Ed.), *Epileptic seizures—behaviour-pain* (pp. 253–258). Berne: Hans Huber.

Reynolds, E.H. (1983). Mental effects of antiepileptic medication: A review. *Epilepsia*, *24*, 585–595.

Reynolds, E.H., & Travers, R.D. (1974). Serum anticonvulsant concentrations in epileptic patients with mental symptoms. *British Journal of Psychiatry*, *124*, 440–445.

Richardson, S.A., Katz, M., Koller, H., & McLaren, J. (1979). Some characteristics of a population of mentally retarded young adults in a British city. *Journal of Mental Deficiency Research*, *23*, 275–287.

Rivinus, T.M. (1982). Psychiatric effects of anticonvulsant regimens. *Journal of Clinical Psychopharmacology*, *2*, 165–192.

Rutter, M. (1970). Autistic children: Infancy to childhood. *Seminars in Psychiatry*, *2*, 435–450.

Schain, R.J., Ward, J.W., & Guthrie, D. (1977). Carbamazepine as an anticonvulsant in children. *Neurology*, *27*, 476–480.

Sheppard, L.C., Ballinger, B.R., & Fenton, G.W. (1987). Anticonvulsant medication in a mental hospital: 1977–1982. *British Journal of Psychiatry*, *150*, 513–517.

Stores, G. (1978). Antiepileptics (Anticonvulsants). In J.S. Werry (Ed.), *Pediatric psychopharmacology: The use of behavior modifying drugs in children* (pp. 274–315). New York: Brunner/Mazel.

Stores, G. (1985a). Clinical and EEG evaluation of seizures and seizure-like disorders. *Journal of the American Academy of Child Psychiatry, 24*, 10–16.

Stores, G. (1985b). Behavioural effects of antiepileptic drugs in children. In M. Dam, L. Gram, B. Pedersen, & H. Orum (Eds.), *Modern approach to antiepileptic drug treatment* (pp. 33–44). Hvidore: Danish Epilepsy Society.

Stores, G. (1986). Nonconvulsive status epilepticus in children. In T.A. Pedley & B.S. Meldrum (Eds.), *Recent advances in epilepsy* (Vol. 3, pp. 295–310). London: Churchill Livingstone.

Stores, G. (in press). Effect of subclinical seizure discharge on learning. In A.P. Aldenkamp, W.C.J. Alpherts, H. Meinardi, & G. Stores (Eds.), *Education and epilepsy*. Lisse: Swets & Zeitlinger.

Stores, G., & Hart, J. (1976). Reading skills of children with generalised or focal epilepsy attending ordinary school. *Developmental Medicine and Child Neurology, 18*, 705–716.

Stores, G., Hart, J.A., & Piran, N. (1978). Inattentiveness in school-children with epilepsy. *Epilepsia, 19*, 169–175.

Thompson, P.J., & Trimble, M.R. (1983). The effect of anticonvulsant drugs on cognitive function: relation to serum levels. *Journal of Neurology, Neurosurgery and Psychiatry, 46*, 227–233.

Trimble, M.R. (1983). Benzodiazepines in epilepsy. In M.R. Trimble (Ed.), *Benzodiazepines divided* (pp. 277–290). Chichester: Wiley.

Trimble, M.R., & Reynolds, E.H. (1984). Neuropsychiatric toxicity of anticonvulsant drugs. In W.B. Matthews & G.H. Glaser (Eds.), *Recent advances in clinical neurology* (Vol. 4, pp. 261–280). Edinburgh: Churchill Livingstone.

Trimble, M.R., & Thompson, P.J. (1984). Sodium valproate and cognitive function. *Epilepsia, 25* (Suppl. 1) S60–S64.

Vallarta, J.M., Bell, D.B., & Reichert, A. (1974). Progressive encephalopathy due to chronic hydantoin intoxication. *American Journal of Diseases in Children, 128*, 27–34.

Wilkinson, I.A., Murphy, J.V., Georgeson, R., & D'Souza, B.J. (1982). On-site seizure clinic impact on the welfare of mentally retarded, institutionalised patients. *Archives of Neurology, 39*, 41–43.

Wolf, P. (1980). Psychic disorders in epilepsy. In R. Canger, F. Angeleri, & J.F. Penry (Eds.), *Advances in epilepsy* (pp. 159–160). New York: Raven Press.

Wolfe, S.M., & Forsythe, A. (1978). Behavior disturbance, phenobarbital and febrile seizures. *Pediatrics, 61*, 728–731.

6
Other Psychotropic Drugs: Stimulants, Antidepressants, the Anxiolytics, and Lithium Carbonate

Mark Chandler, C.T. Gualtieri, and Jeffrey J. Fahs

Abstract

This chapter is really four small papers about medications that have received comparatively little attention in the mental retardation literature. However, this relative in attention should not be taken as a measure of the weakness of the agents or of their limited utility. They all may be of benefit when properly prescribed and managed. In view of a shallow research base, however, prescription must be guided as the writers are guided by clinical experience and the collective wisdom of colleagues in practice, as well as by research from other areas of psychopharmacology.

Stimulants

Hyperactivity is a common behavior problem in mentally retarded populations (Phillips & Williams, 1975, 1977; Rutter, 1975). On the basis of surveys, symptoms of attention deficit/hyperactivity (AD/HA) appear to be more prevalent in retarded people than in populations of normal IQ children. However, the use of stimulant medication has been infrequent among retarded patients, especially in public residential facilities (Cohen & Sprague, 1977; Lipman, 1970). This contrasts with a large community survey of drug prescription among trainable mentally retarded children, where stimulant drugs, although not frequently used, were much more prominent (Gadow & Kalachnik, 1981).

Stimulants are the preferred medical treatment for AD/HA, and they are well known to improve behavior problems, and to improve attention and memory in the short term (Evans, Gualtieri, & Amara, 1986). There have also been reports that they may improve academic classroom learning in children of normal intelligence (Pelham, Bender, Caddell, Booth, & Moorer, 1985), although much of the literature does not suggest long-term academic gains due to the stimulants (e.g., Aman, 1980, 1982b; Barkley & Cunningham, 1978). The effective dose range is low to moderate (Sprague & Sleator, 1977) and there are virtually no known long-term side effects

(Evans & Gualtieri, in press). Stimulant treatment for AD/HA—dating back to 1937 (Bradley, 1937)—is the oldest continuing tradition in psychopharmacology, and one of the most dramatically successful. Why, then, has it been consigned such a low priority in the treatment of hyperactive retarded people, at least in institutions? Severely retarded people who are hyperactive, impulsive, excitable, distractible, or aggressive may be treated with virtually any psychotropic drug, but hardly ever a psychostimulant. This requires explanation.

There have been a number of studies of stimulant medications in retarded persons (Alexandris & Lundell, 1968; Aman & Singh, 1982; Anton & Greer, 1969; Bell & Zubek, 1961; Blacklidge & Ekblad, 1971; Christiansen, 1975; Clausen, Fineman, Henry, & Wohl, 1960; Cutler, Little, & Strauss, 1940–1941; Davis, Sprague, & Werry, 1969; Lobb, 1968; McConnell, Cromwell, Bialer, & Son, 1964; Morris, MacGillivray, & Mathieson, 1955; Spencer, 1980; Varley & Trupin, 1982). A small minority of these studies (Alexandris & Lundell, 1968; Blacklidge & Ekblad, 1971; Christiansen, 1975; Cutler et al., 1940–1941; Varley & Trupin, 1982) have shown isolated areas of improvement. However, the most typical finding has been a lack of drug effects. Some studies (Bell & Zubek, 1961; Lobb, 1968) have actually documented worsening of behavior, especially on learning-related tasks.

Most of these stimulant studies have used double-blind, placebo-controlled designs and acceptable statistical analyses (see Aman, 1982a). Their results, therefore, have to be taken seriously. Overall, the evidence relating to stimulant effects in retarded people must be regarded as negative. However, a note of caution is called for in interpreting this research. Studies that have demonstrated improvement were usually done with mildly or moderately retarded children (Alexandris & Lundell, 1968; Blacklidge & Ekblad, 1971; Cutler et al., 1940–1914; Varley & Trupin, 1982). In contrast, many of the remaining studies were conducted with severely handicapped individuals or with older subjects. Furthermore, as argued by Aman (1985), the overwhelming preponderance of drug research in mental retardation has been done in institutions, and the studies of stimulant medication are no exception to this rule. As mildly and moderately retarded youngsters living in the community make up the majority of all mentally retarded children, the relevance of the available literature can be questioned. In addition, many of the negative studies selected subjects for generic, acting-out problems rather than for a primary complaint of inattention or hyperactivity.

Stimulant drugs have not received extensive evaluation in autistic children. However, the studies that have been done indicate that stimulants are not effective in this group either and, in fact, suggest that they are contraindicated (Campbell, 1975; Campbell et al., 1976; Campbell, Fish, David, et al., 1972). Campbell et al.'s studies showed slight improvements due to stimulant treatments in certain behaviors such as hyperactivity and language production. However, dextroamphetamine caused a variety of serious untoward effects, including irritability, worsening of withdrawal, and motor retardation. Dextroamphetamine and levodopa (both dopamine antagonists) caused a worsening of stereotypies and the emergence of stereotypies de novo in these children.

An amphetamine derivative, fenfluramine, has been proposed as a possible treatment for autistic children (Geller, Ritvo, Freeman, & Yuwiler, 1982; see also Chapter 7). Once again, it appears that high IQ autistic children may be more likely than low IQ subjects to respond favorably (Leventhal, 1985). However, serious concerns have been raised over the potential neurotoxicity of fenfluramine (Gualtieri, 1986), and hence use of this drug must be viewed with caution.

While stimulants appear to effect a consistent enhancement of performance in normal and hyperactive children as well as in normal adults (see Rapoport et al., 1980), most researchers and clinicians tend to agree that the more retarded a subject is, the less likely it is that he or she will respond to stimulant medication. The only published data to the contrary appear in a study by Poling and Breuning (1983), who reported improved operant responding and ratings of behavior in response to the psychostimulant methylphenidate by severely mentally retarded inpatients. Their research showed positive effects on behavior rating scales and a quadratic response on operant measures, a pattern that was first noted by Sprague and Sleator (1977) in normally intelligent AD/HA children. Unfortunately, these data have not been replicated, and serious doubts have been raised concerning their authenticity (Gualtieri, 1987; Holden, 1986, 1987; Sprague, 1987).

The lack of response to stimulants by autistic and severely retarded patients may be explained by the following ideas:

1. Retarded and autistic people are characterized by an overly "narrow" or constricted attentional range. Attention may be even further constricted by stimulant treatment (Aman, 1982a; Lyon & Robbins, 1975).
2. Stimulants are known to increase stereotyped behavior in autistic (and perhaps some retarded) individuals (Aman, 1982a). Furthermore, stereotypies can interfere with learning (Koegel & Covert, 1972) and possibly with social behavior as well (e.g., Aman & Singh, 1982).
3. Stimulant drugs operate therapeutically on frontal lobe structures and therefore require an intact frontal system, especially the mesocortical dopamine system (Evans & Gualtieri, in press; Evans, Gualtieri, & Hicks, 1986). Cortical hypoplasia is a commonly observed neuropathic finding in severely retarded individuals. Therefore, in retarded people, there may not be an adequate neural substrate upon which stimulants can exert a beneficial effect.

On the basis of clinical experience, as much as published research, we conclude that psychostimulant drugs are of limited utility in severely and profoundly retarded people, but that they may be more effective as functional level improves. Preliminary data from a recent study support this position (Aman, Marks, Wilsher, Turbott, & Merry, 1988). Retarded people who respond well to stimulants are likelier to be: (a) young; (b) only mildly to moderately retarded; (c) without previous evidence of stereotypy or of perseverative behavior; and (d) affected by relatively straightforward behavioral symptoms, like hyperactivity, inattention, or distractibility. However, more research is needed to assess stimulant medications in individuals both with and without these characteristics to determine whether this is a valid conclusion.

Antidepressants

Although antidepressants (tricyclic antidepressants [TCAs], monoamine oxidase inhibitors [MAOIs], and the "novel antidepressants") are important agents in adult psychiatry, their use in developmentally disabled persons has not been the subject of systematic study. In Lipman's survey of psychoactive drug use in institutionalized retarded persons, fewer than 4% of the residents were treated with TCAs (Lipman, 1970). In the review of 184 studies of psychoactive drug treatment of persons with mental retardation by Lipman, DiMascio, Reatig, and Kirson (1978), only 12 (7%) were concerned with TCAs, and none involved MAOIs or novel antidepressants. Rimland (1977) reported the use of only one tricyclic (nortriptyline) in 71 (out of 2,000) autistic children who were taking psychotropic drugs, while neuroleptics had been used in almost half of those on medication.

The question is whether these medications are underused and underresearched or whether the paucity of available information speaks to their limited efficacy for retarded people. We agree with Sovner and Hurley (1983) that affective symptoms are underrecognized in mentally retarded people. Therefore, we feel that antidepressants and lithium are underemployed for retarded patients, whereas neuroleptic drugs are probably overprescribed.

Tricyclic antidepressants have been prescribed for a variety of disorders. In addition to their use in depression, TCAs are also regarded as the drugs of choice for panic disorder with concurrent depressive symptoms (Curtis, 1985). The tricyclic imipramine is sometimes used in the treatment of enuresis, nocturnal type, although the effect of the drug for this disorder is probably related to its effects on autonomic regulation of bladder function rather than to any psychotropic mechanism (Blackwell & Currah, 1973). TCAs have also been used in attention deficit disorder as alternatives to stimulants, and the tricyclic desipramine may be an appropriate second choice to stimulants in refractory patients (Biederman & Jellinek, 1984; Donnelly et al., 1986). Among normal IQ adults, tricyclics may also be useful in the prophylaxis of migraine (Couch & Hassanein, 1979), and in the management of chronic pain syndromes, such as pain associated with peripheral neuropathy in diabetes (Spiegel, Kalb, & Pasternak, 1983). Tricyclics have also been prescribed for night terrors, head banging, and encopresis (Gualtieri, 1977). The major utility of antidepressant drugs, however, is in the treatment of major depressive disorders, characterized by genetic predisposition, signs of physiological impairment (psychomotor retardation, sleep disturbance, weight change, constipation), and recurrent depressive episodes. Their proper use in retarded individuals, therefore, will ultimately be a function of accurate diagnosis of affective disorders.

In a review of literature on depression in mentally retarded individuals, Gardner (1967) proposed that the condition tends to be underdiagnosed. If such is the situation, one would expect that improved diagnostic skills and psychiatric management of mentally retarded patients will ultimately lead to more frequent use of antidepressant drugs. Unfortunately, the diagnois of affective disorder may be problematic in retarded patients who are non-verbal, or whose limited ability to conceptualize and convey a mood state compromises the validity of self-report. There are no tested grounds for establishing a diagnosis of major affective disorder in retarded people. Thus far, alleged "tests" for major affective disorder, such as the de-xamethasone suppression test, appear to be less valid in retarded individuals (Sireling, 1986) than in nonretarded people. Given our current knowledge, one must rely on the sensitivity of caregivers to appreciate a low mood state or an anhedonic condition. This evaluation is the essential element of diagnosis; clinically it is easier to recognize affective disorder in this population if the patient has experienced a *change* in mood and harder if the patient has been chronically depressed for several years.

There are, however, some behavioral clues to the diagnosis: a low energy level, lack of interest in events, loss of capacity to enjoy things that were once pleasing, and change in performance at school or work. There are also vegetative signs of affective illness: insomnia or hypersomnia, anorexia or hyperphagia, weight loss or weight gain, constipation, and increased susceptibility to minor infections. Finally there are indirect signs, as if the patient were "acting out" a dysphoric mood state: agitation, anxiety, irritability, destructiveness, and aggression. Social withdrawal is a key symptom. An additional clue may be the cyclic nature of a patient's behavior problems: weeks or months of agitated, hyperactive behavior alternating with cycles of normal behavior or of anergy. With a reliable clinical history of such signs and symptoms, verbal self-report of depressed mood may not be necessary, and treatment should be undertaken following the standard approaches of psychiatric practice.

Studies of Tricyclic Antidepressants with Mentally Retarded Persons

Psychoactive drug treatment in mentally retarded people traditionally has been aimed at controlling disturbing or troublesome behavior rather than at modifying withdrawal, inhibition, psychomotor retardation, or sadness. Although TCAs are sometimes used to control behavior disorders in mentally retarded persons, empirical data to support their efficacy and safety in this capacity are lacking (Gualtieri & Hawk, 1982). However, several case reports of positive effects in this population exist. Keegan, Pettigrew, and Parker (1974) described two adults with Down syndrome who presented with features of psychotic deterioration but who failed to respond to neuroleptic drugs. Both responded favorably to amitriptyline. Kraft, Ardali, Duffy, Hart, and Pearce (1966) found that amitriptyline was useful in the treatment of four out of five mentally retarded boys who had behavior disorders.

Although it was once proposed that imipramine and the MAOIs helped withdrawn, autistic children, Campbell, Fish, Shapiro, and Floyd (1971) were unable to confirm these findings. Carter (1966) found that nortriptyline was effective as a "standard sedative or tranquilizer in the control of disturbed behavior" in mentally retarded patients ages 4 to 70. However, in this study, placebo also exerted a sedative effect and the authors' conceptualization of improvement (i.e., in terms of sedation) may well not fit in with modern views of a therapeutic effect.

Pilkington (1962) divided 30 mentally retarded children into two groups: "affective (cyclothymic)" and "non-affective." In this uncontrolled study, half of the first group improved on imipramine, while all of the second group were made worse by the medication.

Field, Aman, White, and Vaithianathan (1986) reported a single-subject study with a moderately retarded woman with clinical characteristics suggestive of depression. As compared with placebo, repeated administrations of imipramine produced a consistent decrease in crying and in screaming outbursts and an increase in food consumption.

Using a double-blind, placebo-controlled, crossover design, Aman, White, Vaithianathan, and Teehan (1986) assessed the effects of imipramine (3 mg/kg/day) in profoundly retarded residents selected for either depressive symptoms or acting-out behaviors. The results indicated significant behavioral deterioration on variables measuring irritability, social withdrawal, and activity level, regardless of whether the subjects initially presented with depressive or acting-out symptoms. As the study was carried out with profoundly retarded subjects, this suggests that severity of retardation may be a factor in determining clinical response, although the effect of IQ has not been formally evaluated in any study so far.

Anxiety disorders are well studied in adult psychiatric populations, but there is little information on their occurrence in mentally handicapped people. Panic disorder is characterized by attacks of autonomic overactivity not precipitated by a specific phobic stimulus. Symptoms include dyspnea, palpitations, sweating, trembling, and fears of dying, going crazy, or doing something uncontrolled during an attack. In adult psychiatric patients, the disorder may be complicated by agoraphobia and substance abuse.

While there are no studies of anxiety disorders in the mentally retarded popluation, many troublesome symptoms (anxiety, agitation) in this group may be manifestations of an anxiety disorder. If there is a family history of panic disorder, caffeine sensitivity, an episodic course to the behavioral difficulties, and prominent symptoms of anxiety, then it may be appropriate to consider therapy with low doses of TCAs. However, time will be required to evaluate such a practice, as empirical data are lacking both in regards to the validity of these selection criteria and clinical efficacy of the TCAs in such retarded individuals.

Studies of Monoamine Oxidase Inhibitors with Developmentally Disabled Persons

Although the MAOIs antedated the TCAs by several years, their use in North America is almost negligible because of toxicity when given in combination with certain tyramine-containing foods. At this point, MAOIs seem to be used by a minority of psychiatrists, and the usual indications are 'atypical depression'' or panic attacks (Sheehan, 1985). Occasionally, severely depressed individuals are treated with a combination of a TCA and a MAOI, but this is a potentially dangerous combination and should only be used by experienced clinicians in inpatient settings, and only in the gravest circumstances. Very little has been written concerning MAOIs in the treatment of children or developmentally handicapped individuals.

Soblen and Saunders (1961) found that phenelzine alleviated apathy, withdrawal, low motor activity, and flattened affect in 15 out of 20 schizophrenic and behavior disorder adolescents. Heaton-Ward (1961) reported that nialamide had no influence on mental age or behavior of 51 mentally retarded persons. Carter (1960) found that residents treated with isocarboxazid showed greater alertness, responsiveness, sociability, and increased weight gain. However, the validity of the findings of these poorly controlled studies is open to serious question.

Studies of Novel Antidepressants in Mentally Retarded Persons

There are, to the authors' knowledge, neither controlled studies nor anecdotal reports on the use of novel antidepressants in retarded patients. It is not clear what impact drugs like amoxapine, maprotiline, alprazolam, and trazodone will have on the future practice of psychopharmacology, since the risk-to-benefit ratio may not be as favorable as originally hoped. Amoxapine, for example, may cause tardive dyskinesia, and maprotiline has a serious proclivity to lower the seizure threshold—a major drawback for retarded patients, many of whom have seizure disorders. Alprazolam appears to have antidepressant and antipanic efficacy. Like other benzodiazepines to which it is related, alprazolam may cause behavioral disinhibition, hyperactivity, irritability, aggression, and addiction. Trazodone (a triazolopyridine derivative chemically unrelated to tricyclic and tetra-cyclic antidepressants) can be very sedating, can cause priapism, and tends to have an idiosyncratic efficacy profile.

Guidelines for Treatment with Antidepressants

Treatment of depressed patients with TCAs usually begins with low doses, ranging from 25 to 50 mg/day, with gradual upward titration to doses between 150 and 300 mg/day for adults. Plasma level determinations may be obtained and are often helpful when the physician is faced with questions of noncompliance, with lack of therapeutic responsiveness, or with the potential for adverse reactions in high-risk patients. While "therapeutic levels" have been determined for some TCAs (e.g., desipramine, nortriptyline), for others the relationship between plasma levels and clinical response is much less clear (see also Chapter 3).

Commonly used doses of TCAs can range from 50 to 300 mg/day; doses in the range of 800–1,000 mg can be fatal. This extremely low therapeutic-to-lethal dose ratio should clearly limit the use of TCAs only to circumstances where the most careful supervision of drug administration is possible.

It is now widely accepted that imipramine possesses antipanic activity in a variety of panic-related disorders (Liebowitz, 1985) and is probably the pharmacological treatment of choice for this type of anxiety. In the treatment of panic disorder, tricyclic medications are begun at a low dose (10 mg/day then increased to 30 or 40 mg/day) while carefully tracking affective symptoms, as some patients report anxiety and worsening of panic attacks if the dose is started too high or increased too quickly. Once 50 mg/day is reached, the treatment course can proceed as in treating depression. Treatment of hyperkinesis and enuresis usually requires much lower doses, and correspondingly lower serum levels, than the treatment of depression. The drugs seem to exert an immediate effect in these disorders, whereas their effect on depressive symptoms can be delayed 2 to 3 weeks.

The potential cardiotoxicity of TCAs requires that the physician carefully monitor medication use in patients with cardiac disease. While TCAs may be safely used in such patients, it is best to choose one with a favorable cardiotoxic profile, such as doxepin or desipramine; the novel antidepressants, maprotiline and trazodone, may carry even less risk. Nortriptyline may be less likely to lower blood pressure if postural hypotension is a problem.

In light of cardiotoxicity of TCAs, careful monitoring of the patient's cardiac status prior to treatment and during the titration of dose to proper levels is recommended. An EKG should usually be done before starting the drug. Blood pressure and pulse should also be measured because hypotension or tachycardia can occur. These drugs can cause a variety of systemic toxic effects, such as dry mouth, gastrointestinal symptoms, and weight gain, and are known to lower the seizure threshold.

In the treatment of a depressive episode, symptoms usually clear within 3 to 6 weeks after medication achieves therapeutic levels. Often the medication can be continued for 6 months and then gradually tapered over 2 to 4 weeks (to prevent withdrawal, which is characterized by anxiety symptoms) with no maintenance antidepressant therapy required. The same strategy is true for TCA use in panic disorder.

The only unequivocal indication for the use of antidepressants in mentally retarded individuals is unipolar depression, characterized by the signs and symptoms listed earlier. Panic disorder is another reasonable indication for imipramine, but this problem is not frequently described in the mentally retarded population. Although imipramine is effective in the treatment of enuresis, we do not recommend its routine application for this disorder. There are certain sleep disorders that are appropriately treated with TCAs. The use of imipramine or other TCAs for the routine treatment of hyperactivity and other behavior problems should be discouraged, although there may be exceptional cases where the application of an antidepressant may be warranted.

Antianxiety and Sedative-Hypnotic Agents

In many respects, antianxiety drugs and the sedative/hypnotics are indistinguishable except in terms of the intent of the prescribing clinician. Antianxiety agents are used for the treatment of anxiety, whereas sedative/hypnotic agents are used for the treatment of insomnia. However, the actual drug choice may be identical and is most commonly a benzodiazepine. The distinction between the two indications has often been made on the basis of marketing strategies of pharmaceutical companies and subsequently reinforced by their use in clinical practice. In fact, antianxiety agents are sedating and may be used as sedative/hypnotic agents, and sedative/hypnotic agents have a calming effect and may be used as antianxiety agents.

Anxiolytics and sedative/hypnotics are the most widely prescribed medications in the United States, and they are commonly used in mentally retarded people. However, the scientific literature concerning their use with the mentally retarded population is a virtual desert. The reason for this investigative neglect is not entirely clear, though it may be related to diagnostic difficulties. A reasoned approach to the use of these agents is necessary, while further research is to be greatly encouraged and supported.

Prevalence of Use

In Lipman's (1970) widely cited survey, about 8% of the institutionalized mentally retarded people in the United States were receiving anxiolytics, or minor tranquilizers, making this class of agents a distant second to the neuroleptics in terms of psychotropic drug use. Two benzodiazepines, diazepam (Valium) and chlordiazepoxide (Librium), were the most commonly used, followed by meprobamate (Miltown) and hydroxyzine (Vistaril and Atarax).

Subsequent surveys of drug use (e.g., Silva, 1979; Tu, 1979) have yielded similar results. Of psychotropic drugs, antianxiety agents are still second only to the neuroleptics in frequency of employment in mentally retarded persons.[1] In a recently published national survey Hill, Balow, and Bruininks (1985) found that 5.4% of the institutionalized population and 3.8% of the community sample were receiving antianxiety agents. In both populations, benzodiazepines comprised the bulk of these agents. Intagliata and Rinck (1985) reported a prevalence usage rate of minor tranquilizers of 16.9% and 5.5% for their institutional and community samples, respectively, again with benzodiazepines comprising the bulk.

Antianxiety Agents (Anxiolytics)

INDICATIONS AND THERAPEUTIC USE

Despite this evidence of their widespread use in the mentally retarded population, the guidelines for prescription of anxiolytic agents in this population are unclear. There are no studies that examine their use in retarded individuals for their primary indication of anxiety, and very few that have examined their use at all. As Intagliata and Rinck (1985) found, anxiolytics appear to be given to mentally retarded persons primarily to control hyperactive, agitated, aggressive, or otherwise disruptive behaviors. However, the available research seems to indicate that anxiolytics have limited usefulness for these types of behaviors. In fact, the few available well-controlled studies show that these behaviors do not improve, and indeed often worsen, with the administration of antianxiety agents. For example, Zrull, Westman, Arthur, and Bell (1963) found no improvement in the behavior of "hyperkinetic" children with the administration of chlordiazepoxide, and this group found similar results with the use of diazepam (Zrull, Westman, Arthur, & Rice, 1964). Furthermore, LaVeck and Buckley (1961), in a study of chlordiazepoxide, and Walters, Singh, and Beale 1977), in their evaluation of lorazepam, reported that these benzodiazepines actually worsened many of the targeted behaviors and improved none. Therefore, at the present time it must be concluded that there is no scientific foundation to support the use of antianxiety agents for suppressing acting-out behavior in this population. Any use of these agents for the

---

[1]Readers should bear in mind that the authors are referring to agents strictly defined as *psychotropic drugs* here. In most mental retardation institutions, antiepileptic drugs are easily the second most commonly prescribed medications, and among developmentally disabled people (especially children) in community settings, antiepileptic drugs may supersede even the neuroleptics in prevalence of use (see Chapter 1).

control of hyperactive or aggressive behaviors must be subject to careful scrutiny and cautious interpretation of perceived benefit; it even seems reasonable to recommend placebo-controlled, double-blind conditions for clinical use in this respect.

There are no studies available that examine the use of antianxiety agents in mentally retarded persons for their *primary* indication, namely, the short-term treatment of anxiety. This situation is probably attributable to a general underrecognition of anxiety disorders in mentally retarded individuals. There does not appear to be any reason to suspect that these agents would not be effective for this indication, just as they are in the intellectually normal, though in some individuals with obvious or presumed brain damage, the well-recognized "paradoxical" effect may be found with their use (see the next section).

BENZODIAZEPINES

Since their introduction in the 1960s, benzodiazepines have continued to be regarded as extremely safe and effective in the treatment of anxiety disorders, and they remain the drugs of choice in this clinical situation. They have essentially replaced the barbiturates and nonbarbiturate, non-benzodiazepine agents (e.g, propanediols, such as meprobamate), largely because of their superior safety profile and equal or greater therapeutic effectiveness. Some clinicians, especially in the field of mental retardation, continue to prefer hydroxyzine (Atarax, Vistaril), although this drug is less efficacious in decreasing anxiety than the benzodiazepines, and it lowers the seizure threshold. However, it does have the advantage of not producing physical dependence.

The benzodiazepines probably exert their therapeutic effects by interacting with an endogenous benzodiazepine receptor, which is widespread throughout the brain, and which, in turn, interacts with γ-aminobutyric acid (GABA) receptors as well as with other neuromodulators (Gray, 1983; Guidotti, 1978; Tallman, Paul, Skolnick, & Gallager, 1980). The several drugs in this family are quite similar to each other, differing primarily in onset of action and half-life (duration of action). For example, diazepam (Valium) has a rapid onset of action as well as a long half-life, which may make it preferable in certain situations, whereas oxazepam (Serax), with its slower onset of action and short half-life, may be preferable in others.

The most common untoward effects of the benzodiazepines, including drowsiness and sedation, represent extensions of their pharmacological actions. In addition, ataxia and psychomotor impairment may appear in some individuals, especially at higher dosages and may constitute a serious limitation in settings requiring sustained attention and coordination (e.g., vocational workshop).

Increasing concern about the use of benzodiazepines has surfaced over the past several years with the recognition of tolerance and withdrawal reactions to these agents. It is now recognized that such reactions may occur following long-term use of even standard therapeutic dosages as well as following short-term use of high dosages (Hallstrom & Lader, 1981). However, well-monitored use poses little danger to the patient.

BENZODIAZEPINES AS ANTICONVULSANTS (see also Chapter 5)

Benzodiazepines have an important, but limited, role in the treatment of seizure disorders (Schmidt, 1983; Trimble, 1983; Adams & Victor, 1985). Intravenously administered diazepam continues to play a significant part in the emergency treatment of status epilepticus. Furthermore, orally administered clonazepam has a role in the treatment of certain types of epilepsy, particularly generalized absence and myoclonic seizures. It is possible that nitrazepam has a function similar to that of clonazepam, though its use is much less accepted and the drug is not available in the United States. However, beyond these rather specific exceptions, benzodiazepines appear to have little to contribute to the treatment of epilepsy.

Nevertheless, several investigators have noted that the prevalence of diazepam in retarded people as a psychotropic agent may be artifically inflated because it is frequently used as an anticonvulsant. If this is the case, then it speaks to another problem in the pharmacotherapy of mentally retarded people that has yet to be adequately addressed (see Chapter 5). In short, since orally administered diazepam has little or no efficacy as a long-term anticonvulsant in epileptic patients of normal IQ, there appears to be little reason for this to be otherwise in mentally retarded patients. The questions that arise include whether epilepsy in mentally retarded individual is significantly different such that diazepam does play an important role as an anticonvulsant, or whether this is yet another instance of inappropriate administration of medication in people with mental retardation.

OTHER ANTIANXIETY AGENTS

Diphenhydramine (Benadryl) and hydoxyzine (Atarax, Vistaril) continue to enjoy a certain amount of popularity as anxiolytics among clinicians prescribing for mentally retarded individuals. However, despite their relative safety, there is little in the literature to support their efficacy as antianxiety agents in mentally retarded persons (Freeman, 1970; Rivinus, 1980). Therefore, any such use should be carefully monitored and scrutinized.

The role of the tricyclic antidepressant and MAOI drugs for suppressing panic attacks is discussed earlier in this chapter. In addition, beta-adrenergic blocking drugs, particularly propranolol, appear to be effective in the treatment of the somatic aspects of anxiety (e.g., tachycardia), and may therefore have a special role in those patients in whom such complaints are most prominent (Gualtieri, Golden, & Fahs, 1983; Greenblatt

& Shader, 1978; Noyes, 1985; see Chapter 7). However, they are clearly inferior to the benzodiazepines as general antianxiety agents.

SUMMARY

Antianxiety agents constitute a commonly employed class of psychotropic agents among mentally retarded persons. Although it is difficult to tell from the available surveys, it is likely that they are frequently used to control hyperactive and aggressive behaviors, for which their effectiveness has not been demonstrated. In fact, it has usually been shown that they worsen these behaviors. On the other hand, their use in the treatment of anxiety has yet to be empirically examined in mentally retarded people, though it may be expected that these agents do have a limited role in this situation. Principles of use in this respect would appear to be identical to those in the nonretarded population.

Sedative/Hypnotic Agents

The pattern of use of sedative/hypnotic agents is somewhat more difficult to ascertain from published reports than that of the antianxiety agents. For example, in Lipman's (1970) survey, sedative/hypnotics were not mentioned as a separate category. Although it is probable that the use of different anxiolytics often differs only in the intent of the prescribing clinician, in the reporting of survey data this intent is usually not indicated. Therefore, whether benzodiazephines, barbiturates, or hydroxyzine are to be viewed as anxiolytics, as sedative/hypnotics, or even (as in the case of phenobarbital) as anticonvulsants is often not clear. However, in the well-reported and recent studies of Hill et al. (1985) and Intagliata and Rinck (1985), prevalence rates for the use of sedative/hypnotic agents were indicated. In their national study of both community and institutional settings, Hill and colleagues (1985) found that 3.9% of the community sample and 7.3% of the institutional sample were receiving sedative/hypnotic agents. Similarly, Intagliata and Rinck (1985) reported that 4.3% of the community sample and 9.4% of the institutional sample were receiving sedative/hypnotic agents in their survey in Missouri. The two most commonly prescribed agents were chloral hydrate and flurazepam (Dalmane). Whether these rates are changing cannot be stated with confidence, since the methodological difficulties already mentioned make comparison with earlier studies impossible. Nevertheless, it would appear that sedative/hypnotic agents comprise a commonly used class of psychotropic agents among mentally retarded individuals.

INDICATIONS AND THERAPEUTIC USE

The indication for the use of sedative/hypnotic agents is relatively straightforward, and consists of a desire for short-term sedation, usually in symptomatic treatment of insomnia. In addition, it is a common practice among clinicians who work with mentally retarded individuals to use these agents for short-term sedation during physical examinations and other diagnostic investigations. Beyond these, there would appear to be little role for their use. There is essentially no relevant professional literature that speaks to their use in mentally retarded people, and therefore, any guidelines must be drawn largely from their use in the general population (Fahs, 1985; Gelenberg, 1983).

Since drugs play a relatively minor role in the rational treatment of insomnia, management of this symptom should begin with a careful evaluation. When pharmacological treatment is indicated, it should generally occur within the context of concurrent nonbiological approaches. As with the antianxiety agents, benzodiazepines are easily the preferred class of drugs for the pharmacological treatment of insomnia, as well as for other situations in which short-term sedation is indicated. There are several other possible choices, but probably the only acceptable alternatives would be the chloral derivatives (e.g., chloral hydrate) and diphenhydramine (e.g., Benadryl). However, if the patient is already taking one of the traditional antianxiety agents (e.g., one of the "nonhypnotic" benzodiazepines or hydroxyzine) for the daytime treatment of anxiety, then the dose or scheduling of that agent may be shifted in order to exploit its sedative effects at bedtime rather than adding another medication.

There are currently three benzodiazepines available in the United States that are designated specifically for use as sedative/hypnotic agents: flurazepam (Dalmane), temazepam (Restoril), and triazolam (Halcion). These agents differ primarily in length of half-life, with flurazepam being the longest and triazolam being the shortest. Treatment may be initiated with any of these agents at their lower dosage taken about 30 minutes before retiring. With flurazepam, one may expect greater hypnotic efficacy on the second and subsequent nights of administration as the drug accumulates, while with the shorter-acting agents, the maximum hypnotic response may be seen on the first night. A transient worsening of sleep may occur following discontinuation of any of the hypnotics, even after short-term administration. In addition, daytime sedation with impairment of cognitive and psychomotor function is frequent with the long-acting flurazepam due to its accumulation, and daytime anxiety as a result of repeated withdrawal due to the short half-life of triazolam has also been reported. Therefore, it is probable that the intermediate half-life of temazepam is to be perferred as a hypnotic (Oswald, 1983).

The cautions with regard to withdrawal and dependence apply to all of the benzodiazepines, and continuous long-term use is to be discouraged. Therefore, these drugs must be prescribed judiciously, for only short periods (usually no more than 2 weeks), and monitored carefully lest the patient's difficulty be exacerbated.

"PARADOXICAL" RESPONSE TO SEDATIVE/HYPNOTIC AGENTS

It is well known that some mentally retarded patients respond to the administration of sedative/hypnotic agents with increased levels of motor activity, restlessness, or other forms of agitated behavior, termed the "paradoxical" response. This response is also observed in elderly patients with dementia, in children, and in patients with a variety of forms of brain damage. This observation has led many clinicians to caution against the use of these agents in mentally retarded patients, and, indeed, it is an important factor to take into account. However, the recent work of Barron and Sandman (Barron & Sandmann, 1983, 1984, 1985; Sandman, Datta, & Barron, 1983) suggests some intriguing possibilities stemming from this phenomenon. They describe a constellation of factors related to the presence of a "paradoxical" response in mentally retarded patients, including a history of perinatal trauma, the presence of self-injurious behavior and stereotypy, and a beneficial response of their self-injurious behavior to the administration of the opiate antagonist, naloxone. While these findings have yet to be replicated and further extended, the implications are clear: there may be a subgroup of mentally retarded individuals whose self-injurious behavior is etiologically related to an impaired endogenous opiate system and in whom a paradoxical response to sedative/hypnotic agents may serve as a "pharmacological marker." Should this prove to the case, treatment approaches involving manipulation of the opiate system would appear to be quite specific.

Lithium Carbonate

Knowledge about the proper use of lithium in retarded people is derived almost entirely from research and clinical experience in nonretarded patients. For normal IQ people, lithium is specifically indicated for treatment of bipolar disorder and for the prophylaxis of recurrent unipolar depression. It may also have indications for the treatment of certain forms of aggression, for "augmentation" of antidepressant action in refractory depression, and occasionally in the treatment of schizophrenia and "cyclothymic personality disorder." It has also been used to treat virtually any severe behavior problem that has not responded to alternative treatments.

Bipolar Disorder

Lithium is prescribed mainly for bipolar affective disorder, an illness characterized by severe mood swings and various accessory symptoms such as paranoia, delusions, and hallucinations. Patients with this disorder have manic episodes characterized by elation or irritability, overtalkativeness, increased motor activity, and decreased need for sleep. They may also have depressive episodes marked by depression of mood, mental and motor slowing, fatigue, anhedonia, and suicidal ideation. Although sleeplessness and weight loss can be prominent symptoms, the depressions of patients with bipolar affective disorder may be characterized by hyperphagia, hypersomnolence, perplexity, and stupor.

There has been little research on bipolar illness in mentally retarded people, perhaps because this disorder, like the other affective disorders, is felt to be difficult to diagnose in this population. However, when Sovner and Hurley (1983) reviewed reports of affective illness in the mentally retarded population, they found that the full range of diagnoses, including bipolar illness, was represented. They concluded that vegetative signs, family history, and behavioral changes were most useful for making the diagnosis in patients with severe or profound mental retardation. In addition, the presence of overactivity, noisiness, obscene language, suicide threats, and delusions of bodily malfunction could alert the clinician to possible affective disorder. Despite the difficulty in arriving at such a diagnosis in this population, there is no known reason to consider retarded people as immune from bipolar disorder. There is also no reason to consider lithium as less effective in the treatment of this disorder in retarded people than in cognitively normal persons.

Hasan and Mooney (1979) reported three cases of manic-depressive illness in mentally retarded adults. These patients had quite different symptom complexes and were variously characterized by depression, bursts of restlessness, manic behavior, tantrums, and aggression to staff. Lithium was prescribed (in one case in conjunction with fluphenazine) and the presenting problems generally remitted, leading to discharge, with a successful adjustment at home in two of the cases.

Reid and Leonard (1977) reported on a mildly retarded woman who experienced vomiting when she was depressed, and who had brief bouts of talkativeness and excessive friendliness. Her behavior was compared in the first year, during which she received prochlorperazine and chlorpromazine, with that in the second year when lithium was added. Striking reductions in depression, vomiting, and elation were noted in the second year. Kelly, Koch, and Buegel (1976) described a mildly retarded woman who displayed a "cyclothymic" behavior pattern since early childhood. At 15 years of age she was diagnosed as manic-depressive and subsequently she received chlorpromazine, haloperidol, and physical restraint, but without improvement. Lithium monotherapy was then initiated and her behavior became more controlled, with a "leveling" of cyclical behavior and increased prosocial behavior, which persisted to follow-up 4 years later.

Unfortunately, the bulk of the literature concerned with bipolar disorders and lithium in mentally retarded persons is composed of such case reports and uncontrolled studies. Naylor, Donald, LePoidevin, and Reid (1974), however, conducted a placebo-controlled, double-blind study of 14 retarded patients, all of whom had a history of cyclical behavior changes. Each spent a year on lithium and a year on placebo, with order assigned randomly. Based on clinical knowledge and familiarity with the patient, interviewers rated the subjects as "normal" or "ill" each week. The number of "ill" ratings were found to be significantly fewer during lithium therapy than during the placebo condition.

Aggression

Lithium has been found to be effective in reducing experimentally induced aggression in laboratory animals (Sheard, 1970a, 1970b), leading to its subsequent use with aggressive human beings, such as assaultive male prisoners (Sheard, 1975). Campbell et al. (1984) reported a double-blind study of lithium carbonate, haloperidol, and placebo in 61 children, ages 6–12 years, with Conduct Disorder, undersocialized aggressive type. Lithium was found to be significantly superior to placebo on psychiatrists' ratings of hyperactivity, aggression, hostility, and unresponsiveness. A few studies have explored the effects of lithium on the aggressive behavior of mentally retarded and autistic persons.

Three case studies have described therapeutic effects with lithium in mentally retarded individuals who were either aggressive to themselves or others. Cooper and Fowlie (1973) used lithium in a self-injurious girl and reported cessation of self-injury together with increased cooperative behavior and greater interest in other people. Lion, Hill, and Madden (1975) found that lithium produced a reduction in presenting symptoms (consisting of cyclical temper outbursts, psychomotor agitation, and verbal threats) in a mentally retarded man. Finally, Goetzl, Grunberg, and Berkowitz (1977) described three young mentally retarded adults with a variety of symptoms, including aggressive/disruptive behavior, fighting, insommia, agitation, hyperactivity, labile mood, and pressured speech. Lithium treatment produced a marked reduction in symptoms and, sometimes, a successful return from the hospital to the community.

Dostal and Zvolsky (1970) treated 14 aggressive, hyperactive, phenothiazine-resistant severely retarded adolescents with lithium. Subjects received their usual neuroleptic medication plus lithium at low blood levels (0.3 mEq/L) during Phase 1, lithium alone during Phase 2, and lithium at mean levels of 0.9 mEq/l in Phase 3. There were improvements in affectivity, aggressiveness, psychomotor activity, restlessness, and undisciplined behavior during the latter two phases.

Micev and Lynch (1974) reported results of a 12-week, nonblind trial of lithium in 10 severely retarded patients. All displayed aggressive and self-injurious behavior. Rating scales were used and serum levels were maintained at 0.6 mEq/L. Five of the nine aggressive patients showed "significant" improvement; three improved slightly and one showed no change. Of the eight patients who engaged in self-injurious behavior, six showed cessation of such behavior, one showed some improvement, and one showed no change.

Worrall, Moody, and Naylor (1975) conducted a double-blind, placebo-controlled study in eight severely retarded women. Nurses rated aggressive behavior during lithium or placebo treatment in 4-week blocks over 16 weeks. Two patients had to be withdrawn from the study because of severe toxic effects. Maintenance doses of previously prescribed psychoactive drugs were continued throughout the study. Three patients became less aggressive on lithium, one was more aggressive, and two showed no change.

Tyrer, Walsh, Edwards, Berney, and Stephens (1984) examined factors associated with a good response to lithium in 25 aggressive mentally handicapped patients whom they had treated. Characteristics associated with a good clinical response included the following: less than one aggressive episode per week before treatment, overactivity, stereotypic behavior, female sex, and epilepsy.

Finally, Campbell, Fish, Korein, et al. (1972) conducted what may be the only controlled study of lithium treatment in autistic children with a variety of acting-out behavior problems. They compared lithium with chlorpromazine on a double-blind basis, but placebo was not incorporated in the design. In general, neither of the drugs was therapeutically effective, and lithium was less so than chlorpromazine. However, one child with severe self-mutilation, explosive affect, and violent temper tantrums showed marked improvements.

Recommended Clinical Indications for Lithium

Lithium may prove to be a useful agent in the management of severely aggressive or self-injurious patients of normal or below-normal intelligence, who cannot be controlled with less restrictive approaches. However, it is difficult to generalize on the basis of anecdotal reports and (for the most part) poorly controlled studies. For the individual patient, the clinician may do well to consider lithium in circumstances where pharmacological control is essential and other measures have failed.

Lithium is sometimes used in schizophrenic patients who ordinarily would be treated with neuroleptics but who have developed tardive dyskinesia or transient withdrawal dyskinesia and for whom continued neuroleptic treatment is ill-advised. Therefore, it may also be a reasonable alternative for retarded patients with tardive dyskinesia. We know of no lithium trials in specific syndromic groups within the mentally retarded population such as Down Syndrome, Lesch-Nyhan syndrome, Prader-Willi syndrome, or patients with Fragile-X chromosome.

The treating physician must be aware of the physiological effects lithium may manifest. Some of the more commonly reported include the following: EEG abnormalities (lithium is known to lower the seizure threshold); cardiovascular changes, such as pulse irregularities and hypotension; gastrointestinal effects, in the form of diarrhea, constipation, dry mouth, anorexia, nausea, and vomiting; neuromuscular effects, like tremor, ataxia, dyskinesia, and hyperactive reflexes; endocrine effects, like goiter (hypothyroidism), and a hematological effect, a reversible leukocytosis, sometimes with white blood cell counts over 15,000 per cubic millimeter.

Lithium has a number of effects related to the kidneys. It may alter transport of electrolytes or cause reversible nephrogenic diabetes insipidus or polyuria with secondary polydipsia. The incidence of nephrotoxic effects of lithium remains unclear. Bendz (1983) reviewed 23 studies of kidney function in lithium-treated patients and concluded that in a small proportion of patients treated long term, a partly irreversible reduction in tubular function occurred. The review found no increased risk of kidney damage associated with combined treatment with neuroleptics. The clinical salience of lithium nephrotoxicity is probably not very high, and periodic monitoring of physiological parameters (serum creatinine and BUN, urine specific gravity) is usually sufficient to prevent serious consequences.

There have been few studies of lithium's effect on neuropsychological tests, but most studies find a subtle, reversible decline in functioning (e.g., Platt, Campbell, Green, Perry, & Cohen, 1981). Patients may complain of memory loss, physical discomfort, and dysphoric effects. Side effects such as fatigue, tremor, and muscle weakness may contribute to lowered scores in tests requiring motor performance.

In mentally retarded persons with an unequivocal diagnosis of bipolar disorder or of recurrent unipolar depression, lithium is the treatment of choice. Lithium may be considered as a treatment measure for patients in the following categories:

1. Mentally retarded patients with nonspecific behavior disorders who have a strong family pedigree of bipolar affective disorder and/or lithium response
2. Patients with severe behavior disorders that are characterized by cyclicity or a strong "affective flavor"
3. Patients with explosive aggressive behavior

It is also reasonable to try lithium in cases of the most severe behavior problems, simply because all other treatment approaches have failed.

Lithium treatment is usually begun gradually, starting with one tablet (300 mg) and increasing the dose every few days, until therapeutic serum levels are achieved. Lithium blood levels have been found to correlate highly with clinical efficacy. After 3 or 4 days on a given dose, a blood sample is measured 8 to 12 hours after the last dose of lithium. If the blood lithium level is subtherapeutic, the dose can be increased. Therapeutic levels are between 0.7 and 1.0 mEq/L, and in adults an oral dose of 900 to 1,500 mg/day is usually required to achieve these concentrations (see also Chapter 3). Occasionally, a patient will respond to "subtherapeutic" levels.

Levels higher than 2 mEq/L can be dangerous. The early signs of lithium overdose include anorexia, gastric discomfort, diarrhea, vomiting, thirst, polyuria, hyperreflexia, and hand tremor. Toxic effects associated with high blood levels are more serious, and may include muscle fasciculations and twitching, ataxia, somnolence, confusion, dysarthria, and seizures. Although blood levels must be determined every 3–5 days during initial treatment with lithium, during maintenance treatment blood levels need only be determined on a monthly basis, while remaining alert to signs and symptoms of toxicity. Periodic evaluation of the patient's renal, thyroid, and electrolyte status is recommended for patients on chronic lithium treatment because of possible long-term adverse effects.

One must be alert for signs of an organic brain syndrome due to drug interaction when using lithium in combination with any neuroleptic. The population of mentally retarded patients present special problems in monitoring lithium. If the patient is noncommunicative, the clinician must be especially alert to physical manifestations of toxicity.

Considering the potential toxicity of the drug, and the paucity of good research concerning its use in mentally retarded persons, it is reasonable practice to confine lithium treatment only to the most severe cases, where behavior management, appropriate programing, and a proper environment are inadequate for control of behavior problems. It is likely, however, that lithium will prove to be preferable to the neuroleptic drugs in the treatment of such patients.

Conclusion

Despite an unsatisfactory data base, some very general conclusions can be drawn about each of these four drug groups. The available studies on the stimulant drugs do not support their application in severely and profoundly retarded institutionalized patients or in autistic children. On the other hand, these drugs have not been well studied among mildly and moderately retarded children, residing in the community, who have been selected for symptoms related to hyperactivity, and it may eventually prove to be the case that a sizable proportion of these children can benefit from such therapy. The principal indication for the antidepressants is major depressive disorder, although these drugs may be of value in treating certain anxiety disorders (such as panic disorder) and some severe behavior disorders in this population. There is no good evidence that the anxiolytics are effective in managing acting-out behaviors among mentally retarded persons, but (as in normal IQ populations) they are probably effective on a short-term basis in treating anxiety-based disorders and insomnia. Finally, the principal indication for lithium is bipolar disorder, although it may also be useful for managing severe aggressive and/or self-injurious behavior as well as behavior disorders of a cyclic nature or where there is a strong family pedigree of bipolar affective disorder.

It is interesting to note that, with the exception of the stimulants in the institutional context, none of these drugs has received adequate assessment among mentally retarded individuals. Hence, even the above guidelines must be treated as very tentative at this time. It is also of interest that the principal indications for some of these drugs involve sadness, withdrawal, inhibition, anxiety, and so forth—symptoms that appear most obviously to distress the person concerned rather than society. It is difficult to escape the impression that there may have been a bias in the psychopharmacological research toward the suppression of troublesome behavior to the neglect of an array of "silent" disorders in this population. Also implicit in this whole discussion is the assumption that psychopathology is expressed in essentially the same manner (although often in much more subtle ways) among intellectually handicapped people as in people of normal IQ. This premise needs to be tested through systematic study to determine whether we are identifying and labeling symptoms correctly (especially among severely and profoundly retarded patients) and if not, to determine what modifications should be made. Finally, it is apparent that the potential array of disorders that might be treated with these drugs is considerable. However, because of a virtual absence of relevant drug research with developmentally disabled subjects, we are forced, during much of this chapter, to make recommendations by reference to psycopharmacology in the normal IQ population. It is clear that a great deal more research needs to be done before the place of these agents in the psychopharmacology of persons with developmental disabilities is properly understood.

References

Adams, R.D., & Victor, M. (1985). *Principles of neurology* (3rd ed.). New York: McGraw-Hill.

Alexandris, A., & Lundell, F.W. (1968). Effect of thioridazine, amphetamine and placebo on the hyperkinetic syndrome and cognitive area in mentally deficient children. *Canadian Medical Associate Journal, 98*, 92–96.

Aman, M.G. (1980). Psychotropic drugs and learning problems—A selective review. *Journal of Learning Disabilities, 13*, 87–96.

Aman, M.G. (1982a). Psychoactive drug effects in developmental disorders and hyperactivity: Toward a resolution of disparate findings. *Journal of Autism and Developmental Disabilities, 12*, 385–398.

Aman, M.G. (1982b). Psychotropic drugs in the treatment of reading disorders. In R.N. Malatesha & P.G. Aaron (Eds.), *Reading disorders: Varieties and treatments* (pp. 453–471). New York: Academic Press.

Aman, M.G. (1985). Drugs in mental retardation: Treatment or tragedy?. *Australia and New Zealand Journal of Developmental Disabilities, 10*, 215–226.

Aman, M.G., Marks, R., Wilsher, C.P., Turbott, S.H., & Merry, S. (1988). *The clinical effects of methylphenidate and thioridazine in intellectually subaverage children with behavior disorders.* Unpublished manuscript in preparation, Ohio State University.

Aman, M.G., & Singh, N.N. (1982). Methylphenidate in severely retarded residents and the clinical significance of stereotypic behavior. *Applied Research in Mental Retardation, 3*, 345–358.

Aman, M.G., White, A.J., Vaithianathan, D., & Teehan, C.J. (1986). Preliminary study of imipramine in profoundly retarded residents. *Journal of Autism and Developmental Disorders, 16*, 263–273.

Anton, A.H., & Greer, M. (1969). Dextroamphetamine, catecholamines and behavior. *Archives of Neurology, 21*, 248–252.

Barkley, R.A., & Cunningham, C.E. (1978). Do stimulant drugs improve the academic performance of hyperkinetic children? A review of outcome research. *Clinical Pediatrics, 17*, 85–92.

Barron, J., & Sandman, C.A. (1983). Relationship of sedative/hypnotic response to self-injurious behavior and stereotypy by mentally retarded clients. *American Journal of Mental Deficiency, 88*, 177–186.

Barron, J., & Sandman, C.A. (1984). Self-injurious behavior and stereotypy in an institutionalized mentally retarded population. *Applied Research in Mental Retardation, 5*, 499–511.

Barron, J., & Sandman, C.A. (1985). Paradoxical excitement to sedative/hypnotics in mentally retarded clients. *American Journal of Mental Deficiency, 90*, 124–129.

Bell, A., & Zubek, J.P. (1961). Effects of deanol on the intellectual performance of mental defectives. *Canadian Journal of Psychology, 15*, 172–175.

Bendz, H. (1983). Kidney function in lithium-treated patients. *Acta Psychiatrica Scandinavica, 68*, 303–324.

Biederman, J., & Jellinek, M.S. (1984). Current concepts: Psychopharmacology in children. *New England Journal of Medicine, 310*, 968–972.

Blacklidge, V.Y., & Ekblad, R.L. (1971). The effectiveness of methylphenidate hydrochloride (Ritalin) on learning and behavior in public school educable mentally retarded children. *Pediatrics, 47*, 923–926.

Blackwell, B., & Currah, J. (1973). The psychopharmacology of nocturnal enuresis. In I. Kolvin, R. McKeith, & S. Meadow (Eds.), *Clinics in developmental medicine: Bladder control and enuresis*, (pp. 231–257). London: Heinemann.

Bradley, C. (1937). The behavior of children receiving benzedrine. *American Journal of Psychiatry, 94*, 577–585.

Campbell, M. (1975). Pharmacotherapy in early infantile autism. *Biological Psychiatry, 10*, 399–423.

Campbell, M., Fish, B., David, R., Shapiro, T., Collins, P., & Koh, C. (1972). Response to tri-iodothyronine and dextroamphetamine: A study of preschool schizophrenic children. *Journal of Autism and Childhood Schizophrenia, 2*, 343–358.

Campbell, M. Fish, B., Korein, J., Shapiro, T., Collins, P., & Koh, C. (1972). Lithium and chlorpromazine: A controlled crossover study of hyperactive severely disturbed young children. *Journal of Autism and Childhood Schizophrenia, 2*, 234–263.

Campbell, M., Fish, B., Shapiro, T., & Floyd, A. (1971). Imipramine in preschool autistic and schizophrenic children. *Journal of Autism and Childhood Schizophrenia, 1*, 267–282.

Campbell, M., Small, A.M., Collins, P.J., Friedman, E., David, R., & Genieser, N. (1976). Levodopa and levoamphetaine: A crossover study in young schizophrenic children. *Current Therapeutic Research, 19*, 70–86.

Campbell, M., Small, A.M., Green, W.H., Jennings, S.J., Perry, R., Bennett,

W.G., & Anderson, L. (1984). Behavioral efficacy of haloperidol and lithium carbonate. A comparison of hospitalized aggressive children with conduct disorder. *Archives of General Psychiatry, 41*, 650–656.

Carter, C. (1960). Isocarboxazid in the institutionalized mentally retarded. *Diseases of the Nervous System, 21*, 568–570.

Carter, C. (1966). Nortriptyline HCL as a tranquilizer for disturbed mentally retarded patients: A controlled study. *American Journal of Medical Sciences, 251*, 465–467.

Christiansen, D.E. (1975). Effects of combining methylphenidate and a classroom token system in modifying hyperactive behavior. *American Journal of Mental Deficiency, 80*, 266–276.

Clausen, J., Fineman, M., Henry, C.E., & Wohl, N. (1960). The effect of deaner (2-dimethyl-aminoethanol) on mentally retarded subjects. *Training School Bulletin, 57*, 3–12.

Cohen M.N., & Sprague, R.L. (1977, March). *Survey of drug usage in two midwestern institutions for the retarded.* Paper presented at the Gatlinburg Conference on Research in Mental Retardation, Gatlinburg, Tennessee.

Cooper, A.F., & Fowlie, H.C. (1973). Control of gross self-mutilation with lithium carbonate. *British Journal of Psychiatry, 22*, 370–371.

Couch, J.R., & Hassanein, R.S. (1979). Amitriptyline in migraine prophylaxis. *Archives of Neurology, 36*, 695–699.

Curtis, G.C. (1985). New findings in anxiety: A synthesis for clinical practice in 1985. *Psychiatric Clinics of North America, 8*, 169–175.

Cutler, M., Little, J.W., & Strauss, A.A. (1940–1941). The effect of Benzedrine on mentally deficient children. *American Journal of Mental Deficiency, 45*, 59–65.

Davis, K.V., Sprague, R.L., & Werry, J.S. (1969). Stereotyped behavior and activity level in severe retardates: The effect of drugs. *American Journal of Mental Deficiency, 72*, 721–727.

Donnelly, M., Zametkin, A.J., Rapoport, J.L., Ismon, D.R., Weingartner, H., Lane, E., Oliver, J., & Linnolla, M. (1986). Treatment of childhood hyperactivity with desipramine: Plasma drug concentration, cardiovascular effects, plasma and urinary catecholamine levels and clinical response. *Clinical Pharmacology, 37*, 72–81.

Dostal, T., & Zvolsky, P. (1970). Anti-aggressive effect of lithium salts in severe mentally retarded adolescents. *International Psychopsychiatry, 5*, 302–307.

Evans, R.W., & Gualtieri, C.T. (in press). New developments in pediatric psychopharmacology: Psychostimulants and alternative drugs. In B. Goldberg & K. Wojakowski (Eds.), *Proceedings of the Annual CPRI Symposium.*

Evans, R.W., Gualtieri, C.T., & Amera, I. (1986). Methylphenidate and memory: Dissociated effects in hyperactive children. *Psychopharmacology, 90*, 211–216.

Evans, R.W., Gualtieri, C.T., & Hicks, R.E. (1986). Neuropathic substrate for stimulant drug effects in hyperactive children. *Clinical Neuropharmacology, 9*, 264–281.

Fahs, J.J. (1985). Insomnia. In L. Dornbrand, A.J. Hoole, R.H. Fletcher, & C.G. Pickard (Eds.), *Manual of clinical problems in adult ambulatory care.* Boston: Little, Brown.

Field, C.J., Aman, M.G., White, A.J., & Vaithianathan, C. (1986). Single-subject study of imipramine in a mentally retarded woman with depressive symptoms. *Journal of Mental Deficiency Research, 30*, 191–198.

Freeman, R.D. (1970) Psychopharmacology and the retarded child. In F.J. Meno-

Iascino (Ed.), *Psychiatric approaches to mental retardation* (pp. 294–368). New York: Basic Books.

Gadow, K.D., & Kalachnick, J. (1981). Prevalence and pattern of drug treatment for behavior and seizure disorders of TMR students. *American Journal of Mental Deficiency*, *73*, 588–595.

Gardner, W.I. (1967). Occurrence of severe depressive reactions in the mentally retarded. *American Journal of Psychiatry*, *124*, 386–388.

Gelenberg, A.J. (1983). Anxiety. In E.L. Bassuk, S.C. Schoonover, & A.J. Gelenberg (Eds.), *The practitioner's guide to psychoactive drugs* (2nd ed., pp. 167–201). New York: Plenum Press.

Geller, E., Ritvo, E.R., Freeman, B.J., & Yuwiler, A. (1982). Preliminary observations on the effect of fenfluramine on blood serotonin and symptoms in three autistic boys. *New England Journal of Medicine*, *307*, 165–169.

Goetzl, U., Grunberg, F., & Berkowitz, B. (1977). Lithium carbonate in the management of hyperactive aggressive behavior of the mentally retarded. *Comprehensive Psychiatry*, *18*, 599–606.

Gray, J.A. (1983). Gamma-aminobutyrate, the benzodiazepines and the septohippocampal system. In M.R. Trimble (Ed.), *Benzodiazepines divided: A multidisciplinary review* (pp. 101–126). New York: Wiley.

Greenblatt, D.J., & Shader, R.I. (1978) Pharmacotherapy of anxiety with benzodiazepines and beta-adrenergic blockers. In M.A. Lipton, A. DiMascio, & K.F. Killam (Eds.), *Psychopharmacology: A generation of progress*, (pp. 1381–1390). New York: Raven Press.

Gualtieri, C.T. (1977). Imipramine and children: A review and some speculations about the mechanism of drug action. *Diseases of the Nervous System*, *38*, 368–375.

Gualtieri, C.T. (1986). Fenfluramine and autism: Careful reappraisal is in order. *The Journal of Pediatrics*, *108*, 417–419.

Gualtieri, C.T. (1987). Re: M.G. Aman & N.N. Singh, "A critical apparaisal of recent drug research in mental retardation: the Coldwater studies." [Letter to the editor]. *Journal of Mental Deficiency Research*, *31*, 222–223.

Gualtieri, C.T., Golden, R.N., & Fahs, J.J. (1983). New developments in pediatric psychopharmacology. *Journal of Developmental and Behavioral Pediatrics*, *4*, 202–209.

Gualtieri, C.T., & Hawk, B. (1982). Antidepressant and antimanic drugs. In S.E. Breuning & A.D. Poling (Eds.), *Drugs and mental retardation* (pp. 215–234). Springfield, IL: Thomas.

Guidotti, A. (1978). Synaptic mechanisms in the action of benzodiazepines. In M.A. Lipton, A. DiMascio, & K.F. Killam (Eds.), *Psychopharmoacology: A generation of progress* (pp. 1349–1357). New York: Raven Press.

Hallstrom, C., & Lader, M.H. (1981). Benzodiazapine withdrawal phenomena. *International Pharmacopsychiatry*, *16*, 235–244.

Hasan, M.K., & Mooney, R.P. (1979). Three cases of manic/depressive illness in mentally retarded adults. *American Journal of Psychiatry*, *36*, 1069–1071.

Heaton-Ward, W.A. (1961). Inference and suggestion in a clinical trial (Niamid in mongolism). *Journal of Mental Science*, *107*, 115–118.

Hill, B.K., Balow, E.A., & Bruininks, R.H. (1985). A national study of prescribed drugs in institutions and community residential facilities for mentally retarded people. *Psychopharmacology Bulletin*, *21*, 279–284.

Holden, C. (1986). NIMH review of fraud charge moves slowly. *Science, 234*, 1488–1489.

Holden, C. (1987). NIMH finds a case of "serious misconduct". *Science, 235*, 1566–1567.

Itagliata, J., & Rinck, C. (1985). Psychoactive drug use in public and community residential facilities for mentally retarded persons. *Psychopharmacology Bulletin, 21*, 268–278.

Keegan, D.L., Pettigrew, A., & Parker, Z. (1974). Psychosis in Down's syndrome treated with amitriptyline. *Canadian Medical Association Journal, 110*, 1128–1129.

Kelly, J.T., Koch, M., & Buegel, D. (1976). Lithium carbonate in juvenile manic/depressive illness. *Diseases of the Nervous System, 37*, 90–92.

Koegel, R.L., & Covert, A. (1972). The relationship of self-stimulation to learning in autistic children. *Journal of Applied Behavior Analysis, 5*, 381–387.

Kraft, I.A., Ardali, C., Duffy, J., Hart, J., & Pearce, P. R. (1966). Use of amitriptyline in childhood behavior disturbances. *International Journal of Neuropsychiatry, 2*, 611–614.

LaVeck, G.D., & Buckley, P. (1961). The use of psychopharmacologic agents in retarded children with behavior disorders. *Journal of Chronic Diseases, 13*, 174–183.

Leventhal, B.L. (1985, May). *Fenfluramine administration to autistic children: Effect on behavior and biogenic amines.* New Clinical Drug Evaluation Unit Annual Meeting Proceedings, Key Biscayne, FL.

Liebowitz, M.R. (1985). Imipramine in the treatment of panic disorder and its complications. *Psychiatric Clinics of North America, 8*, 37–47.

Lion, J.R., Hill, J., & Madden, D.J. (1975). Lithium carbonate and aggression: A preliminary report. *Diseases of the Nervous System, 36*, 97–98.

Lipman, R.S. (1970). The use of psychopharmacological agents in residential facilities for the retarded. In F.J. Menolascino (Ed.), *Psychiatric approaches to mental retardation* (pp. 387–398). New York: Basic Books.

Lipman, R.S., DiMascio, A., Reatig, N., & Kirson, T. (1978). Psychotropic drugs and mentally retarded children. In M. A. Lipton, A. DiMascio, & K.F. Killam (Eds.), (pp. 1437–1449). *Psychopharmacology: A generation of progress.* New York: Raven Press.

Lobb, H. (1968). Trace GSR conditioning with Benzedrine in mentally defective and normal adults. *American Journal of Mental Deficiency, 73*, 239–246.

Lyon, M., & Robbins, T. (1975). The action of central nervous system stimulant drugs: A general theory concerning amphetamine effects. In W.B. Essman & L. Valzelli (Eds.), *Current developments in psychopharmacology (Vol. 2).* New York: Spectrum.

McConnell, T.R., Cromwell, R.L., Bialer, I., & Son, C.D. (1964). Studies in activity level: VII. Effects of amphetamine drug administration on the activity level of retarded children. *American Journal of Mental Deficiency, 68*, 647–651.

Micev, V., & Lynch, D.M. (1974). Effect of lithium on disturbed severely mentally retarded patients. *British Journal of Psychiatry, 125*, 110.

Morris, J.V., MacGillivray, R.C., & Mathieson, C.M. (1955). The results of the experimental administration of amphetamine sulfate in oligophrenia. *Journal of Mental Science/British Journal of Psychiatry, 101*, 131–140.

Naylor, G.J., Donald, J.M., LePoidevin, D., & Reid, A.H. (1974). A double-blind trial of long-term lithium therapy in mental defectives. *British Journal of Psychiatry*, *124*, 52–57.

Noyes, R. (1985). Beta-adrenergic blocking drugs in anxiety and stress. *Psychiatric Clinics of North America*, *8*, 119–132.

Oswald, I. (1983). Benzodiazepines and sleep. In M.R. Trimble (Ed.), *Benzodiazepines divided: A multidisciplinary review* (pp. 261–274). New York: Wiley.

Pelham, W.E., Bender, M.E., Caddell, J., Booth, S., & Moorer, S.H. (1985). Methylphenidate and children with Attention Deficit Disorder: Dose effects on classroom, academic and social behavior. *Archives of General Psychiatry*, *42*, 948–952.

Phillips, I., & Williams, N. (1975). Psychopathology and mental retardation: A study of 100 mentally retarded childredn: I. Psychopathology. *American Journal of Psychiatry*, *132*, 1265–1271.

Phillips, I., & Williams, N. (1977). Psychopathology and mental retardation: A statistical study of 100 mentally retarded children treated at a psychiatric clinic: II. Hyperactivity. *American Journal of Psychiatry*, *134*, 418–419.

Pilkington, T.L. (1962). A report on "Tofranil" in mental deficiency. *American Journal of Mental Deficiency*, *66*, 729–732.

Platt, J.E., Campbell, M., Green, W.H., Perry, R., & Cohen, I.L. (1981). Effects of lithium carbonate and haloperidol on cognition in aggressive hospitalized school aged children. *Journal of Clinical Psychopharmacology*, *1*, 8–13.

Poling, A., & Breuning, S.E. (1983). Effects of methylphenidate on the fixed ratio performance of mentally retarded children. *Pharmacology, Biochemistry and Behavior*, *18*, 541–544.

Rapoport, J.L., Buchsbaum, M.S., Weingartner, H., Zahn, T.P., Ludlow, C., & Mikkelsen, E.J. (1980). Dextroamphetamine—Its cognitive and behavioral effects in normal and hyperactive boys and normal men. *Archives of General Psychiatry*, *37*, 933–943.

Reid, A.J., & Leonard, A. (1977). Lithium treatment of cyclical vomiting in a mentally defective patient. *British Journal of Psychiatry*, *130*, 316.

Rimland, B. (1977). *Comparative effects of treatment on child's behavior*. San Diego: Institute of Child Behavior.

Rivinus, T.M. (1980). Psychopharmacology and the mentally retarded patient. In L.S. Szymanski & P.E. Tanguay (Eds.), *Emotional disorders of mentally retarded persons* (pp. 195–221). Baltimore: University Park Press.

Rutter, M.L. (1975). Psychiatric disorder and intellectual impairment in childhood. *British Journal of Psychiatry*, *SP #9*, 344–348.

Sandman, C.A., Datta, P., & Barron, J. (1983). Naloxone attenuates self-abusive behavior in developmentally disabled clients. *Applied Research in Mental Retardation*, *3*, 5–11.

Schmidt, D. (1983). How to use benzodiazepines. In P.L. Morselli, C.E. Pippinger, & J.K. Penry (Eds.), *Antiepileptic drug therapy in pediatrics* (pp. 271–280). New York: Raven Press.

Sheard, M.H. (1970a). Behavioral effects of p-chlorophenylalanine: Inhibition by lithium. *Behavioral Biology*, *5*, 71–73.

Sheard, M.H. (1970b). Effect of lithium on footshock aggression in rats. *Nature*, *228*, 284–285.

Sheard, M.H. (1975). Lithium in the treatment of aggression. *The Journal of Nervous and Mental Disease*, *160*, 108–118.

Sheehan, D.V. (1985). Monoamine oxidase inhibitors and alprazolam in the treatment of panic disorder and agoraphobia. *Psychiatric Clinics of North America, 8,* 49–62.

Silva, D.A. (1979). The use of medication in a residential institution for mentally retarded persons. *Mental Retardation, 17,* 285–288.

Sireling, L. (1986). Depression in mentally handicapped patients: Diagnostic and neuroendocrine evaluation. *British Journal of Psychiatry, 149,* 274–278.

Soblen, R.A., & Saunders, J.C. (1961). Monoamine oxidase inhibitor therapy in adolescent psychiatry. *Diseases of the Nervous System, 22,* 96–100.

Sovner, R., & Hurley, A.D. (1983). Do the mentally retarded suffer from affective illness. *Archives of General Psychiatry, 40,* 61–67.

Speigel, K., Kalb, R., & Pasternak, G.W. (1983). Analgesic activity of tricyclic antidepressants. *Annals of Neurology, 13,* 462–465.

Spencer, D.A. (1980). Ronyl (pemoline) in overactive mentally subnormal children. *British Journal of Psychology, 8,* 491–500.

Sprague, R.L. (1987). [Letter to the editor]. *Journal of Mental Deficiency Research, 31,* 223–225.

Sprague, R.L., & Sleator, E.K. (1977). Methylphenidate in hyperkinetic children: Differences in dose effects on learning and social behavior. *Science, 198,* 1274–1276.

Tallman, J.F., Paul, S.M., Skolnick, P., & Gallager, D.W. (1980). Receptors for the age of anxiety: Pharmacology of the benzodiazepines. *Science, 207,* 274–281.

Trimble, M.R. (1983). Benzodiazepines in epilepsy. In M.R. Trimble (Ed.), *Benzodiazepines divided: A multidisciplinary review* (pp. 277–288). New York: Wiley.

Tu, J.B. (1979). A survey of psychotropic medication in mental retardation facilities. *Journal of Clinical Psychiatry, 40,* 125–128.

Tyrer, S.P., Walsh, A., Edwards, D.E., Berney, T.P., & Stephens, D.A. (1984). Factors associated with a good response to lithium in aggressive mentally handicapped subjects. *Progress in Neuropsychopharmacology, Biology and Psychiatry, 8,* 751–755.

Varley, C.K., & Trupin, E.W. (1982). Double-blind administration of methylphenidate to mentally retarded children with attention deficit disorder: A double-blind study. *American Journal of Mental Deficiency, 86,* 560–566.

Walters, A., Singh, N., & Beale, I.L. (1977). Effects of lorazepam on hyperactivity in retarded children. *New Zealand Medical Journal, 86,* 473–475.

Worrall, E.P., Moody, J.P., & Naylor, G.J. (1975) Lithium in non-manic depressives: Antiaggressive effect and red blood cell lithium values. *British Journal of Psychiatry, 126,* 464–468.

Zrull, J.P., Westman, J.C., Arthur, B., & Bell, W.A. (1963). A comparison of chlordiazepoxide, d-amphetamine and placebo in the treatment of hyperkinetic syndrome in children. *American Journal of Psychiatry, 120,* 590–591.

Zrull, J.P., Westman, J.C., Arthur, B., & Rice, D.L. (1964). A comparison of diazepam, d-amphetamine and placebo in the treatment of hyperkinetic syndrome in children. *American Journal of Psychiatry, 121,* 388–389.

7
Novel Psychoactive Agents in the Treatment of Developmental Disorders

MAE S. SOKOL AND MAGDA CAMPBELL

Abstract

The rationale for the search for novel drugs in infantile autism, mental retardation associated with behavioral symptoms (including self-mutilation), Tourette syndrome, Down syndrome, and Lesch-Nyhan syndrome is presented. The literature on the use of fenfluramine, naloxone, naltrexone, clonidine, clonazepam, propranolol, and 5-hydroxytryptophan is reviewed. Efficacy and safety, the two main concerns in the use of pharmacotherapy in children with developmental disabilities, are discussed. The relationship between abnormalities of neurotransmitters and a rational intervention with neuropsychopharmacological agents has yet to be elucidated. Much work remains to be done in the treatment of these severely, and often multiply, handicapped children.

Introduction

There are two fundamental concerns when prescribing psychoactive agents to individuals with developmental disabilities whose behavioral, motor, or other symptoms may respond to a drug. These are efficacy and safety. Some symptoms of developmentally disabled individuals are particularly unresponsive to various pharmacological approaches, including the currently available standard drugs. Among these are aggressiveness directed against others and a particularly disturbing behavioral problem, self-mutilation. Both clinical experience and carefully designed studies show that not all patients within a diagnostic category respond, even to a well-established and therapeutically effective drug.

Furthermore, drugs that are effective in decreasing behavioral symptoms may have adverse effects on cognition and learning (Campbell et al., 1984; Werry & Aman, 1975), a very serious issue in children, and particularly in

---

At the time of the writing of this paper, Dr. Sokol was a Clinical Instructor in Psychiatry and a Fellow in Child and Adolescent Psychiatry, Department of Psychiatry, New York University Medical Center, 550 First Avenue, New York, New York 10016.

those who already function on a retarded level and/or have learning disabilities. Even drugs that are effective in reducing or controlling behavioral symptoms and facilitate learning in the laboratory at the same doses (Anderson et al., 1984; Campbell et al., 1978) may be associated with the development of untoward effects when given over prolonged periods of time (Campbell, Grega, Green, & Bennett, 1983; Campbell, Perry, et al., 1983; Golden, Campbell, & Perry, 1987; Gualtieri, Quade, Hicks, Mayo, & Schroeder, 1984; Perry et al., 1985). Since learning, cognitive problems, and subnormal intellectual functioning are usually prominent features in developmental disabilities, drugs that may enhance learning or promote the development of functions that are rudimentary or absent (e.g., language, adaptive skills), while at the same time treating basic behavior problems, are considered highly desirable. Finally, some drugs are effective in terms of statistical significance, but their clinical efficacy is modest at best (Sprague, 1978). Thus, when seeking novel drugs for this field, a heavy emphasis should be placed on efficacy and safety, while at the same time ensuring that the agent does not disrupt cognitive performance.

In recent years, considerable progress has been made in disclosing biochemical abnormalities associated with behavioral, motor, and cognitive phenomena in developmentally disabled people. Several attempts have been made to determine whether the administration of drugs with certain biochemical and pharmacological action, and the potential for correcting biochemical (e.g., neurotransmitter) abnormalities, is associated with a decrease or control of corresponding symptoms (see Campbell, Perry, Small, & Green, 1987). Neurotransmitters are chemical agents that transmit impulses between nerve cells. Many of the actions of drugs used to alter central nervous system (CNS) function imitate or alter the actions of these neurotransmitters (see also Chapter 10). This is the rationale for exploring novel drugs in these populations (see also Table 7.1, which summarizes drug effects in terms of neurochemical profiles in various clinical conditions).

Fenfluramine

Claims for a strong therapeutic effect of fenfluramine and potentially positive effects on IQ and antiserotonergic effects in autistic children were first reported in 1982 by Geller, Ritvo, Freeman, and Yuwiler. This enthusiastic report was based on a study of three outpatients and was followed by a large multicenter study (18 centers), individual studies, and clinical use of this drug.

Fenfluramine is a drug structurally similar to amphetamine. It is a mild antidopaminergic agent and a powerful antiserotonergic drug (Costa, Gropetti, & Revuelta, 1971), which has both stimulating and tranquilizing effects. It is an anorectogenic drug and thus is used in obese individuals in the United States and especially in Europe. However, it has also been

TABLE 7.1. Novel therapeutic agents for developmental disabilities.

Psychoactive agent	Clinical condition	Rationale	Efficacy
Fenfluramine	Infantile autism	Increased serotonin in 30% of autistic children; fenfluramine is a potent antiserotonergic agent	Inconclusive results: may decrease hyperactivity, stereotypies, and echolalia; may increase eye contact, language, and enhance cognitive functions
Opiate antagonists (naloxone, naltrexone)	Mental retardation—associated with self-mutilation	Endogenous opioids reduce pain Abnormalities of endogenous opioid system may be involved in the neurochemical basis of infantile autism	Some positive but inconclusive findings so far
	Infantile autism—to decrease self-mutilation and increase social behaviors, etc.	Opiate antagonists decrease the pain threshold and therefore increase pain sensitivity	
5-Hydroxytryptophan	Down syndrome	5-HTP is a precursor of serotonin; decreased serotonin levels are found in some Down syndrome patients	Negative results
	Lesch-Nyhan syndrome	Self-mutilation and aggression possibly related to decreased serotonin levels	Equivocal effects on self-mutilation with 5-HTP
	Infantile autism	Dysregulation of serotonergic system postulated in the pathogenesis of autism	
	Tourette syndrome	Hypoactive serotonergic functioning	Decreased symptoms in one subject
Propranolol	Violent and explosive behaviors in mental retardation	Propranolol is a β-adrenergic blocking agent which decreases sympathetic discharge	Favorable results in early, uncontrolled studies
Clonidine	Tourette syndrome	Clonidine decreases adrenergic tone; adrenaline may affect symptoms of TS	Good second-line drug; best for alleviating compulsive, aggressive, behavioral, and attentional problems
Clonazepam	Tourette syndrome	Clonazepam increases glutamate release (as does haloperidol)	Not of therapeutic value alone, but may be a useful adjunct to other drugs

TS = Tourette syndrome; 5-HTP = 5-hydroxytryptophan; serotonin = a neurotransmitter that mediates certain behaviors and physiological and cognitive functions; endogenous opioids = endorphins, enkephalins, and dynorphins—the body's own supply of opiates or morphine-like substances, which mediate pain control; neurotransmitter = chemical substance that transmits impulses across synapses and neuroeffector junctions in the nervous system.

explored in adult patients with a variety of psychiatric disorders (Raich, Rickels, & Raab, 1966; Shore, Korpi, Bigelow, Zec, & Wyatt, 1985). In certain laboratory animals, both short- and long-term administration of this drug results in depletion of brain serotonin with return to previous values after its discontinuation (Dehault & Boulanger, 1977). However, depletion with possible long-term or irreversible changes has also been reported (Schuster, Lewis, & Seiden, 1986). At this stage, the implications of animal studies to clinical work are unclear.

Fenfluramine has been studied in autistic children because of its anti-serotonergic effects. Abnormalities of the serotonergic system, specifically high serotonin levels, have been reported in about 30% of autistic children (Campbell et al., 1975; Ritvo et al., 1970). The neurotransmitter serotonin has been implicated in various functions, which include certain behaviors and physiological and cognitive functions (see Young, Kavanagh, Anderson, Shaywitz, & Cohen, 1982). Ritvo and associates (Geller et al., 1982) hypothesized that if serotonin is elevated in the brains of autistic persons who have hyperserotonemia, then lowering of serotonin with administration of fenfluramine may be associated with decreases of certain related behavioral symptoms.

The positive effects of fenfluramine reported in the Geller et al. (1982) study were replicated in 14 autistic outpatients, ages 3 to 18 years, under double-blind and placebo-controlled conditions, with a fixed dose of 1.5 mg/kg/day (Ritvo, Freeman, Geller, & Yuwiler, 1983). In all subjects, a 2-week open placebo baseline was followed by 1-month placebo, 4 months of drug, and, finally, by a 2-month placebo period. Behavioral ratings and IQ testings were performed monthly. Marked decreases of hyperactivity, stereotypies, and echolalia were rated, as well as increases of eye contact, socialization, social awareness, spontaneous and appropriate language, and improved sleep pattern. Nine children gained weight during the 4-month administration of fenfluramine, whereas one 5-year-old child lost 2 pounds and an 18-year-old lost 6 pounds. In six subjects, significant rises in verbal and performance IQs were measured on age-appropriate Wechsler Intelligence Scales; however, the performance IQs continued to show significant increases even 2 months after drug discontinuation, suggesting that a practice effect was operative (Kaufman, 1979). Fenfluramine administration was accompanied by significant decreases of serotonin in blood (an average of 51% after 1 month), which returned to baseline 1 month after discontinuation of drug.

The subjects from the preceding study resumed fenfluramine treatment for another 8 months, which was followed by a 2-month placebo period (Ritvo et al., 1984). The results of this 10-month trial were combined with those in the previous study. Again, the effects of fenfluramine on behavioral symptoms, IQ, and serotonin were replicated. During treatment, eight patients lost weight that they regained during the final placebo period (at 17 months).

August, Raz, and Baird (1985) reported similar behavioral improvements with fenfluramine. However, they did not find increases in IQs in their sample of nine autistic children using the same study design. Most children had transient mild to moderate weight loss. Leventhal (1985) also employed the same design and found that fenfluramine administration was accompanied by significant decreases of serotonin without therapeutic effects in 16 children. Klykylo, Feldis, O'Grady, Ross, and Halloran (1985), who were also participants of Ritvo's multicenter study, reported their findings with 10 subjects. Two, or possibly three, responded beneficially to the drug, with calming effects most prominent; no changes in IQs were found. Weight loss and transient lethargy were the only side effects reported. Groden et al. (1987) found that fenfluramine improved activity level and scores on the sensory response subscale of the Real Life Rating Scale, but there were no net changes on cognitive performance measures.

Of the 18 centers participating in the multicenter study under Ritvo's direction, nine have pooled and analyzed their data involving 81 patients, ages 2 to 24 years (Ritvo et al., 1986). Thirty-three percent of the subjects were considered strong responders. Furthermore, a significant inverse correlation was found between baseline serotonin levels and clinical response, on the one hand, and baseline serotonin levels and IQs on the other.

An independent open pilot study involved 10 autistic inpatients, ages 3 to 5 years (Campbell et al., 1986). Therapeutic doses of fenfluramine ranged from 1.09 to 1.79 mg/kg/day (mean, 1.41). Both calming and stimulating therapeutic effects were noted: four low IQ children improved markedly. At the end of 1 month of fenfluramine administration, most children had weight loss, followed by weight gain at the end of a 2nd month on drug. Above optimal doses, drowsiness, lethargy, and uncontrollable irritability were most common. All laboratory studies including electrocardiogram remained within normal limits. In some patients the positive effects were transient, suggesting a serious limitation of this drug.

Although these early findings are encouraging, it should be noted that the collaborative study by Ritvo et al. (1986) had some methodological flaws. Drug order was not balanced in the sense that drug-placebo periods were of unequal duration. Hence, practice was confounded with drug condition, and IQ scores could have increased due to practice alone. We are presently carrying out a between-groups, double-blind, and placebo-controlled study of fenfluramine with autistic children. The effects of fenfluramine on behavioral symptoms, side effects, and discrimination learning in an automated laboratory are being assessed in what will ultimately be a large group of autistic children. Preliminary analyses involving 11 inpatients suggest that fenfluramine is not statistically superior to placebo, and that it may even have adverse effects on discrimination learning (Campbell, Small, et al., 1987). A larger sample size of this carefully designed clinical trial will help to establish the role of fenfluramine in the treatment of infantile autism. Only by properly controlled studies, utilizing sensitive clinical and performance measures, will the clinical advantages and limitations of this drug be properly established.

Naloxone and Naltrexone

The opiate antagonists are being explored in persons with mental retardation because of their possible effect in blocking or diminishing aggressiveness directed against self, which may be related to the role that endogenous opioids play in the regulation of pain. The rationale for the use of these drugs in infantile autism is that there is some evidence that a dysregulation of the endogenous opioid system may exist in this condition and that these drugs may normalize abnormalities that underlie some of the clinical manifestations of this syndrome (see Deutsch, 1986).

Specific binding sites or receptors for opiates in the brain of man and animals have been shown to exist (Simon, Hiller, & Edelman, 1973). Furthermore, the existence of endogenous ligands for these opiate receptors were found in the brain and in other tissues, which were identified as peptides (Terenius, 1973; see Verebey, Volavka, & Clouet, 1978). These endogenous opioids or morphine-like substances are called enkephalins and endorphins. They are thought to be neuroregulators influencing other neurotransmitters (serotonin, dopamine, and norepinephrine) and a variety of physiological and behavioral functions, such as attention, social behavior, mood, cognition, memory, perception, appreciation of pain, respiration, and growth hormone. Furthermore, there is supportive evidence that abnormalities or imbalances of the endogenous opioid system exist in subgroups of patients and may play a role in schizophrenia and major affective disorder (Berger et al., 1980; Brambilla, Facchinetti, Petraglia, Vanzulli, & Genazzani, 1984; Terenius, Wahlström, & Agren, 1977; Wahlström, Johansson, & Terenius, 1976; see Verebey et al., 1978), self-mutilation (Coid, Allolio, & Rees, 1983), and infantile autism (Gillberg, Terenius, & Lönnerholm, 1985; Weizman et al., 1984).

Kalat (1978), Panksepp (1979), and Sandyk and Gillman (1986) have all hypothesized that abnormalities of the endogenous opioid system may be the neurochemical basis of infantile autism and that behavioral and other abnormalities associated with this syndrome are analogous to opiate addiction. Panksepp (1979; Panksepp & Sahley, 1987) suggested that administration of an opiate antagonist (e.g., naloxone or naltrexone) should be associated with simultaneous decrease of endogenous opiates and related behavioral and other dysfunctions.

Naltrexone is a potent opiate antagonist, relatively free of side effects and with rapid onset of action (Willette & Barnett, 1981). It was explored in autistic children, by two groups of researchers independently employing acute dose range designs with baseline and posttreatment assessments

(Campbell et al., 1988; Herman, Hammock, Arthur-Smith, Egan, Chatoor, Zelnik, Appelgate, & Boeckx, 1986). A single morning dose of naltrexone was given, once a week, in ascending doses (0.5, 1.0, and 2.0 mg/kg/day). A variety of measures were used by multiple raters under a variety of conditions, and with careful laboratory and behavioral monitoring. Significant decreases of stereotypies and increases of positive social behaviors were rated, as well as increases of verbal production. In general, therapeutic effects were both tranquilizing (e.g. decreases in hyperactivity) and stimulating (e.g., increased attention span, language production). Mild sedation was the only untoward effect (Campbell et al., 1988). Positive effects were observed as late as 24 hours after dosing. All laboratory tests, including those for liver profile and electrocardiogram, remained within normal limits (Campbell et al., 1988). Interestingly, in this sample of patients, naltrexone did not seem to have an effect on aggressiveness directed against self. Even though different assessment instruments were used in the two trials, the results were in agreement. These results justify further studies of naltrexone where its efficacy and safety can be assessed under more controlled conditions.

Serious self-injury can be a major problem in a subgroup of mentally retarded individuals, some of whom are autistic (Schroeder, Schroeder, Smith, & Dalldorf, 1978). This behavioral aberration, which has been reported in 8–14% of residents, is often resistant to both behavioral and traditional pharmacological treatment approaches. As noted above, there is some suggestive evidence that aggressiveness directed against self is a correlate or manifestation of abnormalities in the endogenous opioid system (Buchsbaum, Davis, & Bunney, 1977; Coid et al., 1983). Furthermore, an increased release of endorphins in response to induced pain has been reported (Willer, Dehen, & Cambier, 1981), resulting in elevation of pain threshold and hypoalgesia.

The analgesic effects of opiates such as morphine and heroin are well known; the endogenous opioids, and more specifically the endorphins, may have similar properties (Pert, Pert, Davis, & Bunney, 1981). Increased activity or levels of endogenous opioids may be associated with insensitivity to pain (Coid et al., 1983) and, therefore, directly lead to self-injurious behavior. At alternative interpretation of self-injurious behavior has also been proposed. Painful stimulation yields release of endorphins (Akil, Richardson, Hughes, & Barchas, 1978), which may have reinforcing properties (Belluzzi & Stein, 1977). Accordingly, self-injurious behavior will increase the release of endorphins, which in turn would create a euphoric state that would further reinforce self-mutilation (Sandman et al., 1983). Thus self-injurious behavior may be a manifestation of addiction to some of the endogenous opioid-like endorphins and enkephalins. The hyperalgesic properties of opiate antagonists (Buchsbaum et al., 1977) and their ability to eliminate the possible reinforcing effects of the endogenous opioids (Belluzzi & Stein, 1977; Kelsey, Belluzzi, & Stein, 1984) provide a rational basis for assessing the efficacy of opiate antagonists, such as naloxone and naltrexone, in individuals with prominent features of self-mutilation.

Sandman et al. (1983) administered naloxone to two profoundly retarded nonverbal adults, with a long history of severe self-mutilating behavior. After a stable baseline, three doses of naloxone (0.1, 0.2, and 0.4 mg/kg/day) were given intramuscularly in a double-blind and crossover design. Dosing was on alternate days, and the order of treatment condition was reversed during the 2nd week of treatment. The subjects were videotaped at fixed intervals and the tapes were rated by four raters independently. In one subject, naloxone took effect in 10 minutes, but by 70 to 80 minutes its effects began to diminish. At 0.1 mg/kg, self-injurious episodes were reported as dramatically decreased, with measures of self-restraint reduced to a lesser degree. In the other subject there was also a dramatic change, with self-injury and restraint practically eliminated.

In an open clinical trial, naloxone was given intravenously, for 2 consecutive days, following a 1-day baseline, to a 15-year-old mentally retarded boy with a 10- to 12-year history of severe and treatment-resistant self-mutilation (Richardson & Zaleski, 1983). Naloxone infusion was given over a 6-hour period in two doses: 1 mg/30 ml on the 2nd day, and 2 mg/30 ml on the 3rd day of the study. Self-mutilation actually doubled during the intravenous infusion of the drug but, in the evening and for 2 days poststudy, there was a marked decrease of such behavior as compared to baseline.

The efficacy of naloxone in reducing self-injurious behavior was also explored in an 8-year-old severely retarded boy with a history of severe head-banging (approximately 200–250/hour) of 2 years' duration (Davidson, Kleene, Carroll, & Rockowitz, 1983). As in the report of Richardson and Zaleski (1983), and unlike the Sandman et al. (1983) study, baseline observations were carried out. The study was double-blind, placebo controlled, with randomization and two dosage levels of naloxone over a period of 5 days. Behavioral ratings were done at fixed intervals and interrater reliability was 96%. Head-banging showed no quantitative change, though it seemed to be less intensive in response to naloxone. Two case reports by Bernstein and her associates are more encouraging and suggest the need for further studies (Bernstein, Hughes, & Thompson, 1984; Bernstein, Hughes, Mitchell, & Thompson, 1985). However, in a placebo-controlled and double-blind procedure involving two profoundly retarded individuals, naloxone failed to have an effect on self-injurious behavior (Beckwith, Couk, & Schumacher, 1986).

While naloxone's effects are short-lived, naltrexone is both potent and long-acting and, therefore, perhaps a more appropriate drug for treating self-injurious behavior. For two of three subjects at doses of 0.5–1.5 mg/kg/day, given orally, naltrexone was significantly superior to placebo in reducing self-injurious behavior (Herman, Hammock, Arthur-Smith,

Egan, Chatoor, Zelnik & Boeckx, 1986). These are encouraging preliminary results and require systematic studies of naltrexone in this population.

5-Hydroxytryptophan

The administration of 5-hydroxytryptophan (5-HTP) has been reported to be an effective treatment in several conditions in which there are purportedly low serotonin levels. In adults, these include depression (van Praag & Korf, 1974) and schizophrenia (Wyatt, Vaughan, Galanter, Kaplan, & Green, 1972). In children, there is inconclusive evidence that 5-HTP is useful in Down syndrome (Bazelon et al., 1967), Lesch-Nyhan syndrome (Mizuno & Yugari, 1974), and Tourette syndrome (TS) (Van Woert, Yip, & Balis, 1977). Five-HTP is a precursor of the CNS neurotransmitter serotonin (5-hydroxytryptamine). Serotonin is synthesized from the amino acid, tryptophan. Endogenous serotonin is believed to be involved in pain perception, sleep, and various normal and abnormal behaviors, associated with affective disorders (Douglas, 1985) and infantile autism (Campbell et al., 1975; Ritvo et al., 1970; see Young et al., 1982).

Down Syndrome

The therapeutic efficacy of 5-HTP in Down syndrome was explored following the finding that trisomy 21 Down syndrome patients had decreased peripheral blood levels of serotonin (Rosner, Ong, Paine, & Mahanand, 1965). It has been reported that in a Down syndrome patient, decreased platelet serotonin correlated with a variety of symptoms, including degree of hypotonia, decreased activity level, and buccolingual dyskinesia (Coleman, 1971).

Bazelon et al. (1967) administered 5-HTP orally to 14 Down syndrome infants with hypotonia. Administration of oral 5-HTP was started between 2 and 102 days after birth. Eleven subjects received *d-l*, 5-HTP and three were given *l*, 5-HTP. Hypotonicity was used as a guideline for adjusting 5-HTP dosage. Improved muscle tone was reported, but no inferences about intelligence could be made from this study. Adverse effects included motor restlessness, vomiting, diarrhea, opisthotonos, hypertension, and cutaneous flushing.

Partington, MacDonald and Tu (1971) performed a short-term, placebo-controlled study of 5-HTP in Down syndrome children. Subjects were 12 mentally retarded children, six with nonspecific forms of trisomy 21, and six with severe mental retardation. Reports of motor activity and behavior were collected from nurses and scored on a 5-point scale. A neurological examination was standardized for this study with particular attention to motor activity measured by an actometer, protrusion of tongue, and muscle tone. No behavioral or neurological changes were found.

Weise, Koch, Shaw, and Rosenfeld (1974) gave 5-HTP to 26 Down syndrome infants and found no developmental improvement as measured by the Gesell Developmental Schedules, and no improvement in muscle tone. Medication was given from early infancy until age 3 to 4 years; 19 of the 26 subjects completed the trial. Three of the patients developed loose stools.

Pueschel, Reed, Cronk, and Goldstein (1980) reported a double-blind study of 89 Down syndrome children in which patients were randomly assigned to placebo, pyridoxine, 5-HTP, or 5-HTP plus pyridoxine (the coenzyme needed in 5-HTP's decarboxylation to serotonin). Pyridoxine was employed because it reportedly increases serotonin levels in Down syndrome children (see also Chapter 8). All three active treatments raised serotonin blood levels equally well in about 40% of patients. Initial analyses showed that 5-HTP enhanced adaptive function, with significant increments observed on the Vineland Social Maturity Scale. However, when parental compliance in administering medication was taken into account, there was no longer any significant difference between the treatment group in regard to cognitive and adaptive functioning.

It should be noted that little is known about 5-HTP and serotonin transport across the blood-brain barrier or how administration of these compounds affects the various functions of the brain (Pueschel et al., 1980). In any case, these studies failed to demonstrate any improvement in behavior or muscle tone when 5-HTP was administered to Down syndrome patients.

Lesch-Nyhan Syndrome

The Lesch-Nyhan syndrome results from an inborn error of metabolism in which self-mutilation is prominent (Lesch & Nyhan, 1964; Nyhan, 1976). Mental retardation, cerebral palsy, and choreoathetosis may be associated with this condition (Nyhan, Johnson, Kaufman, & Jones, 1980). Biting, usually starting in infancy when teeth first erupt, causes a distinctive tissue loss of lips and fingers. Animal models and human studies suggest that aggressive and self-mutilative behaviors are related to hyposerotonemia (Cataldo & Harris, 1982; Nyhan et al., 1980). This has led to therapeutic strategies to decrease self-mutilation in humans by increasing serotonin levels.

In an open trial, Mizuno and Yugari (1974) administered oral 5-HTP, serotonin's immediate precursor, to four Lesch-Nyhan syndrome patients, ages 1 to 12 years. Five-HTP was administered for 36 weeks; mutilation ceased in all four subjects and reappeared within 12 to 15 hours of discontinuing 5-HTP. Nyhan et al. (1980) treated nine Lesch-Nyhan patients, ages 5 to 14 years, with 5-HTP and concurrent carbidopa. Imipramine was added to the regimen, the rationale being to increase serotonin's central action. Though the drugs were administered in an open fashion, the patients were videotaped, and the tapes were judged by raters who were blind to the treatment. Self-mutilation was significantly reduced in seven patients, but tolerance developed within 1 to 3 months. However, Mizuno and Yugari (1974) did not observe tolerance phenomena during 36 weeks of 5-HTP administration, without the peripheral decarboxylase inhibitor carbidopa. Others have failed to obtain positive results with 5-HTP (Anderson, Herrmann, & Dancis, 1976; Ciaranello, Anders, Barchas, Berger, & Cann, 1976). Overall, the results of 5-HTP use for control of self-mutilation in Lesch-Nyhan syndrome seem equivocal. Even in studies where a positive effect was seen, tolerance was often reported.

Infantile Autism

In contrast to Down syndrome subjects, about one third of autistic children have elevated serotonin levels in peripheral blood (Ritvo et al., 1970), particularly those with low IQs (Campbell et al., 1975). However, a subgroup of autistic children with high IQs appears to have low serotonin concentrations (Ritvo et al, 1986). Nevertheless, two reports of 5-HTP treatment in autistic children failed to show therepeutic effects (Sverd, Kupietz, & Winsberg, 1978; Zarcone et al., 1973), and 5-HTP does not appear to be of value in treating this disorder.

Tourette Syndrome

Finally, hypoactive serotonergic functioning has been postulated in Tourette syndrome (TS) (Butler, Koslow, Seifert, Caprioli, & Singer, 1979; Cohen, Shaywitz, Caparulo, Young, & Bowers, 1978; Lal, Allen, Etienne, Sourkes, & Humphreys, 1977). A serotonin antagonist, cyproheptadine, when given in open fashion, aggravated motor and phonic tics in a 10-year-old male with TS. Immediate partial relief of tics occurred after discontinuing cyproheptadine. Van Woert et al. (1977) reported that the serotonin precursor 5-HTP decreased symptoms in a 15-year-old male TS patient in whom self-mutilation was the major symptom. L-5-HTP in combination with carbidopa controlled the motor and phonic tics and self-mutilation.

Conclusion

Although much hope has been placed on 5-HTP's usefulness in conditions with low serotonin levels, its efficacy has not been substantiated. There is no evidence that individuals with Down syndrome and infantile autism are helped by this medication, whereas there is equivocal evidence for its efficacy in Lesch-Nyhan and Tourette syndromes.

Propranolol

Violence is one of the most difficult management problems faced by those who work with developmentally disabled persons. The mainstay of pharmacotherapy for violent behavior has been the neuroleptics, but lithium salts, benzodiazepines, and anticonvulsants have also been used. The fact that these agents are often ineffective or cause troublesome side effects has led to a search for medications with greater efficacy and safety.

Propranolol is one such agent under investigation. There is an increasing body of data that indicates that propranolol is effective in numerous psychopathological conditions, including violent and explosive behaviors in patients with organic brain damage (Elliott, 1977; Mattes, Rosenberg, & Mays, 1984; Ratey, Morrill, & Oxenkrug, 1983; Williams, Mehl, Yudofsky, Adams & Roseman, 1982; Yudofsky, Williams, & Gorman, 1981).

Propranolol is a β-adrenergic blocking agent used widely in the treatment of hypertension. Both brain and peripheral β-adrenergic receptors are subject to its effects. It interferes with the function of the sympathetic nervous system by blocking receptors on effector organs in a competitive fashion, thereby inhibiting the ability of sympathomimetic amines such as noradrenaline to act (Weiner, 1985). Thus, sympathetic discharge, which prepares the organism for "fight or flight" and mediates stress and anxiety, can be modulated by propranolol. In psychiatric disorders, there is not yet clear evidence of propranolol's mode of action. Speculation that propranolol alters mood and behavior mainly by its actions on the brain has been disputed (see Elliott, 1977; Yudofsky et al., 1981).

Treating aggressive symptoms with propranolol in psychiatric patients usually requires higher doses (up to 20 mg/kg/day) than those used in hypertension (2–4 mg/kg/day). Careful monitoring of vital signs in an inpatient setting and dosage increment of 20 mg or less per day can help to reach high therapeutic propranolol levels safely.

A retrospective study suggests that propranolol may be useful in treating rage outbursts that had begun in childhood or adolescence (Williams et al., 1982). Thirty patients, 7 to 35 years of age, who failed to respond to stimulants, neuroleptics, anticonvulsants, or combinations of these, received 50 to 1,600 mg/day (median 161 mg/day) of propranolol in an open fashion. More than 75% of these patients improved moderately to markedly on propranolol. Adverse effects included somnolence, lethargy, hypotension, bradycardia, and depression. All side effects were transient and reversible. Moreover, propranolol's efficacy-to-adverse-effect ratio was clearly more favorable than that of neuroleptics, anticonvulsants, and stimulants.

A recent open clinical trial of propranolol treatment in 19 severely to profoundly retarded patients with unmanageable behavior yielded favorable results (Ratey et al., 1986). A substantial decrease in aggressive and self-abusive behavior was demonstrated in 12 of the subjects. Four others showed moderate improvements, and three did not respond. The mean dose of 120 mg/day (range 40–240 mg/day) was much lower than in studies of subjects having normal IQ. The authors pointed out that prolonged therapy at a given dose may augment the chances of observing therapeutic effects. Hypotension and/or bradycardia occurred at low doses in seven of these patients, who were therefore not able to receive more than 100 mg/

day. Two of these subjects were among the three who showed no improvement from the medication.

Controlled prospective studies with concomitant neurochemical evaluations are critical to assess further propranolol's efficacy and mode of action in violent behavior.

Clonidine

Clonidine hydrochloride has recently been found to be effective in the treatment of Tourette syndrome, a condition characterized by motor and vocal tics as well as attentional difficulties, hyperactivity, compulsions, and obsessions. It is now well established clinically that many TS patients are relieved of symptoms by haloperidol, a potent dopamine receptor blocking agent. This led to the hypothesis that overactivity of one or more central dopaminergic neurotransmitter systems is involved in TS, a position largely supported by many pharmacological studies. However, adrenergic, cholinergic, and serotonergic systems have also been implicated in TS (Friedhoff & Chase, 1982).

Haloperidol is the first drug found to be effective for TS and remains the drug of choice (Bruun, 1984; Shapiro & Shapiro, 1982a). It relieves symptoms of up to 80% of patients but, because of side effects, only about 20% choose to continue haloperidol therapy for long periods (Cohen, Detlor, Young, & Shaywitz, 1980). Side effects include short-term untoward effects, such as extrapyramidal, anticholinergic, sedative, and hypotensive effects, as well as interference with cognitive performance and mood (Baldessarini, 1985; Borison et al., 1982; Cohen et al., 1980). The long-term side effect, tardive dyskinesia, is of greater concern (see Chapter 9). The use of other neuroleptics, such as pimozide, poses the same problems. This has led to a search for newer, safer medications, such as clonidine, to treat TS.

Clonidine seems to have fewer side effects than haloperidol, and no severe adverse effects have been reported. It is an alpha-adrenergic agonist that decreases central adrenergic tone. It is often used in the treatment of hypertension (see Rudd & Blaschke, 1985). Cohen, Young, Nathanson, and Shaywitz (1979) administered clonidine (2–3 μg/kg/day) to eight children having severe TS symptoms, who had failed to respond to haloperidol or could not tolerate its side effects. Decreases were observed in the severity of tics as well as psychiatric symptoms. Leckman et al. (1982) have suggested that factors possibly predictive of outcome with clonidine administration may include sex, age, age of onset, family history, and response to clonidine by other family members. Borison et al. (1982) found that patients (age range 8–44 years, $M = 18$ years) who responded to haloperidol also tended to respond to clonidine, and they hypothesized that this may indicate that both drugs work through similar mechanisms.

Of the first nine trials of clonidine between 1979 and 1982, six were conducted without double-blind or placebo-controlled conditions. Four found favorable results, with at least 50% of patients benefiting (Leckman et al., 1982). Results were similar in subsequent placebo-controlled, double-blind trials. Some recent studies have indicated that clonidine is affective in 25% to 70% of TS patients (Selinger et al., 1984), whereas Cohen et al. (1980) reported that more than 70% of TS patients respond to clonidine.

Bruun (1984) reported that in her clinical experience 34 of 72 patients (47%) responded satisfactorily to clonidine, and 11 had a better response to haloperidol and clonidine combined than to haloperidol alone. Bruun considered clonidine successful if patients preferred to remain on the medication and there was a 50% or greater reduction of tics. The patients reported improvement in mood, concentration, and motivation on clonidine, but tics were not reduced as dramatically as with haloperidol. Thirty-eight of the 72 patients did not have a satisfactory response to clonidine, either because of a lack of a therapeutic response or adverse effects (irritability, insomnia, racing thoughts, nightmares) or both. It is noteworthy that only 7 of these 72 patients had not received haloperidol in the past, and these 7 all improved on clonidine; however, they all had mild symptomatology.

Clonidine seems less effective than haloperidol in decreasing the motor and vocal tics of TS, but more effective in alleviating compulsive, aggressive, behavioral, and attentional problems. Patients often report, however, that they feel less concerned about their tics while on clonidine (Cohen et al., 1980; Bruun, 1984; Leckman et al., 1982). There is evidence that clonidine remains effective in reducing the symptoms of patients with TS when administered over a period of up to 4 years. The results of Leckman et al. (1982) are consistent with earlier reports (Cohen, Young, et al., 1979; Cohen et al., 1980). Patients who responded initially to clonidine continued to do so with long-term treatment and in some cases even showed increased improvement. Children with extremely severe TS have benefited over this length of time and have required only slight increments in dosage (Cohen, Leckman, & Shaywitz, 1985).

Clonidine appears to be a safe and effective *second-line* treatment for TS. It may also be a useful adjunct to haloperidol in certain cases. Although it is less effective than haloperidol in alleviating motor and vocal tics, patients often feel less bothered by their tics while on clonidine.

Clonazepam

There is evidence that clonazepam may be an effective therapeutic agent in several clinical conditions (Chouinard, 1985; Chouinard, Young, & Annable, 1983; Falk, 1986; Victor, Link, Binder, & Bell, 1984). It is beneficial in the treatment of several types of epileptic seizures (absence, atypical absence, infantile spasm, myoclonic, and atonic) and has been approved in the United States for this purpose since 1960 (Browne, 1976, 1978). More recent reports indicate that this drug given alone, or in conjunction with haloperidol or clonidine, has therapeutic value in some patients with TS (Bruun, 1984).

Clonazepam is a high-potency benzodiazepine, having antianxiety, sedative, hypnotic, and antiseizure properties. The benzodiazepines exert mainly presynaptic, and some postsynaptic, inhibition in the central nervous system (CNS), which simulates the action of γ-aminobutyric acid (GABA), and enhances GABA-induced glutamate release (Harvey, 1985). GABA, glutamate, and glycine are amino acids that act as neurotransmitters in the CNS. It is of note that haloperidol (the drug of choice in TS) and benzodiazepines both increase glutamate release (Browne, 1976).

Gonce and Barbeau (1977) conducted an open pilot study of clonazepam in seven patients with TS. They found partial improvement, mainly in vocalizations, but also in motor tics in three patients; two of these patients improved on 2 mg twice a day with no further improvement at higher doses. The third patient showing improvement received clonazepam 3.5 mg/day combined with haloperidol and biperiden hydrochloride. However, although this patient showed decreased frequency and intensity of barks as well as fewer motor tics, an old symptom (facial grimaces) reappeared with clonazepam administration. Two other patients of the seven had equivocal results. Shapiro and Shapiro (1981, 1982b) had inconclusive results with clonazepam in TS, and Bruun (1984) reported that it may be useful only in conjunction with haloperidol or clonidine.

Thus, clonazepam may be useful as an adjunct to other drugs in TS, but does not appear to be of therapeutic value when used alone. It is impossible at this time to make definitive conclusions about clonazepam's efficacy because of the naturally fluctuating course of the syndrome as well as the small number of subjects studied. Placebo-controlled, double-blind, and carefully designed studies are needed to assess further the role of clonazepam in TS (Caine, 1985).

Conclusion

The research with novel psychoactive agents exemplifies strategies that may be used in seeking useful pharmacological intervention for specific conditions. In many cases, biochemical or neurochemical features associated with a given disorder have suggested the use of a particular agent that theoretically might be expected to correct the observed imbalance and hence to have a therapeutic effect. This has led to work with numerous different agents, seven of which are described in this chapter. Although not all of this work was strictly formulated in such a logical context, as a group this work suggests a rational, scientific basis for extending our knowledge of both therapeutic modalities and the pathophysiology of the developmental disabilities. Unfortunately, these attempts have not always met with therapeutic success. Nevertheless, it is likely that this method will be more successful than the hit-or-miss approach that often characterized early drug research with developmentally disabled individuals, and it is to be hoped that researchers of the future will continue to refine this strategy.

Acknowledgments. This work was supported in part by NIMH Grants MH-32212 and MH-40177, by a grant from Stallone Fund for Autism Research, and by Social and Behavioral Sciences Research Grant 12-108 from March of Dimes Birth Defects Foundation (Dr. Campbell).

References

Akil, H., Richardson, D.E., Hughes, J., & Barchas, J.D. (1978). Enkephalin-like material in ventricular cerebrospinal fluid of pain patients after analgetic focal stimulation. *Science*, *201*, 463–465.

Anderson, L.T., Campbell, M., Grega, D.M., Perry, R., Small, A.M., & Green, W.H. (1984). Haloperidol in infantile autism: Effects on learning and behavioral symptoms. *American Journal of Psychiatry*, *141*, 1195–1202.

Anderson, L.T., Herrmann, L., & Dancis, J. (1976). The effects of L-5-hydroxytryptophan on self-mutilation in Lesch-Nyhan disease: A negative report. *Neuropadiatrie*, *7*, 439–442.

August, G.J., Raz, N., & Baird, T.D. (1985). Brief report: Effects of fenfluramine on behavioral, cognitive, and affective disturbances in autistic children. *Journal of Autism and Developmental Disorders*, *15*, 97–107.

Baldessarini, R.J. (1985). Drugs and the treatment of psychiatric disorders. In A.G. Gilman, L.S. Goodman, T.W. Rall & F. Murad (Eds.), *The pharmacological basis of therapeutics* (pp. 387–445). New York: Macmillan.

Bazelon, M., Paine, R.S., Cowie, V.A., Hunt, P., Houck, J.C., & Mahanand, D. (1967). Reversal of hypotonia in infants with Down's syndrome by administration of 5-hydroxytryptophan. *Lancet*, *1*, 1130–1133.

Beckwith, B.E., Couk, D.I., & Schumacher, K. (1986). Failure of naloxone to reduce self-injurious behavior in two developmentally disabled females. *Applied Research in Mental Retardation*, *7*, 183–188.

Belluzzi, J.D., & Stein, L. (1977). Enkephalin may mediate euphoria and drive-reduction reward. *Nature*, *26*, 556–558.

Berger, P.A., Watson, S.J., Akil, H., Elliott, G.R., Rubin, R.T., Pfefferbaum, A., Davis, K.L., Barchas, J.D., & Li, C.H. (1980). β-endorphin and schizophrenia. *Archives of General Psychiatry*, *37*, 635–640.

Bernstein, G.A., Hughes, J.R., Mitchell, J.E., & Thompson, T. (1985). Effects of naltrexone on self-injurious behavior: A case study. *Proceedings of the 32nd Annual Meeting of the American Academy of Child Psychiatry*, p. 33.

Bernstein, G.A., Hughes, J.R., & Thompson, T. (1984, October). *Naloxone reduces the self-injurious behavior of a mentally retarded adolescent.* Paper presented at the Annual Meeting of the American Academy of Child Psychiatry and Canadian Academy of Child Psychiatry, Toronto, Canada.

Borison, R.L., Ang, L., Chang, S., Dysken, M., Comaty, J.E., & Davis, J.M. (1982). New pharmacological approaches in the treatment of Tourette syndrome. In A.J. Friedhoff & T.N. Chase (Eds.), *Advances in neurology, Gilles de la Tourette syndrome* (Vol. 35, pp. 377–382). New York: Raven Press.

Brambilla, F., Facchinetti, F., Petraglia, F., Vanzulli, L., & Genazzani, A.R. (1984). Secretion pattern of endogenous opioids in chronic schizophrenia. *American Journal of Psychiatry, 141*, 1183–1189.

Browne, T.R. (1976). Clonazepam: A review of a new anticonvulsant drug. *Archives of Neurology, 33*, 326–332.

Browne, T.R. (1978). Clonazepam. *New England Journal of Medicine, 229*, 812–816.

Bruun, R.D. (1984). Gilles de la Tourette's syndrome: An overview of clinical experience. *Journal of the American Academy of Child Psychiatry, 23*, 126–133.

Buchsbaum, M.S., Davis, G.C., & Bunney, W.E., Jr. (1977). Naloxone alters pain perception and somatosensory evoked potentials in normal subjects. *Nature, 270*, 620–622.

Butler, I.J., Koslow, S.H., Seifert, W.E., Caprioli, R.M., & Singer, H.S. (1979). Biogenic amine metabolism in Tourette syndrome. *Annals of Neurology, 6*, 37–39.

Caine, E.D. (1985). Gilles de la Tourette's syndrome. A review of clinical and research studies and consideration of future directions for investigation. *Archives of Neurology, 42*, 393–397.

Campbell, M., Anderson, L.T., Meier, M., Cohen, I.L., Small, A.M., Samit, C., & Sachar, E.J. (1978). A comparison of haloperidol, behavior therapy and their interaction in autistic children. *Journal of the American Academy of Child Psychiatry, 17*, 640–655.

Campbell, M., Friedman, E., Green, W.H., Collins, P.J., Small, A.M., & Breuer, H. (1975). Blood serotonin in schizophrenic children. A preliminary study. *International Pharmacopsychiatry, 10*, 213–221.

Campbell, M., Grega, D.M., Green, W.H., & Bennett, W.G. (1983). Neuroleptic-induced dyskinesias in children. *Clinical Neuropharmacology, 6*, 207–222.

Campbell, M., Perry, R., Bennett, W.G., Small, A.M., Green, W.H., Grega, D., Schwartz, V., & Anderson, L. (1983). Long-term therapeutic efficacy and drug-related abnormal movements: A prospective study of haloperidol in autistic children. *Psychopharmacology Bulletin, 19*, 80–83.

Campbell, M., Perry, R., Polonsky, B.B., Deutsch, S.I., Palij, M., & Lukashok, D. (1986). Brief report: An open study of fenfluramine in hospitalized young autistic children. *Journal of Autism and Developmental Disorders, 16*, 495–506.

Campbell, M., Perry, R., Small, A.M., & Green, W.H. (1987). Overview of drug treatment in autism. In E. Schopler & G.B. Mesibov (Eds.), *Neurobiological issues in autism* (pp. 341–356). New York: Plenum Press.

Campbell, M., Small, A.M., Green, W.H., Jennings, S.J., Perry, R., Bennett, W.G., & Anderson, L. (1984). Behavioral efficacy of haloperidol and lithium carbonate: A comparison in hospitalized aggressive children with conduct disorder. *Archives of General Psychiatry, 41*, 650–656.

Campbell, M., Small, A.M., Palij, M., Perry, R., Polonsky, B.B., Lukashok, D., & Anderson, L.T. (1987). The efficacy and safety of fenfluramine in autistic children: Preliminary analysis of a double-blind study. *Psychopharmacology Bulletin, 23* (1), 123–127.

Campbell, M., Adams, P., Small, A.M., Tesch, L.McV. & Curren, E.L. (1988). Naltrexone in infantile autism. *Psychopharmacology Bulletin*, *24* (1) (in press).

Cataldo, M.F., & Harris, J. (1982). The biological basis for self-injury in the mentally retarded. *Analysis and Intervention in Developmental Disabilities*, *2*, 21–39.

Chouinard, G. (1985). Antimanic effects of clonazepam. *Psychosomatics*, *26*, (Suppl. 12), 7–12.

Chouinard, G., Young, S.N., & Annable, L. (1983). Antimanic effect of clonazepam. *Biological Psychiatry*, *18*, 451–466.

Ciaranello, R.D., Anders, T.F., Barchas, J.D., Berger, P.A., & Cann, H.M. (1976). The use of 5-hydroxytryptophan in a child with Lesch-Nyhan syndrome. *Child Psychiatry and Human Development*, *7*, 127–133.

Cohen, D.J., Detlor, J., Young, J.G., & Shaywitz, B.A. (1980). Clonidine ameliorates Gilles de la Tourette syndrome. *Archives of General Psychiatry*, *37*, 1350–1357.

Cohen, D.J., Leckman, J.F., & Shaywitz, B.A. (1985). The Tourette syndrome and other tics. In D. Shaffer, A.A. Ehrhardt, & L.L. Greenhill (Eds.), *The clinical guide to child psychiatry* (pp. 3–28). New York: The Free Press.

Cohen, D.J., Shaywitz, B.A., Caparulo, B., Young, J.C., & Bowers, M.B., Jr. (1978). Chronic, multiple tics of Gilles de la Tourette's disease. CSF acid monoamine metabolites after probenecid administration. *Archives of General Psychiatry*, *35*, 245–250.

Cohen, D.J., Young J.G., Nathanson, J.A., & Shaywitz, B.A. (1979). Clonidine in Tourette's syndrome. *Lancet*, *2*, 551–553.

Coid, J., Allolio, B., & Rees, L.H. (1983). Raised plasma metenkephalin in patients who habitually mutilate themselves. *Lancet*, *II*, 545–546.

Coleman, M. (1971). Infantile spasms associated with 5-hydroxytryptophan administration in patients with Down's syndrome. *Neurology*, *21*, 911–919.

Costa, E., Gropetti, A., & Revuelta, A. (1971). Action of fenfluramine on monoamine stores of rat tissues. *British Journal of Pharmacology*, *41*, 57–64.

Davidson, P.W., Kleene, B.M., Carroll, M., & Rockowitz, R.J. (1983). Effects of naloxone on self-injurious behavior: A case study. *Applied Research in Mental Retardation*, *4*, 1–4.

Dehault, J. & Boulanger, M. (1977). Fenfluramine long-term administration and brain serotonin. *European Journal of Pharmacology*, *43*, 203–205.

Deutsch, S.I. (1986). Rationale for the administration of opiate antagonists in treating infantile autism. *American Journal of Mental Deficiency*, *90*, 631–635.

Douglas, W.W. (1985). Histamine and 5-hydroxytryptamine (serotonin) and their antagonists. In A.G. Gilman, L.S, Goodman, T.W. Rall, & F. Murad (Eds.), *The pharmacological basis of therapeutics* (pp. 605–638). New York: Macmillan.

Elliott, F.A. (1977). Propranolol for the control of belligerent behavior following acute brain damage. *Annals of Neurology*, *1*, 489–491.

Falk, W.E. (1986). Clonazepam (Clonapin): A treatment potpourri. *The Massachusetts General Hospital Newsletter: Biological Therapies in Psychiatry*, *9*, 6–7.

Friedhoff, A.J., & Chase, T.N. (Eds.), (1982). *Advances in Neurology, Gilles de la Tourette Syndrome* (Vol. 35). New York: Raven Press.

Geller, E., Ritvo, E.R., Freeman, B.J., & Yuwiler, A. (1982). Preliminary observations on the effects of fenfluramine on blood serotonin and symptoms in three autistic boys. *New England Journal of Medicine*, *307*, 165–169.

Gillberg, C., Terenius, L., & Lönnerholm, G. (1985). Endorphin activity in childhood psychosis: Spinal fluid levels in 24 cases. *Archives of General Psychiatry*, *42*, 780–783.

Golden, R.R., Campbell, M., & Perry, R. (1987). A taxometric method for diagnosis of tardive dyskinesia. *J. Psychiatric Research*, *21*, 233–241.

Gonce, M., & Barbeau, A. (1977). Seven cases of Gilles de la Tourette's syndrome: Partial relief with clonazepam: A pilot study. *The Canadian Journal of Neurological Sciences*, *4*, 279–283.

Groden, G., Groden, J., Dondey, M., Zane, T., Pueschel, S., & Veliceur, W. (1987). Effects of fenfluramine on the behavior of autistic individuals. *Research in Developmental Disabilities*, *8*, 203–211.

Gualtieri, C.T., Quade, D., Hicks, R.E., Mayo, J.P., & Schroeder, S.R. (1984). Tardive dyskinesia and other clinical consequences of neuroleptic treatment in children and adolescents. *American Journal of Psychiatry*, *141*, 20–23.

Harvey, S.C. (1985). Hypnotics and sedatives. In A.G. Gilman, L.S. Goodman, T.W. Rall, & F. Murad (Eds.), *The pharmacological basis of therapeutics* (pp. 339–371). New York: Macmillan.

Herman, B.H., Hammock, M.K., Arthur-Smith, A., Egan, J., Chatoor, I., Zelnik, N., Appelgate, K., Boeckx, R.L. (1986). Effects of naltrexone in autism: Correlation with plasma opioid concentrations. *Scientific Proceedings of the Annual Meeting of the American Academy of Child and Adolescent Psychiatry*, Vol. II, pp. 11–12.

Herman, B.H., Hammock, M.K., Arthur-Smith, A., Egan, J., Chatoor, I., Zelnik, N., & Boeckx, R.L. (1986). A biochemical role for opioid peptides in self-injurious behavior. *Scientific Proceedings of the Annual Meeting of the American Academy of Child and Adolescent Psychiatry*, Vol. II, p. 29.

Kalat, J.W. (1978). Speculations on similarities between autism and opiate addiction [Letter to the editor]. *Journal of Autism and Childhood Schizophrenia*, *8*, 477–479.

Kaufman, A.S. (1979). *Intelligent testing with the WISC-R*. New York: Wiley.

Kelsey, J.E., Belluzzi, J.D., & Stein, L. (1984). Does naloxone suppress self-stimulation by decreasing reward or by increasing aversion? *Brain Research*, *307*, 55–59.

Klykylo, W.M., Feldis, D., O'Grady, D., Ross, D.L., & Halloran C. (1985). Brief report: Clinical effects of fenfluramine in ten autistic subjects. *Journal of Autism and Developmental Disorders*, *15*, 417–423.

Lal, S., Allen, J., Etienne, P., Sourkes, T.L., & Humphreys, P. (1977). Dopaminergic function in Gilles de la Tourette's syndrome, Sydenham's chorea and torsion dystonia. *Clinical Neurology and Neurosurgery*, *79*, 66–69.

Leckman, J.F., Cohen, D.J., Detlor, J., Young, J.G., Harcherik, D., & Shaywitz, B.A. (1982). Clonidine in the treatment of Tourette syndrome: A review of data. In A.J. Friedhoff & T.N. Chase (Eds.) *Advances in neurology, Gilles de la Tourette syndrome* (Vol. 35, pp. 391–401). New York: Raven Press.

Lesch, M., & Nyhan, W.L. (1964). A familial disorder of uric acid metabolism and central nervous system function. *American Journal of Medicine*, *36*, 561–570.

Leventhal, B.L. (1985, May). *Fenfluramine administration to autistic children: Effects on behavior and biogenic amines*. Paper presented at the 25th NCDEU Annual Meeting, Key Biscayne, FL.

Mattes, J.A., Rosenberg, J., & Mays, D. (1984). Carbamazepine versus propranolol in patients with uncontrolled rage outbursts: A random assignment study. *Psychopharmacology Bulletin*, *20* (1), 98–100.

Mizuno, T., & Yugari, Y. (1974). Self-mutilation in Lesch-Nyhan syndrome. *Lancet*, *1*, 761.

Nyhan, W.L. (1976). Behavior in the Lesch-Nyhan syndrome. *Journal of Autism and Childhood Schizophrenia*, *6*, 235–252.

Nyhan, W.L., Johnson, H.G., Kaufman, I.A., & Jones, K.L. (1980). Serotonergic approaches to the modification of behavior in the Lesch-Nyhan syndrome. *Applied Research in Mental Retardation*, *1*, 25–40.

Panksepp, J. (1979). A neurochemical theory of autism. *(TINS) Trends in Neuroscience*, *2*, 174–177.

Panksepp, J., & Sahley, T.L. (1987). Possible brain opioid involvement in disrupted social intent and language development in autism. In E. Schopler & G.B. Mesibov (Eds.), *Neurobiological issues in autism* (pp. 357–372). New York: Plenum Press.

Partington, M.W., MacDonald, M.R.A., & Tu, J.B. (1971). 5-Hydroxytryptophan (5-HTP) in Down's syndrome. *Developmental Medicine and Child Neurology*, *13*, 362–372.

Perry, R., Campbell, M., Green, W.H., Small, A.M., Die Trill, M.L., Meiselas, K., Golden, R.R., & Deutsch, S.I. (1985). Neuroleptic-related dyskinesias in autistic children: A prospective study. *Psychopharmacology Bulletin*, *21* (1), 140–143.

Pert, A., Pert, C.B., Davis, C.G., & Bunney, W.E., Jr. (1981). Opiate peptides and brain function. In H.M. van Praag, M.H. Lader, D.J. Rafaelson, & E.J. Sachar (Eds.), *Handbook of biological psychiatry* (Vol. IV, pp. 547–582). New York: Marcel Dekker.

Pueschel, S.M., Reed, R.B., Cronk, C.E., & Goldstein, B.I. (1980). 5-Hydroxytryptophan and pyridoxine: Their effects in young children with Down's syndrome. *American Journal of Diseases of Children*, *134*, 838–844.

Raich, W.A., Rickels, K., & Raab, E. (1966). A double-blind evaluation of fenfluramine in anxious somatizing neurotic medical clinic patients. *Current therapeutic research*, *8*, 31–33.

Ratey, J.J., Mikkelson, E.J., Smith, G.B., Upadhyaya, A., Zuckerman, H.S., Martell, D., Sorgi, P., Polakoff, S., & Bemporad, J. (1986). β-Blockers in the severely and profoundly mentally retarded. *Journal of Clinical Psychopharmacology*, *6*, 103–107.

Ratey, J.J., Morrill, R., & Oxenkrug, G. (1983). Use of propranolol for provoked and unprovoked episodes of rage. *American Journal of Psychiatry*, *140*, 1356–1357.

Richardson, J.S., & Zaleski, W.A. (1983). Naloxone and self-mutilation. *Biological Psychiatry*, *18*, 99–101.

Ritvo, E.R., Freeman, B.J., Geller, E., & Yuwiler, A. (1983). Effects of fenfluramine on 14 outpatients with the syndrome of autism. *Journal of the American Academy of Child Psychiatry*, *22*, 549–558.

Ritvo, E.R., Freeman, B.J., Yuwiler, A., Geller, E., Schroth, P., Yokota, A., Mason-Brothers, A., August, G.J., Klykylo, W., Leventhal, B., Lewis, K., Piggott, L., Realmuto, G., Stubbs, E.G., & Umansky, R. (1986). Fenfluramine treatment of autism: UCLA Collaborative study of 81 patients at nine medical centers. *Psychopharmacology Bulletin*, *22* (1), 133–147.

Ritvo, E.R., Freeman, B.J., Yuwiler, A., Geller, E., Yokota, A., Schroth, P., & Novak, P. (1984). Study of fenfluramine in outpatients with the syndrome of autism. *Journal of Pediatrics*, *105*, 823–828.

Ritvo, E.R., Yuwiler, A., Geller, E., Ornitz, E.M., Saeger, K., & Plotkin, S. (1970). Increased blood serotonin and platelets in infantile autism. *Archives of General Psychiatry*, *23*, 566–572.

Rosner, F., Ong, B.H., Paine, R.S., & Mahanand, D. (1965). Blood-serotonin activity in tusonic and translocation Down's syndrome. *Lancet*, *1*, 1191–1193.

Rudd, P., & Blaschke, T.F. (1985). Antihypertensive agents and the drug therapy of hypertension. In A.G. Gilman, L.S. Goodman, T.W. Rall, & F. Murad (Eds.), *The pharmacological basis of therapeutics* (7th ed., pp. 784–805). New York: Macmillan.

Sandman, C.A., Datta, P.C., Barron, J., Hoehler, F.K., Williams, C., & Swanson, J.M. (1983). Naloxone attenuates self-abusive behavior in developmentally disabled clients. *Applied Research in Mental Retardation*, *4*, 5–11.

Sandyk, R., & Gillman, M.A. (1986). Infantile autism: a dysfunction of the opioids? *Medical Hypotheses*, *19*, 41–45.

Schroeder, S.R., Schroeder, C.S., Smith, B., & Dalldorf, J. (1978). Prevalence of self-injurious behaviors in a large state facility for the retarded: A three-year follow-up study. *Journal of Autism and Childhood Schizophrenia*, *8*, 261–269.

Schuster, C.R., Lewis, M., & Seiden, L.S. (1986). Fenfluramine: Neurotoxicity. *Psychopharmacology Bulletin*, *22* (1), 148–151.

Selinger, D., Cohen, D.J., Ort, S., Anderson, G.M., Caruso, K.A., & Leckman, J.F. (1984). Partial salivary response to clonidine in Tourette's syndrome: Indicator of adrenergic responsivity. *Journal of the American Academy of Child Psychiatry*, *23*, 392–398.

Shapiro, A.K., & Shapiro, E. (1981). The treatment and etiology of tics and Tourette syndrome. *Comprehensive Psychiatry*, *22*, 193–205.

Shapiro, A.K., & Shapiro, E. (1982a). Clinical efficacy of haloperidol, pimozide, penfluridol, and clonidine in the treatment of Tourette syndrome. In A.J. Friedhoff & T.N. Chase (Eds.), *Advances in Neurology, Gilles de la Tourette syndrome* (Vol. 35, pp. 383–386). New York: Raven Press.

Shapiro, A.K., & Shapiro, E. (1982b). An update on Tourette syndrome. *American Journal of Psychotherapy*, *36*, 379–390.

Shore, D., Korpi, E.R., Bigelow, L.B., Zec, R.F., & Wyatt, R.J. (1985). Fenfluramine and chronic schizophrenia. *Biological Psychiatry*, *20*, 329–352.

Simon, E.J., Hiller, J.M., & Edelman, I. (1973). Stereospecific binding of the potent narcotic analgesic (3H) etorphine to rat-brain homogeneate. *Proceedings of the National Academy of Science USA*, *70*, 1947–1949.

Sprague, R.L. (1978). Principles of clinical trials and social, ethical and legal issues of drug use in children. In J.S. Werry (Ed.), *Pediatric psychopharmacology: The use of behavior modifying drugs in children* (pp. 109–135). New York: Brunner/ Mazel.

Sverd, J., Kupietz, S.S., & Winsberg, B.G. (1978). Effects of L-5-hydroxy-tryptophan in autistic children. *Journal of Autism and Childhood Schizophrenia*, *8*, 171–180.

Terenius, L. (1973). Characteristics of the "receptor" for narcotic analgesics in synaptic plasma membrane fraction from rat brain. *Acta Pharmacologica Toxicologica*, *33*, 377–384.

Terenius, L., Wahlström, A., & Agren, H. (1977), Naloxone (Narcan) treatment in depression: Clinical observations and effects on CSF endorphins and mono-amine metabolites. *Psychopharmacology*, *54*, 31–33.

van Praag, H.M., & Korf, J. (1974). Serotonin metabolism in depression: Clinical application of the probenecid test. *International Pharmacopsychiatry*, *9*, 35–51.

Van Woert, M.H., Yip, L.C., & Balis, M.E. (1977). Purine phosphoribasyl trans-ferase in Gilles de la Tourette syndrome. *New England Journal of Medicine*, *296*, 210–212.

Verebey, K., Volavka, J., & Clouet, D. (1978). Endorphins in psychiatry. *Archives of General Psychiatry*, *35*, 877–888.

Victor, B.S., Link, N.A., Binder, R.L., & Bell, I.R. (1984). Use of clonazepam in mania and schizoaffective disorders. *American Journal of Psychiatry*, *141*, 1111–1112.

Wahlström, A., Johansson, L., & Terenius, L. (1976). Characterization of endor-phins (endogenous morphine-like factors) in human CSF and brain extracts. In H.W. Kosterlitz (Ed.), *Opiates and endogenous opioid peptides* (pp. 49–56). Amsterdam: North Holland.

Weiner, N. (1985). Drugs that inhibit adrenergic nerves and block adrenergic re-ceptors. In A.G. Gilman, L.S. Goodman, T.W. Rall, & F. Murad (Eds.), *The pharmacological basis of therapeutics* (pp. 181–214). New York: Macmillan.

Weise, P., Koch, R., Shaw, K.N.F., & Rosenfeld, M.J. (1974). The use of 5-HTP in the treatment of Down's syndrome. *Pediatrics*, *54*, 165–168.

Weizman, R., Weizman, A., Tyano, S., Szekely, G., Weissman, B.A., & Sarne, Y. (1984). Humoral-endorphin blood levels in autistic, schizophrenic and healthy subjects. *Psychopharmacology*, *82*, 368–370.

Werry, J.S., & Aman, M.G. (1975). Methylphenidate and haloperidol in children. *Archives of General Psychiatry*, *32*, 790–795.

Willer, J.C., Dehen, H., & Cambier, J. (1981). Stress-induced analgesia in humans: Endogenous opioids and naloxone reversible depression of pain reflexes. *Sci-ence*, *212*, 680–691.

Willette, R.E, & Barnett, G. (Eds.). (1981). *Narcotic antagonists: Naltrexone phar-macochemistry and sustained-release preparations*. NIDA Research Monograph 28, Washington, DC, U.S. Government Printing Office.

Williams, D.T., Mehl, R., Yudofsky, S., Adams, D., & Roseman, B. (1982). The effect of propranolol on uncontrolled rage outbursts in children and adolescents with organic brain dysfunction. *Journal of the American Academy of Child Psychiatry*, *21*, 129–135.

Wyatt, R.J., Vaughan, T., Galanter, M., Kaplan, J., & Green, R. (1972). Be-havioral changes of chronic schizophrenic patients given L-5-hydroxytrypto-phan. *Science*, *177*, 1124–1126.

Young, J.G., Kavanagh, M.E., Anderson, G.M., Shaywitz, B.A., & Cohen, D.J. (1982). Clinical neurochemistry of autism and associated disorders. *Journal of Autism and Developmental Disorders*, *12*, 147–165.

Yudofsky, S., Williams, D., & Gorman, J. (1981). Propranolol in the treatment of rage and violent behavior in patients with chronic brain syndromes. *American Journal of Psychiatry*, *138*, 218–220.

Zarcone V., Kales, A., Scharf, M., Tan, T., Simmons, J., & Dement, W.C. (1973). Repeated oral ingestion of 5-hydroxytryptophan: The effect on behavior and sleep processes in two schizophrenic children. *Archives of General Psy-chiatry*, *28*, 843–846.

8
Vitamin, Mineral, and Dietary Treatments

MICHAEL G. AMAN AND NIRBHAY N. SINGH

Abstract

Evidence pointing to nutritional deficiencies among mentally handicapped and autistic people is discussed briefly, followed by a short overview of genetically transmitted metabolic disorders. Some important historical episodes involving nutritional supplements are then summarized, followed by critical reviews of several recent megavitamin therapies. Finally, some of the popular dietary interventions, including those free of refined sugar or food additives and food dyes, are discussed in relation to treating developmentally disabled people.

In this paper we consider various nutritional approaches to the treatment of developmentally disabled people. These include the use of vitamin and mineral supplements, usually in megadoses, and special diets designed to eliminate or minimize substances thought to be behaviorally toxic for certain children. Earlier, "psychotropic drug" was defined as any substance administered for the purpose of producing behavioral, emotional, or cognitive changes (Chapter 1). Given the claims made for certain vitamin/mineral treatments, they would clearly qualify as psychotropic drugs using this definition. In addition, the methods and necessary controls employed for evaluating both nutritional supplements and special diets are nearly identical to those for assessing the more traditional psychotropic drugs. Hence, it is appropriate that a section on nutritional therapies be included within this issue.

This is a very rapidly growing area of research activity. Indeed, we had intended to include this material within Chapter 1 but found that the relevant literature was too large to be accommodated there. In this chapter we briefly discuss some general nutritional considerations as they apply to developmentally disabled persons and some historical experiences in relation to nutritional (and other) therapies. However, most space is reserved for discussions of (a) the Bronson GTC3 vitamin formula claimed to improve adaptive functioning in mentally retarded children (Harrell, Capp, Davis, Peerless, & Ravitz, 1981), (b) vitamin B_6 (pyridoxine) therapy in Down syndrome and autistic children, and (c) use of the Feingold (1975a) diet in handicapped children. Hence, this review is not intended to be an exhaustive coverage of nutritional considerations, but it does summarize some of the research dealing with specific treatments that have been topical in recent years.

Nutritional Deficiencies in Developmentally Disabled Persons

There are a number of reasons why developmentally disabled people may be more disposed to nutritional problems than the general public. The American Dietetic Association (1981) and Cole, Lopez, Epel, Singh, and Cooperman (1985) have summarized several of these as follows. Many developmentally handicapped individuals have physical problems resulting in difficulty in chewing or swallowing. This may lead to the use of soft/overcooked foods depleted of vitamins. Many developmentally disabled persons receive anticonvulsant drugs (see Chapter 1) that, in turn, can cause deficiencies of folic acid, calcium, and vitamin D, and can cause megaloblastic anemia and disturbances in bone metabolism. Neuroleptic and antidepressant drugs commonly cause xerostomia (dry mouth), which may also have nutritional consequences. Likewise, a possible side effect of stimulant drugs, such as dextroamphetamine and methylphenidate, is a reduction of food intake with a possible depression of growth in height and weight (Roche, Lipman, Overall, & Hung, 1979). Last, but certainly not least in importance, many socioculturally mentally retarded children are reared by parents who are themselves mentally retarded and who often have an inadequate grasp of nutritional principles.

Studies that have assessed the intake of mentally retarded children or residents have often found their diets to be deficient in various vitamins and minerals (Ellman et al., 1986; Gouge & Ekvall, 1975; Wilton & Irvine, 1983). Other studies have examined nutrient levels in body fluids or hair samples taken from mentally retarded persons and have again reported deficiencies (Barlow, Sylvester, & Dickerson, 1981; Cole et al., 1985; Matin, Sylvester, Edwards, & Dickerson, 1981; see Sylvester, 1984). Likewise, autistic children have been studied for trace element concentrations in plasma and in hair samples (Gentile, Trentalange, Zamichek, & Coleman, 1983; Jackson & Garrod, 1978; Shearer, Larson, Neuschwander, & Gedney, 1982; Wecker, Miller, Cochran, Dugger, & Johnson, 1985). Differences between autistic and control subjects have been reported in some studies, but most of these differences have been unsupported by the remaining studies. Research into plasma amino acid concentrations (Jackson & Garrod, 1978), plasma levels of folic acid, ascorbic acid, pyridoxine, and riboflavin (Sankar, 1979), as well as nutrient intake (Shearer et al., 1982) has not found marked differences between auistic and normal children.

However, there have been isolated reports of deficient and/or excessive levels of many of these in previous research so that the picture appears to be quite confused.

There are in fact a number of genetically transmitted *metabolic disorders* found among developmentally disabled persons that can be controlled either by reductions or increases in specific nutrients. These include disorders of amino acid metabolism (e.g., maple syrup urine disease and phenylketonuria) and carbohydrate metabolism (e.g., galactosemia) (American Dietetic Association, 1981). These are well-studied and specific conditions, in which aberrations in metabolism result either in a buildup of toxic metabolites or in deficient levels of essential nutrients. The nutritional treatments that have been applied to these disorders are rational and have been scientifically validated. With some disorders, early identification and appropriate dietary intervention can minimize the insult to cognitive and physical development.

Our concern in this paper is not with such established and well-authenticated nutritional interventions. Instead, we focus on some of the more controversial approaches to the treatment of behavior problems in developmental disabilities, such as those that go by the names "ortho-molecular medicine" or "megavitamin therapy." Sometimes these are characterized by a shotgun approach in which a large number of nutritional substances are given in large doses. Major claims have been made for some of these, and they have been much publicized in the lay and professional literature.

Some Historical Experiences

Treatment with developmentally disabled persons has at one time or another moved in virtually every conceivable direction, spurred on perhaps by the seriousness of the disabilities presented by these individuals and a desire to try something, no matter how unproven, in the hope that it will have therapeutic effects. Louttit (1965) and Share (1976) have described a number of the purported therapies that have been used with mentally retarded individuals. These have included treatment with vitamins such as thiamin (B_1) and vitamin E, as well as vitamins given in combination with glutamic acid (discussed below). Another treatment involved the administration of celastrus paniculata, a shrub whose seeds have been used in India as a stimulant for intelligence (Louttit, 1965). Sicca cell therapy, which has been claimed to produce improvements in Down syndrome children, consists of injecting embryonic cells into muscles to stimulate the activity and growth of corresponding cellular tissues (Share, 1976). Thyroid therapy, pituitary extract, and the "U" series (a concoction of 48 vitamins, minerals, enzymes, and common drugs) have all been used in various developmentally disabled populations (Share, 1976). As pointed out by Louttit and

Share, extravagant claims have been made for some of these treatments, but few if any have been demonstrated to be of value in scientifically controlled studies.

One interesting phenomenon, both from an historical and a scientific perspective, is glutamic acid. Glutamic acid (GA) is a nonessential amino acid regarded by some workers (e.g., Zimmerman & Burgemeister, 1959) as a cerebral stimulant and now widely regarded as an important excitatory neurotransmitter in the central nervous system. The experience with GA is interesting because it resulted in a massive research effort totaling *at least 53 studies* with mentally retarded subjects and a minimum of 13 studies with other populations (Vogel, Broverman, Draguns, & Klaiber, 1966).

Gadson (1951) and Waelsch (1948) have chronicled many of the events leading to this bandwagon research effort. In 1943 Price, Waelsch, and Putnam (cited in Waelsch, 1948) studied patients suffering from petit mal epilepsy and anecdotally reported that behavioral "improvement" occurred with GA treatment. Biochemical studies conducted about this time showed that GA increased the synthesis of acetylcholine, one of the first neurotransmitters to be identified. This was followed, in 1944, by an animal study in which GA-treated rats learned mazes in less time than the untreated rats. Shortly thereafter, Albert, Hoch, and Waelsch (1946) and Zimmerman, Burgemeister, and Putnam (1946) (cited in Gadson, 1951) reported that GA brought about substantial IQ gains (5–17 points) in mentally retarded subjects. These early reports resulted in intense interest both professionally and in the media, and they were followed by a rash of over 60 publications, many of which were either poorly controlled or totally uncontrolled.

In 1960, Astin and Ross published a review that was highly critical of this literature. They classified the GA studies first in terms of whether they employed some semblance of control and, second, in terms of whether or not positive results were reported. They found that positive effects occurred disproportionately often among those studies lacking control groups. However, Vogel et al. (1966) subsequently disputed Astin and Ross's conclusions. After reconstructing and adding to their two-way table of positive/negative and controlled/uncontrolled studies, Vogel et al. concluded that there was no statistical association between outcome and the presence of controls, and they concluded that glutamic acid supplementation may have a role to play in cognitive functioning.

At first blush, one of the more compelling pieces of evidence regarding a therapeutic role for GA was the early animal research showing improvements in learning rate due to GA. However, several subsequent animal studies were unable to replicate the early optimistic findings (Glutamic Acid, 1951). To us, the most intriguing question relates to why investigators became interested in GA in the first place. Two of the figures most associated with this work (Waelsch, 1948; Zimmerman & Burgemeister, 1959) have suggested that there was an etiological connection between epilepsy and mental retardation, thereby providing a "rationale" for GA therapy in mentally retarded populations. Thus, it appears that the GA phenomenon was brought about both by a knowledge that it was biologically active and by a mistaken belief that an epileptic-like phenomenon may have been contributing to these children's disability. However, it does not appear that there was any reason to assume that GA (or acetylcholine) was deficient in any of the mentally retarded subgroups included in these studies. One review summed up the situation well:

> The underlying reasoning, not found in the actual papers, is as tempting as it is logically unconvincing: there is lots of the substance in the brain; it *must* have something to do with the brain function; the more, the better; let's feed it. (Glutamic Acid, 1951)

Vitamin Supplementation Studies—Harrell Controversy

In 1981, Harrell et al. reported the results of a trial using large doses of a vitamin/mineral formula in a diagnostically mixed group of mentally retarded children. Harrell and her associates reasoned that some of these children might be suffering from a genetotropic disease—that is, a condition in which the person inherits a need for an augmented supply of one or more nutrients. Harrell et al.'s findings were so dramatic that they attracted widespread comment both in the professional and the lay press, and large numbers of parents of handicapped children sought megavitamin treatment through their physicians (see Bennett, McClelland, Kriegsmann, Andrus, & Sells, 1983).

Briefly, Harrell et al. (1981) conducted a two-phase study that initially involved 22 mentally retarded children. In the first phase, which lasted 4 months, 10 subjects were assigned to the dietary supplement group and 12 subjects to a placebo group. In addition, thyroid supplementation was provided to the entire group (both treatment and control) except for two children whose parents refused this part of the program. At the end of the first phase of treatment, the group receiving dietary supplements was reported to have shown a statistically significant 5-point IQ gain as compared with no change for the control subjects. However, there was serious attrition in this part of the study with five and one subjects dropping out of the treatment and control groups, respectively.

During the second phase of the Harrell et al. study, the original treatment group continued to receive supplementation for an additional 4 months, and 10 of the control subjects received the vitamin/mineral supplement for 8 months. Progress during this period was compared with that in the previous placebo interval and, therefore, this portion of the study was neither controlled nor blind. For the 10 children originally in the control group, Harrell et al. reported stunning IQ gains during treatment, with a mean increase of 16.0 points! In addition, the original treatment group was reported to show an average gain of 14 points over the full 8-month treatment interval. Harrell's group reported other beneficial effects as well, such as significant gains in height and (anecdotally) improved appearance in three Down syndrome children, "improved texture of finger nails, healthier hair or skin, and . . . cessation of hyperactivity" (p. 577). The Down syndrome children were reported to be among those who showed the greatest improvements.

Not suprisingly, the Harrell report generated a great deal of interest on the part of professionals and the public alike and in some quarters the supplementary diet (known as the Bronson GTC3 formula) was enthusiastically embraced. A number of workers set out to replicate the findings of Harrell et al. (1981), and in the last few years several studies examining the Harrell supplement have appeared. These and the Harrell report are summarized according to a number of methodological and outcome characteristics in Table 8.1.

The subsequent studies were all well designed. All incorporated a double-blind, placebo-controlled, between-groups design, and all had *larger* groups than used in the original report. In terms of outcome, not one of these replications found significant gains due to the vitamin/mineral supplements (Bennett et al., 1983; Chanowitz, Ellman, Silverstein, Zingarelli, & Ganger, 1985; Coburn, Schaltenbrand, Mahuren, Clausman, & Townsend, 1983; Ellis & Tomporowski, 1983; Ellman, Silverstein, Zingarelli, Shafter, & Silverstein, 1984; Smith, Spiker, Peterson, Cicchetti, & Justin, 1984; Weathers, 1983). This is in spite of the fact that collectively they examined a wide array of dependent variables, relating to IQ and cognitive development, behavioral adjustment, motor proficiency, electrocortical measures, growth and development, and general health status.

One possible difficulty with these studies, as replications, is that most of them did not utilize thyroid supplements *in combination* with the nutritional supplements as was done by Harrell et al. (1981). However, the study by Chanowitz et al. (1985) was specifically designed to deal with this posiblity, and it incorporated four experimental groups to evaluate every combination of dietary supplement (vitaman versus placebo) and thyroid supplement (thyroid versus placebo). In this study, the thyroid + vitamin group showed a very slight mean gain (1.1 months, N.S.) in mental age over a 4-month interval, whereas the other groups were essentially unchanged. Even if the Chanowitz et al. results were not available, however, it would be difficult to attribute much significance to the presence of thyroid supplementation in the Harrell et al. study. The two children who did not receive thyroid treatment in that study were both reported to show 13-point gains in IQ. Also, it should be noted that other than the Chanowitz et al. study, three of the replications systematically checked thyroid levels of their subjects before treatment and found them to be normal (Bennett et al., 1983; Coburn et al., 1983; Smith et al., 1984). The method for assessing thyroid deficiency in the Harrell et al. study is said to be

TABLE 8.1. Summary of studies of the Bronson GTC3 formula.

Authors	Number of subjects	% Down syndrome in suppl. group	Blind?	Placebo?	Age range[a]	Duration	Results
Harrell et al., 1981	16	40	Y	Y	5–15	4 months	Significant IQ gains (5 points)
	10	22	N	N	5–15	8 months	Significant IQ gains (16 points)
							Significant gains in height
Bennett et al., 1983	20	100	Y	Y	5–13	8 months	No significant group changes in IQ, achievement, language performance, height, weight, appearance, general health, or rating scale
Coburn et al., 1983	38[b]	25	Y	Y	16–30	20 weeks	No group differences in IQ or weight gains
Ellis & Tomporowski, 1983	40	37	Y	Y	21–40	7 months	No group differences in IQ or adaptive behavior
Weathers, 1983	47	100	Y	Y	6–17	16 weeks	No significant differences on IQ, visual motor integration, height, weight, appearance, visual acuity, or parent ratings of behavior
Ellman et al., 1984	20	20	Y	Y	16–23	6 months	No group differences on IQ, visual evoked potential, teacher ratings of behavior, appearance, body weight, or seizure occurrence
Chanowitz et al., 1985	37	?	Y	Y	24–26 (means)	4 months	No group differences in mental age gains
Smith et al., 1984	56	100	Y	Y	7–15	8 months	No group differences in IQ, vocabulary, visual motor integration, or motor proficiency

[a]Expressed in years.
[b]This refers only to the groups receiving placebo and the Harrell et al. (1981) formula.

highly unreliable (Ellman et al., 1984) and it is likely that many of Harrell's subjects were in fact *not* thyroid deficient. Thus, if any of the reported changes in Harrell's study were real, they may have been the result of the potentially psychotropic effects of thyroid supplementation.

Three other points should be made with respect to the Harrell et al. (1981) controversy. First, it has been observed that the vitamin/mineral supplement used in these studies has a distinctive smell and flavor, enabling some caregivers to distinguish active substance from placebo (Bennett et al., 1983; Ellis & Tomporowski, 1983). It is widely acknowledged that a lack of blindness tends to encourage positive findings, and it is possible that this may have been a factor in the original report. Second, we are aware of no clear scientific rationale for the use of this particular nutritional formula other than the seemingly vague belief that some developmentally disabled individuals have constitutionally higher requirements for certain nutrients. This is in contradistinction to several other research efforts both with nutrients and with drugs (see Chapter 7) that have been based on sound reasons for adopting a particular mode of treatment. The third point concerns public and professional attitudes toward nutritional and psychopharmacological treatments. Weathers (1983) reported that most parents in his study wished to continue with the megavitamin treatment despite a lack of evidence of any improvement. We have also informally noted this sort of attitude among some colleagues in the field, many of whom are staunchly against the use of psychotropic drugs. This is a curious position in view of the fact that vitamins and minerals are capable of producing adverse effects, some potentially serious, when used in large quantities (see Weathers, 1983; "Megavitamin Side Effects", this chapter).

In summary, we can find no supporting evidence for the claims of improvement due to this particular vitamin/mineral supplement in mentally retarded children. If the combination therapy has any real impact, which we doubt, this may be due to the thyroid supplements that were given. What is perhaps most surprising about this whole episode is that it attracted as much attention as it did, given our disappointing experiences with drugs in the past (Yannet, 1957).

Vitamin B$_6$ (Pyridoxine) Studies

Recently, vitamin B$_6$ has been investigated for its possible therapeutic value both with Down syndrome and autistic children.

Down Syndrome Subjects

At least three studies have appeared of B$_6$ treatment with Down syndrome children. According to Coleman et al. (1985), research has shown that Down syndrome individuals are deficient in B$_6$ and that they may have a smaller body pool of B_6 as compared with controls. In addition, it is now well established that 5-hydroxytryptamine (serotonin) concentrations in peripheral blood are lower than control values in this population (see Pueschel, Reed, Cronk, & Goldstein, 1980). Both Pueschel et al. (1980) and Coleman et al. (1985) have reasoned that administration of pyridoxine (which, as pyridoxal phosphate, is a coenzyme that participates in the decarboxylation of 5-hydroxytryptophan to 5-hydroxytrytamine) may increase serotonin levels in Down syndrome patients even though this is not normally the rate-limiting step for the synthesis of serotonin.

Pueschel et al. (1980) evaluated the effects of placebo, megadoses of pyridoxine, 5-hydroxytryptophan, and pyridoxine + 5-hydroxytryptophan, given for 3 years, in 89 children with Down syndrome (see also Chapter 7). The study was conducted double-blind, with a placebo control, and objective measures of response. Pyridoxine, 5-hydroxytryptophan, and their combination produced increases in 5-hydroxyindole (end products of serotonin metabolism) concentrations, for about 40% of the subjects. However, there were no treatment effects on a variety of adaptive measures including muscle tone, the Bayley Scales of infant development, Vineland Social Maturity Scale, and language development.

Coleman et al. (1985) compared large doses of pyridoxine with placebo over a 3-year period in Down syndrome infants. A transient increase in 5-hydroxytryptamine was observed for the treatment group at 1 year, but this was no longer significant at later stages of the study. Clinical measures (e.g., height, cranial circumference, tongue protrusion) and adaptive measures (standardized scales of development and social maturity) showed no advantage for the treatment group during the study. However, at 3 years after the study, the treatment group was reported to have a significantly higher social quotient. Coleman also reported on side effects detected in a cohort of 400 Down syndrome children receiving large doses of pyridoxine. Twenty-one subjects developed photosensitive blisters, six experienced vomiting and abdominal pain, and two developed motor and sensory polyneuropathy that remitted when B_6 treatment was stopped.

Finally, in an extension to the study of Coleman et al. (1985), Frager, Barnet, Weiss, and Coleman (1985) examined cortical evoked potentials as a function of pyridoxine treatment. After 3 years of treatment, amplitudes of prominent wave components were reported as decreased (representing a normalization) and latencies were increased in the treatment group. However, the clinical significance, if any, of these changes is unknown.

In summary, few clinical or adaptive changes, which could be unequivocally ascribed to vitamin B_6, were found in these studies. However, improvements in social quotient were found 3 years *after* treatment in one study (Coleman et al., 1985), and changes in certain aspects of the evoked potential were found after 3 years of treatment in another investigation (Frager et al., 1985). These appear to have been well-controlled studies that were based on a biochemical rationale, namely evidence of B_6

deficiency and the possibility that vitamin B_6, a coenzyme precursor of 5-hydroxytryptamine metabolism, may increase concentrations of the latter. As there was a specific underlying reason for these studies, they can be contrasted with much of the other work with popular nutritional therapies. However, these investigations provide little evidence that pyridoxine produces useful clinical changes in Down syndrome children.

Studies with Autistic Subjects

In 1973, Rimland reported a survey of high dosage vitamin use in a mixed group of children having severe mental disorders. Rimland was struck by the extent to which parents, in their trial-and-error efforts, ultimately settled on three or four vitamins, principally niacin, ascorbic acid, and pyridoxine. He also described an uncontrolled study that employed most of these, as well as large doses of other vitamins and minerals, in approximately 200 disturbed children. Rimland reported that 45% of this amorphous group showed definite improvement and another 41% showed possible improvement. Autistic children were thought to show particular benefit, with 59% classed as showing definite improvement, and Rimland attributed the greatest changes to the introduction of vitamin B_6.

This led to a subsequent study of large doses of pyridoxine in 16 children with "autistic-like" symptoms (Rimland, Callaway, & Dreyfus, 1978). The study employed a crossover design in which placebo and B_6 were interspersed between three baseline phases. The treatment phases were of variable duration and pyridoxine was given in whatever doses were previously thought to be effective in these children. As assessed by global judgments of change, the subjects were reported to be significantly improved during active treatment phases as compared with placebo phases ($p < .05$, one-tailed). However, others have criticized this study for a variety of methodological problems (Moss & Broverman, 1978). These included a lack of diagnostic rigor in selecting subjects, unknown reliability of the global judgments, and the highly selected nature of the subjects (i.e., children considered to be pyridoxine responders) which precludes generalization of the results to other, unselected children. In addition, Rimland et al. inappropriately used the t test, a parametric statistic, to analyze their nonparametric data, and rather liberally used a one-tailed test to assess their results.

Callaway (1977) reported a placebo-controlled study in which pyridoxine was withdrawn in blind fashion from children thought to be B_6 responsive. Global ratings of change were reported to show significant deterioration during withdrawal of pyridoxine. However, this report was so devoid of information about the methodological procedures followed (e.g., dosage employed, treatment duration, type of rating scale used, nature of the statistical analysis, and so forth) that it is impossible to assess these claims.

Gualtieri, van Bourgondien, Hartz, Schopler, and Marcus (1981) reported an uncontrolled pilot study of pyridoxine accompanied by a mixture of background nutrient supplements in 15 autistic children. As judged by global impressions, six children responded favorably, seven showed no change, and two had toxic reactions (hyperactivity and irritability), resulting in their terminating the trial. Gualtieri et al. were skeptical that the rate of favorable response was greater than would be achieved with placebo, but they commented that the results were of sufficient interest that they intended to conduct a more extensive investigation in the future.

One study on the effects of vitamin B_6 used alone ($n = 37$), magnesium alone ($n = 35$), and B_6 given in combination with magnesium ($n = 21$) in autistic children was reported in two publications (Barthelemy et al., 1981; Martineau, Barthelemy, Garreau, & Lelord, 1985). Although a placebo treatment phase was included in the design, all statistical comparisons were, rather incongruously, done with respect to the drug-free baseline. As a result, the study was not controlled with respect to temporal effects or rater bias, as raters were presumably aware that the baseline was drug free. The authors reported significant improvement on three dimensions of a seven-domain behavior rating scale and significant normalization of homovanillic acid levels for children in the combined (B_6 + magnesium) treatment group. In addition, the Martineau et al. paper also presented data showing a normalization, with the combined treatment, of evoked potential recordings. However, the absence of the correct statistical comparison mitigates these findings greatly, although there is no reason why the correct treatment/placebo comparisons could not be carried out even today.

Lelord et al. (1981) reported the use of megadoses of pyridoxine, supplemented by magnesium, in children with autistic symptoms. In the first stage of this study, 44 children were observed during an open trial. This entailed a baseline of 8 days, supplementation for an unspecified interval, and a return to baseline. Subject changes were monitored by an 18-item symptom scale and target symptom lists drawn up for each child. Fourteen children (32%) were reported to improve during the supplementation phase and to regress during the second baseline. In the second stage of this report, 13 of the responders and 8 nonresponders from the open trial were involved in a placebo-controlled crossover study. Again using the 18-item symptom scale and target symptoms, the subjects were judged globally as having improved or not under the pyridoxine/magnesium combination. Ten of the 13 responders (77%) were reported as improving, compared with only 2 of 8 nonresponders (25%). Although cited as "proof" of the value of B_6 supplementation in these children, it should be noted that the staff members conducting these evaluations presumably knew the identity of the two groups before the study began and hence there may have been an unwitting bias toward reporting no change in the nonresponder group.

Twelve of the autistic children from the above study (Lelord et al., 1981) and 11 normal controls were studied to determine the effect of pyridoxine and magnesium on evoked potentials and urinary homovanillic acid

(HVA), the major metabolite of dopamine (Martineau, Garreau, Barthelemy, Callaway, & Lelord, 1981). This study appears to have been poorly controlled, with the subjects tested first without supplement and later with pyridoxine and magnesium. Increases in amplitude of middle latency evoked potentials and a decrease of urinary HVA, representing a normalization of values, were observed for the autistic children during treatment.

Finally, Martineau, Barthelemy, Garreau, and Lelord (1986) reported a nonblind case study of an autistic boy treated with pyridoxine/magnesium over an 8-month period. Behavior ratings showed a decrease in symptoms (and subsequent rebound after termination of treatment) on four of seven subscales. One subscale (relating to agitation and stereotypic behavior) suggested a worsening with treatment. In contrast to previous studies by this group, some measures of homovanillic acid increased with treatment. Evoked potential measures suggested improvement for the 1st month of treatment followed by considerable deterioration. Martineau et al. interpreted their results as showing that B_6/magnesium treatment can be effective over substantial intervals, but this impression is diminished by the lack of blindness.

In summary, we know of seven studies using pyridoxine in autistic children, and all have suggested improvement. In Table 8.2 these studies have been summarized in terms of their designs, the measures employed, their principal conclusions, and our criticisms of their methodology. We have serious reservations about the methodology employed in two (Barthelemy et al., 1981; Rimland et al., 1978), another (Callaway, 1977) was so devoid of details as to preclude comment, one was an uncontrolled pilot study (Gualtieri et al., 1981), the physiological study was uncontrolled for time effects, and the case report (Martineau et al., 1986) was not blind. The conclusions of the remaining study (Lelord et al., 1981), which featured a comparison between responders and nonresponders, are weakened because raters had foreknowledge of group membership.

Apparently, Rimland's (1973) initial study was instigated by a report of abnormal tryptophan metabolism in autistic children (see Lelord, Calloway, & Muh, 1982). Sankar (1970) has summarized three of his studies on biogenic amine uptake in 237 children with psychiatric disorders. Initially he found that autistic children consistently had lower levels of uptake of serotonin by platelets than did nonschizophrenic children. However, in a more recent study, Sankar (1979) measured plasma levels of folates, riboflavin, vitamin B_6, and ascorabate in children with schizophrenia, autism, psychosis, and behavior disorders. No differences were found between the diagnostic groups, and all findings were within normal ranges. Martineau et al. (1986) pointed to research suggesting that autism may result from impairment of certain CNS dopamine-related structures. Following on from this, Lelord et al. (1982) commented that, if an abnormality of catecholamine metabolism is implicated in childhood, then a therapeutic role for B_6 should not be surprising, because B_6 is an almost "ubiquitous"

TABLE 8.2. Summary of vitamin B_6 studies in Autism.

Authors	Design	Measures	Findings	Criticisms
Rimland et al., 1978	Crossover, placebo controlled	Global judgments	Significant improvement with B_6	Use of preselected subjects; inappropriate use of parametric statistic; nonstandard scale
Callaway, 1977	Crossover?, placebo controlled	Global ratings	Significant improvement with B_6	Lack of information on dose, treatment duration, type of scale, statistical analysis, etc.
Gualtieri et al., 1981	Open trial	Global impressions + standardized rating scale	6 of 15 subjects regarded as positive responders	Uncontrolled pilot study
Barthelemy et al., 1981	Placebo "controlled", partial crossover	7-domain behavior rating scale	3 of 7 subscales showed significant improvement with B_6	Inappropriate comparison of treatment with baseline rather than placebo
Martineau et al., 1985	B_6 + magnesium (All comparisons with baseline)	HVA concentrations, evoked potential recordings	Normalization to HVA and evoked potentials	Same as Barthelemy et al. (1981) study
Lelord et al., 1981	Open trial, $N = 44$	18-item symptom scale	14 of 44 subjects improved with B_6	Uncontrolled
	Crossover, placebo-controlled study of 13 responders and 8 nonresponders	18-item symptom scale	10 of 13 responders and 2 of 8 nonresponders improved with B_6	Raters had foreknowledge of group membership
Martineau et al., 1981	Crossover, placebo controlled	Evoked potential, HVA concentrations	Normalization of HVA concentrations and increased amplitude of evoked potentials	Treatment confounded with time
Martineau et al., 1986	Case study, $N = 1$	Behavior ratings on 7-domain scale	Behavioral deterioration on 4 of 7 subscales with termination of treatment; HVA increases (i.e., change toward greater abnormality)	Nonblind, inadequate number of reversals for single-subect study

HVA = Homovanillic acid.

coenzyme, playing a role in the metabolism of many neurotransmitters. However, this argument is somewhat self-defeating: as B_6 does not have a unique role in influencing the synthesis of the catecholamines, it could in fact stimulate the metabolism of precursors which may cause either increases *or* decreases, and one has no way of knowing what the net effect may be. However, the most serious weakness with this rationale is the absence of any obvious B_6 deficiency in this clinical population, and hence, it is unlikely that increasing the B_6 coenzyme by using megadoses would have pronounced therapeutic effects.

We are not aware of *any* positive studies in this area that have used double-blind procedures, placebo-controlled design, objective measures of known reliability, and appropriate inferential statistics. Equally serious, in the absence of any obvious B_6 deficiency among autistic children, there appears to be no overriding physiological or biochemical rationale to suggest that vitamin B_6 *should* be used with this population. Obviously, if sound empirical data are forthcoming attesting to the clinical utility of a given treatment, then this treatment must be given credence. As noted, however, the literature on nutritional and biochemical differences among autistic children is far from conclusive. Despite these difficulties, some workers have proclaimed the case as proven and have enthusiastically advocated the use of megadoses of vitamin B_6 for a variety of child psychiatric disorders, including autism (e.g., Rimland, 1982). At this stage we regard the notion that substantial numbers of these children have a B_6 dependency as nothing more than an hypothesis and a weak one at that.

Other Nutrient Supplements in Learning Disabled and Hyperactive Children of Normal IQ

Cott Formula

Cott (1971, 1972, 1974) has claimed marked success in treating behavior disorders and learning disabilities with a combination of a megavitamin diet, high in niacin or niacinamide, ascorbic acid, pyridoxine, and calcium pantothenate, and, where necessary, an antihypoglycemia diet. However, we are not aware of any formal research carried out by Cott to evaluate the treatment. Three well-controlled studies, utilizing numerous objective learning and behavioral measures, have evaluated variations of this vitamin formula with hyperactive or learning disabled children of normal IQ (Arnold, Christopher, Huestis, & Smeltzer, 1978; Haslam, Dalby, & Rademaker, 1984; Kershner & Hawke, 1979). None of these studies observed greater benefit resulting from the vitamin supplements than from placebo. Indeed, one of these reports noted a net pattern of worsening with 25% more disruptive classroom behavior appearing under the megavitamin condition (Haslam et al., 1984). In addition, monitoring of liver function showed a significant elevation of serum transaminase levels during active treatment for 42% of subjects.

Supplementation with Essential Fatty Acids

One of the more recent nutritional approaches to behavior problems in children has concerned the essential fatty acids (EFAs). Colquhoun and Bunday (1981), in a highly speculative article, suggested that hyperactivity in some children of normal IQ may be due to deficiencies of EFAs. They also reported anecdotally that 25 children in the Hyperactive Children's Support Group in England had received an EFA supplement and that "at least half" had responded positively.

There have been at least two studies of EFA serum levels in children who were designated as "maladjusted" (Mitchell, Lewis, & Cutler, 1983) or hyperactive (Mitchell, Aman, Turbott, & Manku, 1987). The results indicated significantly lower levels of some EFAs in the children with behavior problems, but the pattern was not consistent across studies and the extent of the obtained differences was small. Aman, Mitchell, and Turbott (1987) treated 31 hyperactive children with an EFA supplement (evening primrose oil; Efamol R) and found significant changes on only 4 of 42 psychomotor and clinical variables. Gibson, Tao, and Attwood (1987) assessed an EFA supplement (Efamol) in 95 children and observed no significant clinical changes on either parent or teacher behavior rating scales. Thus, the experimental work to date provides little or no support for Colquhoun and Bunday's (1981) suggestion that EFA supplements may have a therapeutic effect in hyperactive children of normal IQ.

Megavitamin Side Effects

It has long been known that large doses of the fat soluble vitamins (A, D, K, and E) can be toxic, because these nutrients cumulate in the fat pools of the body (Alhadeff, Gualtieri, & Lipton, 1984). According to DiPalma and Ritchie (1977), this is especially true of vitamins A and D when used in large doses and, under special circumstances, even with supplemental doses. With vitamin A, the most important toxic effects are increased intracranial pressure, skeletal pain, skin lesions, liver damage, and bony changes (Chaney & Ross, 1971; DiPalma & Ritchie, 1977; Pathophysiological Basis, 1982). Excessive levels of vitamin D can lead to high concentrations of calcium and phosphorus in the blood and excessive excretion in the urine, resulting in calcification of soft tissue, walls of the blood vessels, and kidney tubules (Chaney & Ross, 1971; DiPalma & Ritchie, 1977). It is interesting to note that both of these vitamins were included in the Harrell et al. (1981) formula although, of the two, only vitamin A was used in substantial quantities (15,000 International Units [IU] as compared with a Recommended Daily Allowance [RDA] of 4,500 IU for older children).

Alhadeff et al. (1984) have reviewed the literature on toxic effects resulting from excessive water-soluble vitamins and their metabolites. It was once commonly believed that, because water-soluble vitamins in normal doses are excreted in the urine, they are nontoxic. However, Alhadeff et al. listed adverse effects resulting from megadoses of all except four (riboflavin, pantothenate, cobalamin, and biotin) of the water-soluble vitamins.

Only pyridoxine is discussed further here owing to the attention given it by workers in this field. Schaumburg et al. (1983) reported on a new syndrome arising in seven patients from megadoses of pyridoxine. The patients had consumed 2,000–6,000 mg of B_6 per day (RDA = 2 mg), and they presented with toxicity to the peripheral nervous system. The clinical profile included unstable gait and numb feet, numbness and clumsiness of the hands, and, in some cases, numbness around the mouth. Two of these cases were found to have nonspecific axonal degeneration affecting myelinated nerve fibers. Pyridoxine was withdrawn, and in each case substantial improvement occurred over several months after withdrawal. However, in some cases diminished sensory perception was present even 6 months after pyridoxine discontinuance (see also Coleman et al., 1985; Sensory neuropathy, 1984; Vitamin B_6 Toxicity, 1984). In their review, Alhadeff et al. (1984) also mentioned the possibility that high doses of B_6 may be associated with peptic ulcer disease and with seizures. It is appropriate to point out here that Barthelemy et al. (1981), Lelord et al. (1981), and Martineau et al. (1981) all reported using doses of up to 30 mg/kg/day with their autistic subjects. The adults taking 2 to 6 grams of B_6 would have been receiving 33 to 100 mg/kg/day if one estimates the weight of these adults, most of whom were women, at 60 kg each. It seems a fair question to ask whether the doses given to the autistic children pharmacologically approach those taken by the adult patients seen by Schaumburg et al.

Alhadeff et al. (1984) have discussed other issues, in addition to direct toxic effects, which should be considered where water-soluble vitamins are given in megadoses. These include the following: (a) megadoses may lead to dependency states and withdrawal symptoms upon discontinuance, (b) vitamins may mask symptoms of concurrent disease, (c) pharmacological doses of vitamins may interact with drugs or other vitamins, and (d) intake of high doses of water-soluble vitamins may be unintentionally accompanied by high doses of fat-soluble vitamins, which are considered to be much more toxic (i.e., the two types may be packaged together). Thus, it is clear that therapy with megadoses of nutritional substances is not without risks. As in all other areas of psychopharmacology, any gains from vitamin treatment must be weighed against the risks.

Dietary Treatment

The popular press has given much credence to the widespread belief that there is a strong relationship between behavior disorders in children and the ingestion of certain foods. Although this view is based largely on testimonial evidence rather than scientific research, a large number of parents and family physicians prescribe diets for children to minimize the putative harmful effects of food additives. The most popular of these diets, known as the Feingold diet, is based on the assertion that up to 50% of hyperactive children shown dramatic improvements in their behavior when certain food additives are excluded from their diets.

A number of foods and food additives, including sugar, caffeine, and artificial food flavoring, have been implicated. We will consider the scientific bases for the purported relationship between sugar, caffeine, food allergies, and food additives and behavior disorders in children. In the main, most of these studies involved children who were hyperactive or had specific learning disabilities rather than subjects who were developmentally disabled. However, a small number of studies with this population are available, and these are discussed in detail.

Experimental Design

Two types of experimental design have been used in the evaluation of dietary treatments. It may be useful to consider these briefly before the studies are discussed. The most commonly used design is called the "challenge" design, so-called because the subjects are initially placed on a restrictive diet and are then given specific substances that have been removed from the diet. Subjects may or may not be chosen on the basis of previous exposure to the diet. Those who show favorable changes with the diet are called "responders" and those who do not, "nonresponders." They are maintained on a restricted diet that eliminates the offending substance(s) and are then given, in a blind and counterbalanced order, a challenge diet or placebo.

The alternative is called the "controlled diet" design, which does not require the subjects to be on a restricted diet prior to evaluation. The subjects are maintained on their regualr diets and are then given, in a blind and counterbalanced order, a test diet (e.g., food additive-free diet, or no sugar) or a control (placebo) diet (e.g., food containing additives, or sugar). As in the challenge design, a crossover phase can be included to ensure that each subject is tested under both conditions.

Food Allergies (Various Substances)

There has been a widespread belief that some childhood disorders are caused or exacerbated by children's allergic reactions to certain foods and food additives (Crook, 1973). Thus, artificial food colors and such substances as milk, wheat, oats, rye, eggs, cocoa, and corn are thought to cause behavioral disorders, including hyperactivity in some children. Some individuals are indeed sensitive to synthetic dyes and salicylates (Taylor, 1979) and there are claims up to 10% to 15% of children may have food allergies (Humphrey & White, 1970). However, it has not been established that children with behavioral disorders or hyperactivity have a higher incidence of allergies than their age peers. Although some studies (Rapp, 1978; Trites, Tryphonas, & Ferguson, 1980) have reported a higher prevalence of allergies in hyperactive children, others have not (Mitchell et al., 1987). It is likely that many of these studies did not use a representative sample of such children.

A number of investigators have assessed the effects of elimination and challenge diets on the behavior of food-allergic children. That is, all suspected foods are eliminated from a child's diet for several weeks and then the effects of specific foods are assessed as they are gradually introduced to the child's diet. Uncontrolled studies usually report beneficial effects of elimination diets (Rapp, 1978), but better controlled studies do not bear this out (Trites et al, 1980).

In the only study with a developmentally disabled person, the behavior of a 9-year-old moderately mentally retarded boy was reported to be aggravated by a food allergy, with the offending substance being wheat gluten (Bird, Russo, & Cataldo, 1977). A single-subject design was used to test for the effects of wheat gluten, and it was clearly established that the suspected food allergy did not affect the child's behavior. A behavioral intervention was subsequently implemented by the child's mother that dramatically reduced the child's behavior problems.

In summary, some children do show allergic reactions to various foods, but there is little evidence to suggest that food allergies may be a cause of behavioral disorders. Indeed, as Taylor (1979) has noted, an allergic reaction is "an alteration of the body's response to a substance," producing such symptoms as nasal stuffiness, hives, eczema, rashes, nausea, diarrhea, and asthma. Well-controlled studies that have eliminated the offending substance(s) or used a challenge diet have not reported reductions in children's behavioral problems.

Food Additives and Food Colorings—Feingold Diet

In the mid-1970s a pediatrician, Dr. Benjamin Feingold, popularized the idea that there is a link between food additives and hyperactivity (Feingold, 1975a). He reported that 30% to 50% of hyperactive children placed on diets that eliminated food containing artificial food colors, flavors, and salicylates showed a dramatic improvement in their behavior (Feingold, 1975b). Feingold's contention was that children do not have an allergic reaction to food additives but rather the manifestation of a toxic effect.

That is, the reaction produces a behavioral effect (e.g., short attention span, impulsivity) rather than a physical one (e.g., nasal stuffiness, asthma).

Feingold developed a salicylate-free diet, called the Kaiser-Permanente or K-P diet, which excludes all artificial flavors and colors to be used with hyperactive and learning disabled children. Also excluded are all foods containing natural salicylates such as almonds, apples, and tomatoes, and recently, food preservatives (butylated hydroyanisole and butylated hydroxytoluene) have been added to the list. Like most new forms of treatment, the early clinical reports on the effects of the diet were very positive and supported Feingold's hypothesis. Indeed, parents reported dramatic improvements in their children's behavior when on the diet and a rapid deterioration when the diet was violated. However, subsequent controlled studies have found no causal relationship between food additivies and behavioral disturbance in children. While a very small number of children do show improvements on this diet, the cause of their improvement is not readily apparent, although a simple behavioral explanation has recently been advanced by Zametkin (1985). The experimental literature on the Feingold diet with hyperactive and learning disabled children has been repeatedly reviewed in the past few years, and it is not our intention to add yet another review. Suffice it to say that our own reading of the studies has led us to the same conclusions as those of previous reviewers, namely that the diet does not have a measurable effect in most hyperactive children, although a very small percentage of these youngsters (probably less than 5%) may respond favorably. Readers interested in this area should consult the reviews by Concensus Development Panel (1982), Conners (1980), Harley (1980), Harley et al. (1978), Kavale and Forness (1983), Taylor (1979), Varley (1984), Waksman (1983), and Wender (1986).

In addition to hyperactive and learning disabled children, Feingold also claimed that the behavior of juvenile delinquents and mentally retarded children could be improved by the diet (Wender, 1986). However, neither Feingold nor his supporters provided data to support these claims. Recently two studies have been reported that assessed the effects of the K-P diet on mentally retarded persons and another study, using a mentally retarded boy, assessed its effects on the frequency of uncontrolled seizures.

Harner and Foiles (1980) carried out a double-blind, crossover study with 30 institutionalized mentally retarded persons, ages 4 to 25 years. After a 2-week baseline period, the subjects were divided into two groups of 15 subjects who were given the K-P and a control diet for 6 weeks each and then the conditions were crossed over. Measures of general activity level, excitability, and attention span were taken three times each day, 3 days a week. No statistically significant differences on the three variables were found between the two diets.

Thorley (1984) used a double-blind challenge design to assess the behavioral and cognitive effects of the K-P diet on 10 moderately retarded children. All children were on a K-P diet for 14 consecutive days before being given a challenge of artificial color or placebo during 2 consecutive days over the next 14 days. Three sets of measures were taken: behavior rating scales, psychometric tests, and motor activity measures. No significant differences were found between the two conditions.

In the third study, Haavik, Altman, and Woelk (1979) assessed the effects of the K-P diet plus anticonvulsants on the seizure frequency and activity level of a young mentally retarded boy. A repeated reversal design was used, with the family diet being alternated with the K-P diet and the boy's medication being held constant throughout the trial. Neither the child nor the parents were blind to the experimental conditions. The results showed that the K-P diet resulted in a clinically significant reduction of seizure frequency without affecting the child's activity level. While there is evidence to suggest that ketogenic diets are effective in reducing uncontrolled seizures (Palmer & Ekvall, 1978), this is the first study to suggest that the K-P diet may have a role in the control of seizures. However, it must be remembered that the data were derived from a single-subject study that did not incorporate blind conditions.

In summary, it is clear that the experimental evidence does not support the Feingold hypothesis with developmentally disabled populations and minimally so with hyperactive and learning disabled children. In her review of the literature, Wender (1986) concluded that of the 240 children subjected to the Feingold diet in reported studies, at most three (1%) showed a beneficial response. Even if the success rate were higher, it is important to note that the Feingold diet is unlike any other form of therapy since it requires a complete change in the life-style of the child's family, and even then, the child is likely to violate his or her diet.

Sugar

There has been speculation in the popular press that the consumption of large quantities of refined sugar may contribute to the development or maintenance of learning disabilities and hyperactivity in some children (e.g., Yudkin, 1972). Indeed, parental views of the effects of sugar on their hyperactive children are often reinforced by their family physicians. For example, a recent survey of American primary care physicians has shown that up to 45% of them periodically recommend low-sugar diets for hyperactive children (Bennett & Sherman, 1983).

Overconsumption of refined sugar is thought to result in either overt or subclinical changes in the behavior of some children. These changes may involve either psychological or neurological functions. Buchanan (1984) has suggested that overconsumption of sugar may upset the homeostatic balance necessary for proper metabolism. Buchanan maintains that this occurs mainly in children, as adults are better able to maintain a balanced diet because of their greater cognitive sophistication. While the evidence is rather limited, studies by Prinz, Roberts, and Hantman (1980) and Wolraich, Stumbo, Chenard, and Schultz (1986) clearly suggest that there is no difference in the dietary habits of hyperactive and normal children and that the proportions of energy nutrients eaten by these children are similar to those of adults.

Parental reports on the behavioral toxicity of sugar suggest that its overt effects among responders to sugar-free diets may be dramatic and relatively rapid, occurring within 30 minutes of ingestion (Behar, Rapoport, Adams, Berg, & Cornblath, 1984). Others report a slower but short-lived reaction. Two mechanisms have been advanced that could account for such effects. The first is that sugar has a direct toxic effect on the behavior of some children and the other is that there is a somewhat slower hypoglycemic reaction.

A number of studies have reported on the behavioral effects of sugar in children. In a descriptive study, Prinz et al. (1980) reported a significant correlation between sugar intake and behavior in 28 hyperactive children. They found a direct correlation between the amount of sugar foods eaten and destructive aggressive behaviors in these children. While their findings provided support for parental anecdotes, this study was methodologically flawed, and its findings must be interpreted with caution. In addition to problems of measurement and significance levels, the correlational data presented in this study do not allow one to make causal inferences between the effects of sugar and children's behavior. In a replication of this study with much tighter methodological controls, Barling and Bullen (1984) failed to find a positive correlation between sugar consumption and adverse behavioral reactions.

A number of challenge studies have focused on the relationship between sugar ingestion and the behavior and academic performance of children, especially children with attention deficit disorder (ADD) (see Milich, Wolraich, & Lindgren, in press). While there are minor variations in their findings, the better controlled studies show with a great deal of uniformity that when compared to a placebo, sugar does not significantly impair the behavior or academic performance of these children (Behar et al., 1984; Milich & Pelham, 1986; Wolraich, Milich, Stumbo, & Schultz, 1985). Although some research remains to be undertaken, especially in relation to dosage and age variables, the current findings seriously question the purported relationship between sugar ingestion and behavior in children who are not developmentally disabled.

Only two studies have attempted to test the effects of sugar on the behavior of developmentally disabled children. In an early study, O'Banion, Armstrong, Cummings, and Stange (1978) reported the effects of various foods on the hyperactive and disruptive behavior of an 8-year-old autistic boy. Sugar (along with wheat, corn, tomatoes, mushrooms, and dairy products) was implicated in increasing the disruptive behavior of this boy. However, the study was totally uncontrolled, and its findings must, therefore, be viewed with caution. Kanabay (1984) studied the effects of sugar in a single-subject withdrawal design with an autistic boy. Increased sugar ingestion was correlated with increased levels of disruptive behavior, although the child's attention was not affected. Kanabay (1984) suggested that reactivity to sugar might account for some of the disruptive and aggressive behaviors seen in autistic children.

In summary, the only conclusion that can be drawn from the available research is that sugar does not appear to have a measurable effect on the behavior and academic performance of nondevelopmentally disabled children. If it does have subclinical psychological and/or neurological effects, these have not been amenable to measurement thus far. The data on the effects of sugar with developmentally disabled individuals are almost non-existent, with the two available case reports providing an inadequate basis for drawing any conclusions.

Caffeine

It has been suggested that caffeine and sugar may act synergistically in the development or exacerbation of behavioral disorders in children (Powers, 1973). Caffeine, a methylxanthine, is a central nervous system stimulant commonly found in coffee, tea, and cola drinks. When taken orally, it is absorbed rapidly, reaching peak blood plasma levels within 30 minutes, with a plasma half-life of 2.5 to 4.5 hours (Axelrod & Reichenthal, 1953). In a review of the dietary habits of 50 children with various childhood disorders, Powers (1975) found that these children ingested ". . . a huge amount of caffeinated drinks." A survey by the Federation of American Societies for Experimental Biology (FASEB) (1978) found that children aged between 1 and 5 years consumed 3.0 mg/kg of caffeine per day and those between 6 and 11 years, 2.1 mg/kg per day. It appears that children do in fact consume a substantial amount of caffeine in various forms such as coffee, tea, cola drinks, and chocolate.

In the only study that investigated the effects of caffeine on the behavior of mentally retarded persons (18–30-year-old adults), Podboy and Mallory (1977) found that, when compared to caffeinated coffee, decaffeinated coffee significantly reduced their aggressive behavior as well as reducing their overall coffee consumption. While the data suggest that caffeine may *maintain* behavior problems in mentally retarded persons, this was a clinical study without adequate methodological controls and no firm conclusions can be drawn.

Thus it appears, in the United States at least, that children do consume a considerable amount of caffeine, but there are no data to suggest that hyperactive or developmentally disabled children do so any more than their peers. The data in relation to caffeine and children's behavior problems must be regarded as equivocal at this time. Recent studies (e.g., Rapoport, Berg, Ismond, Zahn, & Neims, 1984) suggest that the effect of caffeine may be moderated by the dietary history of the subject, with heavy and low consumers of caffeine having a differential response to equivalent doses. In addition, there is a dearth of information about the impact of caffeine on developmentally disabled children and adults.

Conclusion

In summary, it is well established that developmentally disabled persons are at risk for nutritional deficiencies. Furthermore, there are a number of genetically transmitted metabolic disorders that can be profitably and legitimately treated by dietary means. At the same time there have been some irrational and even bizarre attempts to treat developmentally disabled people with various concoctions of nutritional substances and hormones. One of the most interesting cases from an historical view involved glutamic acid, once the subject of intense research activity but virtually unheard of today.

In the recent past we have seen enthusiastic claims made for the Bronson GTC3 formula (Harrell et al., 1981), vitamin B_6 in autism (Rimland, 1973, 1982), and a mixture of vitamins for hyperactivity and specific learning disabilities (Cott, 1974). This literature is of very uneven quality, and we note that the large majority of well-designed studies tend to be negative. With the possible exception of pyridoxine in autism we regard these therapies as essentially disproven. Likewise, the literature on dietary treatments, designed to cope with food allergies or to remove refined sugar or food additives, is largely negative, despite numerous uncritical claims made in the popular press. More research of better quality, and preferably carried out by independent workers, will be needed before any of these supplemental or dietary approaches can be regarded as useful treatments for behavior or cognitive disorders in the developmentally disabled population.

Few of the vitamin studies reviewed incorporated objective (biochemical) tests of vitamin status before the trials started. As poor diets are common in developmentally disabled people, many of these individuals could have had preexisting (subclinical) deficiencies and hence would improve even on physiological doses as the deficit was corrected (Birkbeck, 1987). This, of course, would not support multivitamin or megavitamin theories but simply would show that dietary and clinical/biochemical status should always be considered in such individuals.

One question that arises is why the public and some workers have been so zealous in their use of these therapies? Freeman (1978) has suggested that part of the appeal may depend on the "anti-establishment" stance of these treatments, and the fact that there are no barriers (such as requiring a doctor's prescription) to implementing them. Another reason undoubtedly is that some people believe these nutritional approaches to be simply "more of a good thing," which may bestow benefits and can cost nothing in physiological and behavioral terms. The data on side effects accompanying megavitamin therapy, although somewhat scanty at this time, clearly show this to be a false assumption, at least for some supplements.

Acknowledgments. Preparation of this paper was supported in part by a grant from the Medical Research Council of New Zealand to Dr. M.G. Aman. The authors would like to thank Drs. John Birkbeck and Gordon Lees (University of Auckland), Betty Kozlowski (Ohio State University), and George Ellman and Charles Silverstein (Sonoma Developmental Center, California) for their helpful critical comments on this paper. We also thank Mrs. Marsha Aman for typing the manuscript.

References

Alhadeff, L., Gualtieri, C.T., & Lipton, M. (1984). Toxic effects of water-soluble vitamins. *Nutrition Reviews, 42*, 33–46.

Aman, M.G., Mitchell, E.A., & Turbott, S.H. (1987). The effects of essential fatty acid supplementation by Efamol in hyperactive children. *Journal of Abnormal Child Psychology, 15*, 75–90.

American Dietetic Association (1981). Infant and child nutrition: Concerns regarding the developmentally disabled. *Journal of the American Dietetic Association, 17*, 443–452.

Arnold, L.E., Christopher, J., Huestis, R.D., & Smeltzer, D.J. (1978). Megavitamins for minimal brain dysfunction. *Journal of the American Medical Association, 240*, 2642–2643.

Astin, A.W., & Ross, S. (1960). Glutamic acid and human intelligence. *Psychological Bulletin, 57*, 429–434.

Axelrod, J., & Reichenthal, J. (1953). The fate of caffeine in man and a method for estimation in biological material. *Journal of Pharmacology and Experimental Therapeutics, 107*, 519–523.

Barling, J., & Bullen, G. (1984). Dietary factors and hyperactivity. *Journal of Genetic Psychology, 146*, 117–123.

Barlow, P.J., Sylvester, P.E., & Dickerson, J.W.T. (1981). Hair trace metal levels in Down syndrome patients. *Journal of Mental Deficiency Research, 25*, 161–168.

Barthelemy, C., Garreau, B., Leddet, I., Ernouf, D., Muh, J.R., & Lelord, G. (1981). *Magnesium Bulletin, 2*, 150–153.

Behar, D., Rapoport, J., Adams, A., Berg, C., & Cornblath, M. (1984). Sugar challenge testing with children considered behaviorally "sugar-reactive". *Journal of Nutrition and Behavior, 1*, 277–288.

Bennett, F.C., McClelland, Kriegsmann, E.A., Andrus, L.B., & Sells, C.J. (1983). Vitamin and mineral supplementation in Down's syndrome. *Pediatrics, 72*, 707–713.

Bennett, F.C., & Sherman, R. (1983). Management of childhood "hyperactivity" by primary care physicians. *Journal of Developmental and Behavioral Pediatrics, 4*, 88–93.

Bird, B.L., Russo, D.C., & Cataldo, M.F. (1977). Considerations in the analysis and treatment of dietary effects on behavior disorders. *Journal of Autism and Childhood Schizophrenia, 7,* 373–382.

Birkbeck, J. (1987). Introduction. In J. Birkbeck (Ed.), *Are we really what we eat?* Auckland, New Zealand: Dairy Advisory Bureau.

Buchanan, S.R. (1984). The most ubiquitous toxin. *American Psychologist, 39,* 1327–1328.

Callaway, E. (1977). Response of infantile autism to large doses of B_6. *Psychopharmacology Bulletin, 13,* 57–58.

Chaney, M.S., & Ross, M.L. (1971). *Nutrition.* Boston: Houghton, Mifflin.

Chanowitz, J., Ellman, G., Silverstein, C.I., Zingarelli, G., & Ganger, E. (1985). Thyroid and vitamin-mineral supplement fail to improve IQ of mentally retarded adults. *American Journal of Mental Deficiency, 90,* 217–219.

Coburn, S.P., Schaltenbrand, W.E., Mahuren, J.D., Clausman, R.J., & Townsend, D. (1983). Effect of megavitamin treatment on mental performance and plasma vitamin B_6 concentrations in mentally retarded young adults. *American Journal of Clinical Nutrition, 38,* 352–355.

Cole, H.S., Lopez, R., Epel, R., Singh, B.K., & Cooperman, J.M. (1985). Nutritional deficiencies in institutionalized mentally retarded and physically disabled individuals. *American Journal of Mental Deficiency, 89,* 552–555.

Coleman, M., Sobel, S., Bhagavan, H.N., Coursin, D., Marquardt, A., Guay, M., & Hunt, C. (1985). A double blind study of vitamin B_6 in Down's syndrome infants: Part 1. Clinical and biochemical results. *Journal of Mental Deficiency Research, 29,* 233–240.

Colquhoun, I., & Bunday, S. (1981). A lack of essential fatty acids as a possible cause of hyperactivity in children. *Medical Hypotheses, 7,* 673–679.

Concensus Development Panel Cosponsored by the National Institute of Allergy and Infectious Diseases and the National Institute of Child Health and Human Development (1982). Defined diets and childhood hyperactivity. *Journal of the American Medical Association, 248,* 290–292.

Conners, C.K. (1980). *Food additives and hyperactive children.* New York: Plenum Press.

Cott, A. (1971). Orthomolecular approach to the treatment of learning disabilities. *Schizophrenia, 3,* 95–105.

Cott, A. (1972). Megavitamins: The orthomolecular approach to behavioral disorders and learning disabilities. *Academic Therapy, 7,* 245–258.

Cott, A. (1974). Treatment of learning disabilities. *Journal of Orthomolecular Psychiatry, 3,* 343–355.

Crook, W.G. (1973). *Your allergic child.* New York: Medcom.

DiPalma, J.R., & Ritchie, D.M. (1977). Vitamin toxicity. *Annual Review of Pharmacology and Toxicology, 17,* 133–148.

Ellis, N.R., & Tomporowski, P.D. (1983). Vitamin/mineral supplements and intelligence of institutionalized mentally retarded adults. *American Journal of Mental Deficiency, 88,* 211–214.

Ellman, G., Salfi, M., Fong, A., Murphy, P., Silverstein, C.I., Smith, J., & Zingarelli, G. (1986). Vitamin B_6 status measures of an institutionalized mentally retarded population. *American Journal of Mental Deficiency, 91,* 30–34.

Ellman, G., Silverstein, C.I., Zingarelli, G., Schafer, E.W.P., & Silverstein, L. (1984). Vitamin-mineral supplement fails to improve IQ of mentally retarded young adults. *American Journal of Mental Deficiency, 88,* 688–691.

Federation of American Societies for Experimental Biology (1978). *Evaluation of the health aspects of caffeine as a food ingredient.* Washington, DC: National Technical Information Service, U.S. Department of Commerce.

Feingold, B.F. (1975a). *Why your child is hyperactive.* New York: Random House.

Feingold, B.F. (1975b). Hyperkinesis and learning disabilities linked to the ingestion of artificial food colors and flavors. *American Journal of Nursing, 75,* 797–803.

Frager, J., Barnet, A., Weiss, I., & Coleman, M. (1985). A double blind study of vitamin B_6 in Down's syndrome infants: Part 2. Cortical auditory evoked potentials. *Journal of Mental Deficiency Research, 29,* 241–246.

Freeman, R.D. (1978). Introduction: A false dawn? *Journal of Special Education, 12,* 7–8.

Gadson, E.P. (1951). Glutamic acid and mental deficiency—A review. *American Journal of Mental Deficiency, 55,* 521–529.

Gentile, P.S., Trentalange, M.J., Zamichek, W., & Coleman, M. (1983). Brief report: Trace elements in the hair of autistic and control children. *Journal of Autism and Developmental Disorders, 13,* 205–206.

Gibson, R.A., Tao, B.S.K., & Attwood, E. (1987). *Control trial of evening primrose oil in the treatment of Attention Deficit Disorder (hyperactivity).* Flinders Medical Centre.

Glutamic acid and mental functions. (1951). *Nutrition Reviews, 9,* 113–117.

Gouge, A.L., & Ekvall, S.W. (1975). Diets of handicapped children: Physical, psychological and socioeconomic correlations. *American Journal of Mental Deficiency, 80,* 149–157.

Gualtieri, C.T., van Bourgondien, M.E., Hartz, C., Schopler, E., & Marcus, L. (May, 1981). *A pilot study of pyridoxine treatment in autistic children.* Paper presented at the meeting of the American Psychiatric Association, New Orleans, LA.

Haavik, S., Altman, K., & Woelk, C. (1979). Effects of the Feingold diet on seizures and hyperactivity: A single-subject analysis. *Journal of Behavioral Medicine, 2,* 365–374.

Harley, J., Ray, R., Tomasi, L., Eichman, P., Matthews, C., Chun, R., Cleeland, C., & Traisman, E. (1978). Hyperkinesis and food additives: Testing the Feingold hypothesis. *Pediatrics, 61,* 818–828.

Harley, J.P. (1980). Dietary treatment of behavioral disorders. In B.W. Camp (Ed.), *Advances in behavioral pediatrics* (Vol. 1, pp. 129–151). Greenwich, CT: JAI Press.

Harner, I.C., & Foiles, R.A.L. (1980). Effect of Feingold's K-P diet on a residential, mentally handicapped population. *Journal of the American Dietetic Association, 76,* 575–580.

Harrell, R.F., Capp, R.H., Davis, D.R., Peerless, J., & Ravitz, L.R. (1981). Can nutritional supplements help mentally retarded children? An exploratory study. *Proceedings of the National Academy of Science, 78,* 574–578.

Haslam, R.H.A., Dalby, J.T., & Rademaker, A.W. (1984). Effects of megavitamin therapy on children with attention deficit disorders. *Pediatrics, 74,* 103–111.

Humphrey, J.H., & White, R.G. (1970). *Immunology for students of medicine* (3rd ed.). London: Blackwell Scientific Publications.

Jackson, M.J., & Garrod, P.J. (1978). Plasma zinc, copper, and amino acid levels in the blood of autistic children. *Journal of Autism and Childhood Schizophrenia*, *8*, 203–208.

Kanabay, G.P. (1984). The effects of sugar upon the behavior of an autistic child within a structured work situation. *Dissertation Abstracts International*, *45*(2-B), 673.

Kavale, K.A., & Forness, S.R. (1983). Hyperactivity and diet treatment: A meta-analysis of the Feingold hypothesis. *Journal of Learning Disabilities*, *16*, 324–330.

Kershner, J., & Hawke, W. (1979). Megavitamins and learning disorders: A controlled double-blind experiment. *Journal of Nutrition*, *109*, 819–826.

Lelord, G., Callaway, E., & Muh, J.P. (1982). Clinical and biological effects of high doses of vitamin B_6 and magnesium on autistic children. *Acta Vitaminologica et Enzymologica*, *4*, 27–42.

Lelord, G., Muh, J.P., Barthelemy, C., Martineau, J., Garreau, B., & Callaway, E. (1981). Effects of pyridoxine and magnesium on autistic symptoms—Initial observations. *Journal of Autism and Developmental Disorders*, *11*, 219–230.

Louttit, R. (1965). Chemical facilitation of intelligence among the mentally retarded. *American Journal of Mental Deficiency*, *69*, 495–501.

Martineau, J., Barthelemy, C., Garreau, B., & Lelord, G. (1985). Vitamin B_6, magnesium, and combined B_6 - Mg: Therapeutic effects in childhood autism. *Biological Psychiatry*, *20*, 467–478.

Martineau, J., Garreau, B., Barthelemy, C., Callaway, E., & Lelord, G. (1981). Effects of vitamin B_6 on averaged evoked potentials in infantile autism. *Biological Psychiatry*, *16*, 627–641.

Matin, M.A., Sylvester, P.E., Edwards, D., & Dickerson, J.W.T. (1981). Vitamin and zinc status in Down syndrome. *Journal of Mental Deficiency Research*, *25*, 121–126.

Milich, R., & Pelham, W.E. (1986). Effects of sugar ingestion on the classroom and playgroup behavior of attention deficit disordered boys. *Journal of Consulting and Clinical Psychology*, *54*, 714–718.

Milich, R., Wolraich, M., & Lindgren, S. (in press). Sugar and hyperactivity: A critical review of empirical findings. *Clinical Psychology Review*.

Mitchell, E.A., Aman, M.G., Turbott, S.H., & Manku, M. (1987). Clinical characteristics and serum essential fatty acid levels in hyperactive children. *Clinical Pediatrics*, *26*, 406–411.

Mitchell, E.A., Lewis, S., & Cutler, D.R. (1983). Essential fatty acids and maladjusted behavior in children. *Prostalandins, Leukotrienes, and Medicine*, *12*, 281–287.

Moss, N., & Broverman, H. (1978). Megavitamin therapy for autistic children. *American Journal of Psychiatry*, *135*, 1425.

O'Banion, D., Armstrong, B., Cummings, R.A., & Stange, J. (1978). Disruptive behavior: A dietary approach. *Journal of Autism and Childhood Schizophrenia*, *8*, 325–337.

Palmer, S., & Ekvall, S. (1978). *Pediatric nutrition in developmental disorders*. Springfield, IL: Thomas.

Pathophysiological basis of vitamin A toxicity. (1982). *Nutrition Reviews*, *40*, 272–274.

Podboy, J.W., & Mallory, W.A. (1977). Caffeine reduction and behavior change in the severely retarded. *Mental Retardation*, *15*, 40.

Powers, H.W.S. (1973). Dietary measures to improve behavior and achievement. *Academic Therapy*, *9*, 203–214.

Powers, H.W.S. (1975). Caffeine, behavior and the LD child. *Academic Therapy*, *11*, 5–19.

Prinz, R.J., Roberts, W.A., & Hantman, E. (1980). Dietary correlates of hyperactive behavior in children. *Journal of Consulting and Clinical Psychology*, *48*, 760–769.

Pueschel, S.M., Reed, R.B., Cronk, C.E., & Goldstein, B.I. (1980). 5-Hydroxytryptophan and pyridoxine: Their effects in young children with Down's syndrome. *American Journal of Diseases of Childhood*, *134*, 838–844.

Rapoport, J.L., Berg, C.J., Ismond, D.R., Zahn, T.P., & Neims, A. (1984). Behavioral effects of caffeine in children: Relationship between dietary choice and effects of caffeine challenge. *Archives of General Psychiatry*, *41*, 1073–1079.

Rapp, D.J. (1978). Does diet affect hyperactivity. *Journal of Learning Disabilities*, *11*, 56–62.

Rimland, B. (1973). High-dosage levels of certain vitamins in the treatment of children with severe mental disorders. In D. Hawkins & L. Pauling (Eds.), *Orthomolecular psychiatry* (pp. 513–539). New York: W.H. Freeman.

Rimland, B. (1982). *Form letter regarding megavitamin therapy for autism and related disorders (Publication No. 39B)*. San Diego: Institute for Child Behavior Research.

Rimland, B., Callaway, E., & Dreyfus, P. (1978). The effect of high doses of vitamin B$_6$ on autistic children: A double-blind crossover study. *American Journal of Psychiatry*, *135*, 472–475.

Roche, A.F., Lipman, R.S., Overall, J.E., & Hung, W. (1979). The effects of stimulant medication on the growth of hyperkinetic children. *Pediatrics*, *63*, 847–850.

Sankar, D.V.S. (1970). Biogenic amine uptake by blood platelets and RBC in childhood schizophrenia. *Acta Paedopsychiatrica*, *37*, 174–182.

Sankar, D.V.S. (1979). Plasma levels of folates, riboflavin, vitamin B$_6$, and ascorbate in severely disturbed children. *Journal of Autism and Developmental Disorders*, *9*, 73–82.

Schaumburg, H., Kaplan, J., Windebank, N., Vick, S., Rasmus, D., & Brown, M.J. (1983). Sensory neuropathy from pyridoxine abuse: A new megavitamin syndrome. *New England Journal of Medicine*, *309*, 445–448.

Sensory neuropathy from megadoses of pyridoxine. (1984). *Nutrition Reviews*, *42*, 49–51.

Share, J.B. (1976). Review of drug treatment for Down's syndrome persons. *American Journal of Mental Deficiency*, *80*, 388–393.

Shearer, T.R., Larson, K., Neuschwander, J., & Gedney, B. (1982). Minerals in the hair and nutrient intake of autistic children. *Journal of Autism and Developmental Disorders*, *12*, 25–34.

Smith, G.F., Spiker, D., Peterson, C.P., Cicchetti, D., & Justine, P. (1984). Use of megadoses of vitamins with minerals in Down syndrome. *Journal of Pediatrics*, *105*, 228–234.

Sylvester, P.E. (1984). Nutritional aspects of Down's syndrome with special reference to the nervous system. *British Journal of Psychiatry*, *145*, 115–120.

Taylor, E. (1979). Food additives, allergy and hyperkinesis. *Journal of Child Psychology and Psychiatry*, *20*, 357–363.

Thorley, G. (1984). Pilot study to assess behavioural and cognitive effects of artificial food colours in a group of retarded children. *Developmental Medicine and Child Neurology*, 26, 56–61.

Trites, R.L., Tryphonas, J., & Ferguson, H.B. (1980). Diet treatment for hyperactive children with food allergies. In R.M. Knights & D.J. Bakker (Eds.), *Treatment of hyperactive and learning disordered children* (pp. 151–163). Baltimore: University Park Press.

Varley, C.K. (1984). Diet and the behavior of children with attention deficit disorder. *Journal of the American Academy of Child Psychiatry*, 23, 182–185.

Vitamin B_6 toxicity: A new megavitamin syndrome. (1984). *Nutrition Reviews*, 42, 44–46.

Vogel, W., Broverman, D.M., Draguns, J.G., & Klaiber, E.L. (1966). The role of glutamic acid in cognitive behaviors. *Psychological Bulletin*, 65, 367–382.

Waelsch, H. (1984). A biochemical consideration of mental deficiency. The role of glutamic acid. *American Journal of Mental Deficiency*, 52, 305–313.

Waksman, S.A. (1983). Diet and children's behavior disorders: A review of the research. *Clinical Psychology Review*, 3, 201–213.

Weathers, C. (1983). Effects of nutritional supplementation on IQ and certain other variables associated with Down syndrome. *American Journal of Mental Deficiency*, 88, 214–217.

Wecker, L., Miller, S.B., Cochran, S.R., Dugger, D.L., & Johnson, W.D. (1985). Trace element concentrations in hair from autistic children. *Journal of Mental Deficiency Research*, 29, 15–22.

Wender, E.H. (1986). The food additive-free diet in the treatment of behavior disorders: A review. *Journal of Developmental and Behavioral Pediatrics*, 7, 35–42.

Wilton, K.M., & Irvine, J. (1983). Nutritional intakes of socioculturally mentally retarded children vs. children of low and average socioeconomic status. *American Journal of Mental Deficiency*, 88, 79–85.

Wolraich, M., Milich, R., Stumbo, P., & Schultz, F. (1985). Effects of sucrose ingestion on the behavior of hyperactive boys. *Journal of Pediatrics*, 106, 675–682.

Wolraich, M.L., Stumbo, P., Chenard, C., & Schultz, F. (1986). Dietary characteristics of hyperactive and control boys and their behavioral correlates. *Journal of the American Dietetic Association*, 86, 500–504.

Yannet, H. (1957). Research in the field of mental retardation. *Journal of Pediatrics*, 50, 236–239.

Yudkin, J. (1972). *Sweet and dangerous*. New York: Bantam.

Zametkin, A. (1985). The carrot hypothesis. *Journal of the American Academy of Child Psychiatry*, 24, 240–241.

Zimmerman, F.T., & Burgemeister, B.B. (1959). A controlled experiment of glutamic acid therapy. *AMA Archives of Neurology and Psychiatry*, 81, 639–648.

9
Tardive Dyskinesia and Developmental Disabilities

Gerald S. Golden

Abstract

Neuroleptic drugs are commonly used in the management of individuals with mental retardation, autism and other pervasive developmental disorders, and Tourette syndrome. Analysis of the risks and features of tardive dyskinesia in these populations is difficult because of the problems of defining tardive dyskinesia in children, definition of patient populations, a high background level of preexisting involuntary movements, and the frequent use of other medications that also are active on the central nervous system. Review of the literature documents that individuals in all of these patient groups are at risk for the development of tardive dyskinesia, although its prevalence is not clear. As these drugs are effective therapeutically in many circumstances, a detailed cost-benefit analysis must be developed for each patient and combined with regularly scheduled monitoring for the presence of a dyskinesia. It has also been demonstrated that a number of other drugs can cause a syndrome resembling tardive dyskinesia. The situation can only be clarified by appropriate drug withdrawals and challenges.

Tardive dyskinesia (TD) refers to abnormal involuntary movements in an individual resulting from chronic exposure to neuroleptic drugs. This was first described in 1957 (Schonecker, 1957) and the term itself was introduced in 1964 (Faurbye, Rasch, Peterson, Brandborg, & Pakkenberg, 1964). The most common clinical use of neuroleptic drugs is for treating major psychoses in adults. Although millions of patients have been treated, and tardive dyskinesia has been recognized for 25 years, many controversies remain. These include the basic definitions of the disorder, the relationship of the onset of the movements and their persistence to changes in the dose of medication, and assessment of the exact risk for a specific individual. In the adult psychiatric population, the prevalence of TD has been reported as ranging between 0.05% and 65% (American Psychiatric Association, 1979). More recent studies suggest a prevalence of 10% to 20% (Kane & Smith, 1982).

A second group of patients, who frequently are treated with neuroleptic drugs, are children and adults with developmental disabilities. Treatment is directed toward controlling behavior, although the response is usually not as dramatic as that of the psychotic adult. For that reason, high doses of medication are often used for prolonged periods of time. In addition, the specific disabilities and their underlying pathophysiology are diverse and often poorly understood. These variables, and others to be discussed, further complicate full understanding of the problem.

This review summarizes the published data concerning tardive dyskinesia in children and adults with developmental disabilities. Other chronic neuroleptic-induced movement disorders, such as tardive Tourette syndrome, are also reviewed. Finally, although the classic definition of TD requires exposure to *neuroleptic* agents, identical syndromes have been reported following the administration of other drugs of this patient population. Because these drugs are frequently used in the overall treatment of developmentally disabled individuals, and their potential for producing a movement disorder is a confounding issue, this area is reviewed also.

Definition and Classification of Tardive Dyskinesia

As noted, tardive dyskinesia consists of abnormal involuntary movements in a patient who has been chronically exposed to neuroleptic drugs. Two types of abnormal movements are characteristic. The first is the buccolingual masticatory syndrome, which is manifested by involuntary movements about the mouth. Most characteristic are chewing and sucking movements and curling and licking movements of the tongue. The second is choreiform movements of the extremities. Some of these may be of large amplitude and ballistic in nature. Associated findings often include movements of the trunk and diaphragmatic movements that can interfere with speech and respiration in severe cases (Goetz & Klawans, 1984; Gualtieri & Guimond, 1981).

At this time there is no biological marker for TD, and the diagnosis is a clinical one. In an attempt to systematize the diagnosis and allow investigators to provide comparable data, several rating scales have been developed. Many of the available scales, as well as psychometric issues in the assessment of TD, have been discussed in detail by Gardos, Cole, and La Brie (1977) and Kalachnik (1983, 1984). Some of the better known and more popular multi-item scales of TD are as follows: the Abnormal Involuntary Movement Scale (AIMS) (Guy, 1976), the Tardive Dyskinesia Rating Scale (TDRS) (Simpson, Lee, Zoubok, & Gardos, 1979), the Smith Tardive Dyskinesia Scale (see Fann, Smith, Davis, & Domino, 1980), the Withdrawal Emergent Symptom Checklist (WESC) (Polizos, Engelhardt, Hoffman, & Waizer, 1973), and the Dyskinesia Identification System–Coldwater (DIS–CO) (Kalachnik, Kidd-Nielsen, & Harder, 1983; Sprague, 1982), which was specifically developed for mentally retarded individuals. The interested reader is referred to the original papers as well as the critiques by Gardos et al. and Kalachnik for further information on these instruments and other pertinent assessment issues.

Research diagnostic criteria for TD have been developed by Schooler and Kane (1982). These require that neuroleptics be used for at least 90 days before the diagnosis of TD can be considered. In addition, there should be at least moderate abnormal, involuntary movements in one area of the body or mild movements in a least two or more areas. Finally, there should be no other coexisting conditions (such as any choreiform disorders or tics) that are known to result in dyskinesias and, if involuntary movements were present before neuroleptic drugs were introduced, the diagnosis of TD should not be made. This latter criterion presents great difficulties in a group of patients with developmental disabilities, as preexisting dyskinesias are commonly present as well as other peculiar movements such as stereotypies.

A much more difficult problem arises when attempting to define the temporal relationships between changing doses of the neuroleptic and the onset and persistence of movement. Schooler and Kane (1982) distinguish six subgroups.

1. *Probable TD*   The patient meets all of the characteristics of TD, but has been examined and rated on only one occasion.
2. *Masked probable TD*   A patient meets the criteria for probable TD but because of an increase in the dose of neuroleptics, the movements are no longer present.
3. *Transient TD*   Movements typical of TD are present, but disappear in 3 months with no modification in the neuroleptic dose.
4. *Withdrawal TD*   The movements occur when neuroleptics are discontinued, but disappear spontaneously within 3 months.
5. *Persistent TD*   Movements continue for longer than 3 months.
6. *Masked persistent TD*   The movements have continued for longer than 3 months, but disappear following an increase in neuroleptic dose.

Whether or not these syndromes differ in any fundamental way is not clear (Goetz & Klawans, 1984). For the purposes of this review, the data are reported without making assumptions concerning this problem.

Of course, the population of patients with developmental disabilities includes many children, which raises a number of additional issues in the diagnosis of TD. It had long been thought that this disorder rarely occurred in children, but a recent survey of pediatric neurologists indicated that one third had seen patients who fit the clinical definition of TD (Silverstein & Johnston, 1985). The diagnostic difficulties and differences between TD in children and adults have been reviewed by Gualtieri, Barnhill, McGimsey, and Schell (1980). They point out that most of the data at that time consisted of studies of small numbers of individuals. It also was apparent that the medication was often used in conditions in which the children had preexisting abnormal movements or stereotypies. The reported movements ranged from a typical buccolingual masticatory syndrome to facial tics. Other patients had choreoathetoid, ballistic, or myoclonic movements. Posturing, torticollis, and ataxia were also reported.

A more recent review by Campbell, Grega, Green, and Bennett (1983) provides supporting evidence that all forms of TD do occur in children. They felt that the dose and length of exposure to medication were risk factors, as they appear to be in the adult.

To summarize, four problems must be taken into account when reviewing the issue of tardive dyskinesia in individuals with developmental disabilities:

1. The uncertain status of the diagnostic criteria of TD in children
2. The presence of a high background level of preexisting involuntary movements in children and adults with developmental disabilities
3. The high incidence of stereotypies in this population
4. The frequent use of medications other than neuroleptics in this population group, including anticonvulsants, muscle relaxants, drugs to reduce spasticity, and other drugs that may also have effects on the central nervous system

General Aspects of Tardive Dyskinesia

TD is most frequently associated with the chronic use of neuroleptic drugs. There appears to be a relationship between total lifetime exposure to these agents and the risk of occurrence (Gualtieri, Schroeder, Hicks, & Quade, 1986), but symptoms can also occur following relatively brief exposure (Kane & Smith, 1982). A common feature of the drugs associated with TD is that they are potent dopamine blockers (see Chapters 7 and 10). There is some evidence that the development of dopamine receptor supersensitivity is the major pathogenetic factor (Goetz & Klawans, 1984).

Attempts have been made to define those individuals at risk for the development of TD (Tarsy, 1983). Age over 50 years appears to be a consistent risk factor; female gender somewhat less so. Despite early attempts to correlate an increased risk in patients with underlying brain damage, this has not been supported by more recent studies.

Treatment is a difficult problem and is largely unsatisfactory (Goetz & Klawans, 1984). Increasing the dose of the neuroleptic drug, or reinstituting it if it has been discontinued, will control symptoms but with the probable development of more severe TD at a later time. Dopamine-depleting agents or drugs that increase striatal cholinergic activity have been tried, but results are not predictable, and these therapies are not being routinely used.

The best prognosis is found if the drug is discontinued. TD may transiently worsen, but some patients will achieve a remission within months or during the next year or two. In some cases, unfortunately, the underlying psychiatric or behavioral problems may be so severe that medication cannot be withdrawn.

Tardive Dyskinesia and Mental Retardation

In addition to some of the complicating issues listed above, individuals with mental retardation may not be able to cooperate fully with an examination and this may cause problems when attempting to use a rating scale for TD. Kalachanik, Kidd-Nielsen, et al. (1983) demonstrated that decreasing IQ level and decreasing cooperation level both increased the number of nonassessable items on the Dyskinesia Identification System–Coldwater. IQ level and level of cooperation were closely interrelated. The items most likely to be nonassessable, especially in the group with profound mental retardation, included mouth opening to allow viewing of tongue movements, examination of leg and toe movements, walking in place, and gait. They concluded that studies of TD in this population would be improved if the subjects were given behavioral training to open their mouths on cue.

The first study of TD as a possible complication of long-term therapy with phenothiazines in a population of subjects with mental retardation was that of Paulson, Rizvi, and Crane (1975). They examined 2,145 residents of a facility for mental retardation and found 103 children in the 11- to 16-year-old age group who had been treated with long-term use of phenothiazines. Twenty-one of these children had mild to moderate TD. There were 15 boys and 16 girls.

Medication was then discontinued for 3 weeks. Seven patients became worse, and in each case the symptoms abated when the drug was reintroduced. The movements of two patients became less apparent after medication was discontinued. On follow-up 4 years later, symptoms persisted at the same level in six patients, were worse in four patients, and had improved in five. The study did not provide information on drug dose and duration. There were also no details concerning the exact method of assessment of the severity of symptoms or interrater reliability. Despite these problems, it seems quite clear that the authors did define a chronic movement disorder that resulted from the use of phenothiazines.

Bicknell and Blowers (1980) reported the presence of abnormal movements in a group of women in a long-term care facility. They ranged in age from 42 to 87 years with a mean age of 65. No clinical details were given but they had been in the hospital from 2 to 50 years with a mean of 32. It is not clear what the total population of the ward was. In this group, nine had received medication in the past 7 years. Forty-nine percent of the total group had obvious TD and 37% were categorized as mild TD. The movements primarily involved the face, tongue, jaws, and hands. All nine who had recently received drugs had some abnormal movements. It is of note that 25 of 31 residents of the ward who had *not* taken neuroleptic drugs also had abnormal movements. This high background level in untreated patients makes interpretation of the movements in those who had drugs difficult (Kane & Smith, 1982).

Two separate populations (residents in a North Carolina and in a Michigan institution) were studied by Gualtieri, Breuning, Schroeder, and Quade (1982). A total of 95 subjects were referred for trial withdrawal of medication. Entry criteria included an IQ less than 75; AAMD Adaptive Behavior Scales in the mentally retarded range, a stable environment, appropriate educational or workshop placement, good general health, the absence of neurological disease that could cause dyskinesia, and continuous neuroleptic therapy for at least 6 months. The 38 patients in North Carolina were followed with serial examinations for 8 weeks after withdrawal of medication, using the Abnormal Involuntary Movement Scale (AIMS). Examination was carried out weekly for the first 8 weeks. If a dyskinesia was present at that time, the patient was followed monthly.

Only the data from the North Carolina series are presented here. This group consisted of 28 males and 10 females with a mean age of 19.4 years and a range of 5 to 47 years. The mean dose was 239.9 mg of chlorpromazine equivalent, the mean duration of treatment was 8.3 years, and thioridazine was the neuroleptic agent used for 74% of the group. Thirty-two percent of patients had no problems following drug withdrawal, 34% had behavioral problems following discontinuation of the medication, and TD was found in 34% of patients. This was mild in 13%, and moderate to severe in 21%. Eight percent of patients had maintenance-onset TD. The authors found no relationship to a specific drug. The most significant predictive factor for TD was the total lifetime dose. Those patients who had maintenance-onset dyskinesia remained symptomatic at the end of the study.

The majority of studies presented did not have placebo or control groups. An attempt to incorporate a more rigorous design was made by Kalachnik et al. (1984). Subjects were drawn from an institutionalized population of 520 residents. They were assessed with the Dyskinesia Identification System–Coldwater (DIS–CO) and evaluated using the Research Diagnostic Criteria for TD. There were 52 residents who had no history of neuroleptic ingestion, 31 who were maintained on stable doses of medication, and 20 who had their drug dose reduced. Evidence of dyskinesia at 3 months was found in 23.1% of individuals who had not taken medication, 19.4% of the stable dose group, and 35% of the neuroleptic reduction group. By 6 months, the drug-free group had an incidence of dyskinesia of 34.6%, the stable group 32.3%, and the neuroleptic reduction group 65%. At the end of 9 months, 40.4% of patients who had taken no medication had signs of dyskinesia, 32.3% of those on stable doses also had abnormal movements, and TD was present in 85% of the neuroleptic reduction group, 45% higher than the base rate. This study had two striking features.

The first is the extremely high incidence of abnormal movements in a group of patients who had no history of exposure to neuroleptic drugs (Kane & Smith, 1982). The second point concerns the increase in ratings of dyskinesia with time, even for the group receiving no medication. This point is discussed further with the next study. The third feature is the continuous increase in TD in the group undergoing neuroleptic reduction and the fact that 85% of patients were affected 9 months later. These figures appear to be higher than those reported by previous investigators.

Aman and Singh (1985) studied 24 severely and profoundly retarded adolescents and adults. Twelve of these patients had been maintained on doses of 100 mg of chlorpromazine equivalent or more for periods ranging from 2.1 to 11.1 years. The control group consisted of seven patients who had not previously taken neuroleptics and five who had been drug-free for at least 1 year with a mean of 3.26 years. The study instrument was the Dyskinesia Identification System–Coldwater. The subjects were on a full dose of medication for the 1st week of the study, and half-dosage for the 2nd week; after that the medication was completely discontinued. The group undergoing drug withdrawal had significantly higher scores than the control patients on movement of the eyes, lower limbs, and body, and difficulties with ambulation. The total dyskinesia scores were higher than in the control group, but did not reach statistical significance. It is of interest that the control group scored higher on lingual movements than the drug withdrawal group. It should be noted also that the dyskinesia ratings of both the control and drug withdrawal groups increased continuously until the 6-week examination. This is probably an example of consensual observer drift (Aman & White, 1986) and is similar to the increments over time in the control groups of the Kalachnik et al. (1984) study.

In a second phase of the Aman and Singh (1985) experiment, all subjects were challenged with methylphenidate. The control group had higher scores than the neuroleptic group for oral and lingual movements, while the neuroleptic group was rated higher on gross body movements. The results did not reach statistical significance. The authors suggested that the failure to show increased dyskinetic symptoms associated with neuroleptic treatment might have been a dose effect. Other studies, such as that of Kalachnik et al. (1984), utilized subjects who had taken significantly higher dosages of medication. This study indicates the importance of including a drug-free control group before definitive conclusions can be reached.

The prevalence of TD among 721 individuals in a state facility for persons with developmental disabilities was assessed at a single point in time by Richardson, Haugland, Pass, and Craig (1986). The study group was 211 of the 299 residents who had received neuroleptics for at least 1 year in the previous 5 years. Assessment tools were the Simpson Abbreviated Dyskinesia Scale (ADS) and the Abnormal Involuntary Movement Scale (AIMS). The study group was also evaluated on checklists for conditions known to produce mental retardation, causes of mental retardation associated with neuromuscular symptoms, and mannerisms seen in the population with mental retardation. Using the ADS mild-to-severe criterion measure, the prevalence of TD was 29.9%; it was 15.6% using the ADS moderate-to-severe criterion. The AIMS gave a prevalence of 48.8%, but this correlated highly with the presence of rocking stereotypy. Significant positive correlations were found with female gender and disorders of metabolism, nutrition, or growth. Negative correlations were found with psychosocial deprivation, taking neuroleptic drugs at the time of assessment, and total cumulative dose at evaluation. These latter unexpected negative relationships may reflect a prior diagnosis of TD in some of the patients concerned, with an attempt to reduce their exposure to neuroleptics. Another observation, of potential heuristic value, was that six of seven subjects having phenylketonuria who were exposed to neuroleptics actually developed TD.

A systematic neuroleptic withdrawal study involving 38 mentally retarded children, adolescents, and young adults was carried out by Gualtieri et al. (1986). The subjects had received neuroleptics for at least 6 months and had no preexisting disorder that might be associated with dyskinesia. Subjects were assigned to either abrupt or gradual withdrawal groups and evaluated by the AIMS. Nondyskinetic withdrawal symptoms were also recorded. Twelve patients had no withdrawal problems and an additional 13 had nondyskinetic withdrawal problems. Thirteen patients (34%) developed TD; seven had TD only; two developed TD and acute behavioral deterioration; two, TD and other withdrawal symptoms; and two developed TD, acute behavioral deterioration, and other nondyskinetic withdrawal symptoms. In eight cases, the TD was moderate to severe; this correlated strongly with total neuroleptic dose, measured in chlorpromazine equivalents. Three of the patients, all of whom had taken large amounts of neuroleptics, had maintenance-onset TD, that is TD that began while the patient was on a stable dose of medication.

Behavioral responses to withdrawal of neuroleptics in individuals with mental retardation were investigated by Schroeder and Gualtieri (1985). There was some evidence, from group data, that abrupt neuroleptic withdrawal was related to more severe dyskinesias than gradual withdrawal.

In summary, the majority of the studies suggest that somewhere between 20% and 45% of mentally retarded individuals will have the onset or an increase in dyskinetic symptoms during neuroleptic withdrawal. Major problems in analyzing these studies must be resolved, however. The use of control groups (Aman & Singh, 1985; Kalachnik et al., 1984) demonstrates that there is a high background level of abnormal movements in the population of individuals with mental retardation. This may be as high as 35% of subjects who have not received neuroleptics. It is self-evident that individuals with severe and profound levels of mental retardation have brains that are functioning abnormally in cognitive areas and the presence of motor abnormalities should perhaps not be surprising. Furthermore, two studies demonstrated the interesting phenomenon of increasing dys-kinesia scores when the control group was followed over time.

Tardive Dyskinesia in Infantile Autism and Related Disorders

The diagnostic criteria of infantile autism were initially established by Kanner (1943) and are not significantly different from those outlined in the *DSM-III* (American Psychiatric Association, 1980). The other pervasive developmental disorders of childhood are less clearly defined. Rather than attempt to fit patients from previously published studies into newly defined diagnostic categories, the authors' data are presented as they exist.

One of the major clinical features of patients diagnosed as having infan-tile autism or other childhood pervasive developmental disorders is the high incidence of stereotypic and other abnormal movements. This makes analysis of newly acquired movements quite difficult, as any given child's repertory may change over time. In addition, if withdrawal of neuroleptics is associated with behavioral deterioration, an increase in mannerisms and stereotypies could be expected. Finally, mental retardation is frequently part of the clinical picture of children with these disorders. This adds the confounding features noted in the previous section.

McAndrew, Case, and Treffert (1972) reported on a sample of 125 chil-dren, 52 of whom were diagnosed as being psychotic, ranging in age from 4 to 16 years. All 125 patients had received phenothiazines and 10 of the group developed abnormal movements within 3 to 10 days after discon-tinuation of the drug. In all cases the symptoms disappeared within 3 to 12 months. Sixty-four patients had medication withdrawn and did not develop symptoms. This second group had received much lower doses and had been treated for a significantly shorter period of time. There were no other significant differences between the groups. Clinical, neurological, and psychological variables were not related to the development of a dys-kinesia.

Polizos et al. (1973) studied 34 children between ages 6 and 12 years who were diagnosed as having childhood schizophrenia. Neuroleptics had been administered 6 to 15 months, and 1 to 2 weeks after drug withdrawal 32 of the patients had a severe behavioral relapse. Fourteen of the 34 subjects (41%) developed withdrawal emergent syndromes between the first and 15th days. Both dyskinetic movements and ataxia were present. The ataxia involved gait and dysmetria of the extremities with intention tremor, im-paired fine motor movements, and generalized hypotonia. The abnormal movements rarely involved the tongue, mouth, or jaw, which differs from the usual picture in adults. They were choreiform in nature and affected the extremities, trunk, and head. Some patients manifested myoclonic, athetoid, or hemiballistic movements. One half of the affected patients lost their symptoms before neuroleptic agents were reintroduced. The remainder had a remission of the ataxia and dyskinesia 1 to 2 weeks after a new drug was started.

Winsberg, Hurwic, Sverd, and Klutch (1978) reported 11 children between 6 and 14 years of age who had been on psychotropic drugs for periods of 6 months to 3 years. This was a heterogeneous group with diagnoses of autism, mental retardation, and minimal brain dysfunction. Five of the 11 patients showed withdrawal emergent syndromes when medication was stopped. This consisted predominately of oral-facial dyskinesia and choreoathetosis.

A larger series, and one analyzed in greater detail, was presented by Engelhardt and Polizos (1978). A group of 53 children who were diagnosed as having childhood schizophrenia with autistic features underwent single-blind drug withdrawal trials. The authors stated that previous studies had convinced them that the children were not placebo responders. The mean age of the group was 8.8 years with a range of 6 to 12 years and a male-to-female ratio of 5:1. The NIMH Treatment Emergent Symptom Scale was used. The 53 subjects received a variety of medications and doses with a total of 184 drug trials for the group. There were 62 trials that were referred to as "high-dose" trials (i.e., with low-potency neuroleptics), which were carried on for a mean of 28 weeks of therapy. Twenty-nine percent of patients manifested a withdrawal emergent syndrome. This ranged from 10% to 50%, dependent on the specific drug used. Following 122 "low-dose" trials (i.e., with high-potency neuroleptics) for a mean of 28 weeks, 61% of patients had a withdrawal emergent syndrome. This ranged from 25% to 87%, dependent on the specific drugs.

In 90% of the cases, there were choreiform movements of the extremities, head, and trunk. Oral dyskinesia was present in less than 20% and was always mild. Only six patients showed this as the sole symptom. Ataxia was present in 86% of the subjects. There was a latent period of 1–2 weeks following withdrawal of the drug, and 80% of patients who showed symptoms did so within 14 days. A spontaneous remission occurred in 35% of patients with a mean duration of 15 days after the onset of symptoms. Because of behavioral relapse, many patients had the drug reintroduced within 1 week after discontinuation. In these patients the withdrawal emergent syndrome disappeared within 2 weeks. The "high-dose" (i.e., low-potency neuroleptic) group had a 56% probability of remission as compared to 31% for the "low-dose" group. This is not surprising as it is widely believed today (although still unproven) that the high-potency neuroleptics are more likely to cause tardive dyskinesia than are the low-potency neuroleptics (see Kane & Smith, 1982). Furthermore, if all doses are converted to their chlorpromazine equivalent (Davis, 1976), the so-called "high-dose" group was receiving an average of 354 mg per day as compared with 489 mg per day for the "low-dose" group.

The long-term therapeutic efficacy of haloperidol and the prevalence of drug-related abnormal movements in autistic children were studied by Campbell et al. (Campbell, Grega, et al. 1983; Campbell, Perry, et al., 1983). The authors specifically looked at this group of subjects because of the high baseline rate of abnormal movements. The assessment of the patients for stereotypies before any medication was given as a unique and important feature of this study.

The patients were divided into two groups. The first received continuous drug therapy while the second was on a program in which medication was taken for 5 days and placebo given for 2 days of every week. Dosages of haloperidol ranged from 0.5 to 3.0 mg per day. Therapy was interrupted every 6 months with a 4-week trial of placebo. Measurement tools were the AIMS and the Rockland Research Institute Abbreviated Dyskinesia Rating Scale.

Eight of 36 patients developed abnormal movements: 4 of 28 males and 4 of 8 females. Four of these patients were on the continuous regimen and four on the discontinuous. The duration of drug therapy in the group developing dyskinesias ranged from 5 weeks to 16 months. Three of the children began having abnormal movements while taking haloperidol, and five while on placebo. Six developed new movements and two showed only an accentuation of previously existing stereotypies. Movements stopped within 16 days to 9 months. This occurred in two patients while they were on haloperidol, four while they were on a placebo, and two after all medication had been discontinued. The authors did note that the drugs were effective in reducing behavioral symptomatology.

The occurrence of tardive dyskinesia in a group of children withdrawn from long-term neuroleptic treatment was studied by Gualtieri, Quade, Hicks, Mayo, and Schroeder (1984). The 41 subjects formed a mixed group: 15 outpatients at a pediatric pharmacology clinic, 10 inpatients on a hospital child psychiatry service, and 16 long-term residents at an institutional facility for mentally retarded persons. The subjects had a mean age of 12.8 years and a range of 3 to 21 years. Neuroleptic drugs were given for a mean of 49.2 months with a mean daily dose of 127.9 mg of chlorpromazine equivalent. The patients were followed from 3 months to 3 years following drug withdrawal.

Eighteen patients (44%) experienced problems following drug cessation. Three patients developed TD, nine a withdrawal emergent syndrome that had the same symptoms as TD but resolved within 3 months, five nondyskinetic symptoms, four acute behavioral deterioration, and in three cases it was not clear whether they had TD or a withdrawal emergent syndrome. Symptoms always occurred during withdrawal or within 4 weeks of stopping the drug. The withdrawal emergent syndrome, nondyskinetic withdrawal symptoms, and behavioral deterioration lasted no more than 8 weeks. Two of the three cases of TD remitted within 9 months and one still persisted after 1 year follow-up. Drugs were reinstituted in 49% of patients, although some of these had medication discontinued at a later date. Only 29% of the subjects required medication after long-term follow-up.

Neuroleptic-related dyskinesias in autistic children were also studied by Perry et al. (1985). Fifty-eight children were studied. They had all shown significant behavioral improvement in previous double-blind studies. The children were randomly assigned to either continuous or discontinuous (5 days a week on haloperidol and 2 days a week on placebo) medication schedules. Every 6 months a 4-week period of placebo was introduced. Observations were made with behavior rating scales, a scale for stereo-typies, the AIMS, an abridged Simpson Scale (Kalachnik, 1984), the Children's Psychiatric Rating Scale, and the Clinical Global Impressions Scale.

Ages of the subjects ranged from 3.6 to 7.8 years. Haloperidol had been administered from 3.5 to 42.5 months in doses ranging from 0.5 to 3.0 mg. Thirteen children (22%) developed a drug-related dyskinesia. In four the onset of movements was during haloperidol administration and in nine when they were taking placebo. Eleven patients developed new move-ments, while in two there was an increase in previously existing stereo-typies. The most frequently involved areas were the mouth, tongue, and upper extremities. Lower extremities and trunk were each involved in two children. Movements spontaneously disappeared in 10 children over a period of 16 days to 9 months. In three children, medication was reinsti-tuted.

In summary, despite the high background of stereotypies and other abnormal movements in children with infantile autism and other pervasive developmental disorders, the occurrence of withdrawal emergent syndromes and occasional cases of persistent TD appear to be well documented. The majority of studies lack untreated controls, however. As demonstrated in the studies of Kalachnik et al. (1984) and Aman and Singh (1985), with mentally retarded subjects, a drug-free group of patients may be rated by observers as having an increased number of dyskinetic move-ments over time. It seems apparent that neuroleptic drugs are useful com-ponents of the treatment of some autistic children, however, but the data at this point do not allow easy calculation of a risk-benefit ratio.

Tardive Dyskinesia in Tourette Syndrome

Tourette syndrome is another condition in which neuroleptic drugs, speci-fically haloperidol and pimozide, are the most effective treatment. The dis-order is chronic and treatment often continues for a long time, although medication doses tend to be low. Most patients receive less than 5 mg of haloperidol per day, with the mean dose in most series being 2.5 mg per day. The diagnostic problems in differentiating the symptoms of Tourette syndrome from those of TD are obvious. The majority of tics in Tourette syndrome involve the head and face, and mouthing movements often accompany the involuntary vocal tics.

Mizrahi, Holtzman, and Tharp (1980) reported a maintenance-onset dyskinesia in a 7-year-old boy following 5 months of treatment with haloperidol at 1 mg per day. The symptoms disappeared 1 month following the discontinuation of medication. When medicine was first discontinued, the tics of the Tourette syndrome increased.

A withdrawal emergent syndrome in a 13-year-old patient who was psychotic and had Tourette syndrome was reported by Caine, Margolin, Brown, and Ebert (1978). In this case symptoms began 8 days following the discontinuation of haloperidol. An acute dyskinesia in three patients with Tourette syndrome, which followed prolonged administration of haloperidol, was reported by Caine and Polinsky (1981). In two of these cases this appeared to be a withdrawal emergent syndrome and, in the other, it was maintenance onset. In the latter case, symptoms resolved within 6 weeks of discontinuing the drug.

Three additional cases of maintenance-onset TD were reported by Golden (1985). The patients were treated with doses of haloperidol ranging between 2 mg and 6 mg daily, for periods of $3\frac{1}{2}$ to 8 years. The major manifestation in each case was an oral-buccolingual dyskinesia. Symptoms disappeared within several weeks of discontinuing the haloperidol, although the typical features of Tourette syndrome became more prominent.

The situation has become more complex with reports of patients who have been labeled as having tardive Tourette syndrome. In these cases, the long-term administration of neuroleptic drugs to patients who do not have abnormal movements is followed by a dyskinetic syndrome having the typical features of Tourette syndrome, including both motor and vocal tics (DeVeaugh-Geiss, 1980; Fog & Pakkenberg, 1980; Klawans, Falk, Nausieda, & Weiner, 1978; Seeman, Patel, & Pyke, 1981; Stahl, 1980). Mueller and Aminoff (1982) reported a patient with features of both Tourette syndrome and TD.

In summary, it is apparent that TD can occur in patients with Tourette syndrome. It does not appear to be a frequent finding, and the diagnostic difficulties are many. The low doses used for treatment may provide the explanation for why this disorder does not occur more commonly.

Symptoms Resembling Tardive Dyskinesia Following Use of Other Drugs

Any population of developmentally disabled individuals will include a high percentage of patients who are taking a number of drugs that act upon the central nervous system. Up to 29% of children with autism will develop seizures that require treatment (Rutter & Bartak, 1971). Mentally retarded individuals also frequently have seizure disorders and may have associated cerebral palsy. Anticonvulsants are among the most commonly used therapeutic agents in developmentally disabled patients (see Chapter 1). Drugs to reduce spasticity, such as benzodiazepines, are also frequently prescribed. Obviously, this group of drugs is psychoactive, and this and other drugs used in treatment of psychiatric symptoms must be considered if a patient taking neuroleptic drugs develops a dyskinetic reaction.

There is a large literature concerning the development of involuntary movement disorders following the administration of phenytoin to patients with seizure disorders. This has recently been reviewed by Howrie and Crumrine (1985). Choreoathetosis, oral-buccal dyskinesias, facial movements, tremors, dystonia, and parkinsonian symptoms have been described. The report of these authors also shows that similar symptoms can follow the acute intravenous administration of this medication, and that long-term use of the drug is not a necessary prerequisite for prolonged dyskinesias.

Abnormal facial movements including continuous contortions of the mouth, grimacing, and tongue thrusting and gyrations have been reported in a child following administration of phenobarbital (Wiznitzer & Younkin, 1984). This infant also had blepharospasm and torticollis. Symptoms subsided when medication was discontinued and recurred after a challenge dose. A dyskinesia involving movements of the tongue, jaw, face, and extremities has been reported following the use of ethosuximide (Ehyai, Kilroy, & Fenichel, 1978; Kirschburg, 1975). One of these patients, a 15-year-old girl, had oral-facial movements that included tongue protrusion, side-to-side movements, and lip smacking. Choreiform movements of the extremities were present in this patient and others in these reports.

Kaplan and Murkofsky (1978) documented an oral-buccal dyskinesia in a 63-year-old woman with depression who was given a combination of amitriptyline, diazepam, and flurazepam. Because of increasing depression the amitriptyline was increased and fishlike oral-buccal movements developed. These did not disappear after the amitriptyline was discontinued. Thirteen months later the benzodiazepine was stopped and within 72 hours movements ceased. Two challenge doses of 5 mg each again produced the oral-buccal movements. These stopped 72 hours later. Amitriptyline was then given alone and no movements occurred. Following this the patient attempted suicide by ingesting flurazepam and 2 days later the movements recurred and lasted for 4 days.

Two cases of dyskinesia that were associated with tricyclic antidepressants were reported by Fann, Sullivan, and Richman (1976). In each case, challenge with amitriptyline reproduced the symptoms.

Antihistaminic decongestants are frequently used for many indications. Two adults with oral-facial dyskinesia associated with prolonged use of these drugs were studied by Thach, Chase, and Bosma (1975). It is of interest that in both cases the movements continued after the drug was stopped, but like TD following neuroleptic therapy, they could be suppressed with the administration of haloperidol.

These case reports are not numerous and represent a miniscule proportion of the clinical literature. However, they indicate the desirability of controlling for administration of drugs other than neuroleptics. Trials of single agents and challenge studies can help document which drug has caused the dyskinesia.

Discussion

Analysis of the available literature demonstrates that tardive dyskinesia can follow the use of neuroleptic drugs in children and adults with a number of developmental disabilities. These include mental retardation, autism, other major psychiatric disorders of childhood, and Tourette syndrome. Because of difficulties in the definition of patient groups and the use of operational criteria for tardive dyskinesia in patients who have difficulty following detailed instructions, a precise figure for prevalence cannot be established, although it appears to approximate 30% of those on chronic neuroleptic therapy. In addition, preexisting adventitious movements and stereotypies are commonly present in all of the diagnostic groups studied. This is a major confounding issue, as studies such as those of Kalachnik et al. (1984) demonstrated that over a 9-month period of observation dyskinesias in a group of mentally retarded individuals undergoing neuroleptic drug reduction increased from 35% to 85%. In a control group of patients who had not taken medication, dyskinesias were found in 23.1% of the subjects 3 months after the study began and in 40.4% of these patients at the end of 9 months. This is also true, although to a lesser degree, with adult psychiatric patients (Kane & Smith, 1982).

This increase in frequency appears to represent consensual observer shift, an increasing sensitivity over time by the observers to the phenomenon being rated (Aman & White, 1986). To minimize this, it is necessary to check the observers against a predetermined standard or against another well-trained observer, and this should be part of any study.

Even though the data available have some limitations, tentative recommendations for the use of neuroleptic drugs in developmentally disabled patients can be made. The first principle is that the risk of tardive dyskinesia seems to depend, to a large extent, on the total lifetime dose of the drug (Kane & Smith, 1982). Second, although these drugs are useful in behavioral management, they are not as highly specific as when administered to adults with acute schizophrenia. In addition, studies demonstrate that these medications can interfere with performance and, possibly, learning (Aman, 1984). Third, the institution of behavioral programs can limit the need for medication.

Based on these working assumptions and principles, neuroleptic drugs should be prescribed for developmentally disabled individuals only when absolutely necessary and when behavioral methods have proven to be insufficient. The smallest dosage necessary should be used, and this should be given for the shortest length of time possible. Attempts should be made to reassess the need for the drug, and the possible development of tardive dyskinesia, on a periodic basis. Whether or not intermittent administration of medication places the patient at higher risk for the development of the dyskinesia is not clear.

A specific monitoring policy has been recommended by Kalachnik, Larum, and Swanson (1983). Although this policy was developed for a custodial facility, the principles could be applied just as easily to an outpatient setting. All patients should be evaluated with a standardized dyskinesia rating scale at the time of first contact, and on a yearly basis, even if medication is not used. This will provide a baseline if drugs are prescribed in the future, delineate other movements that are not caused by drugs or may be caused by other medications, and help uncover any instances of dyskinesia in those patients who may have had neuroleptic drugs in the past. Any patient who is on medication, or has been on medication previously, should be evaluated every 6 months.

Acknowledgment. This work was partially supported by Grant USPHS–MCJ-000-900-21.

References

Aman, M.G. (1984). Drugs and learning in mentally retarded persons. In G.D. Burrows, & J.S. Werry (Eds.), *Advances in human psychopharmacology* (Vol. 3, pp. 121–163). Greenwich, CT: JAI Press.

Aman, M.G., & Singh, N.N. (1985). Dyskinetic symptoms in profoundly retarded residents following neuroleptic withdrawal and during methylphenidate treatment. *Journal of Mental Deficiency Research, 29*, 187–195.

Aman, M.G., & White, A.J. (1986). Measures of drug change in mental retardation. In K.D. Gadow (Ed.), *Advances in learning and behavioral disabilities* (Vol. 5, pp. 159–205). Greenwich, CT: JAI Press.

American Psychiatric Association (1979). *Task Force Report 18: Tardive dyskinesia.* Washington, DC: American Psychiatric Association.

American Psychiatric Association. (1980). *Diagnostic and statistical manual of mental disorders* (Ed. 3, pp. 86–90). Washington, DC: American Psychiatric Association.

Bicknell, D.J., & Blowers, A.J. (1980). Tardive dyskinesia and the mentally handicapped. *British Journal of Psychiatry, 136*, 315–316.

Caine, E.D., Margolin, D.I., Brown, G.L., & Ebert, M.H. (1978). Gilles de la Tourette's syndrome, tardive dyskinesia, and psychosis in an adolescent. *American Journal of Psychiatry, 135*, 241–243.

Caine, E.D., & Polinsky, R.J. (1981). Tardive dyskinesia in persons with Gilles de la Tourette's disease. *Archives of Neurology*, *38*, 471–472.

Campbell, M., Grega, D.M., Green, W.H., & Bennett, W.G. (1983). Neuroleptic-induced dyskinesias in children. *Clinical Neuropharmacology*, *6*, 207–222.

Campbell, M., Perry, R., Bennett, W.G., Small, A.M., Green, W.H., Grega, D., Schwartz, V., & Anderson, L. (1983). Long-term therapeutic efficiency and drug-related abnormal movements: A prospective study of haloperidol in autistic children. *Psychopharmacology Bulletin*, *19* (1), 80–83.

Davis, J.M. (1976). Comparative doses and costs of antipsychotic medication. *Archives of General Psychiatry*, *33*, 858–861.

DeVeaugh-Geiss, J. (1980). Tardive Tourette syndrome. *Neurology*, *30*, 562–563.

Ehyai, A., Kilroy, A.W., & Fenichel, G.M. (1978). Dyskinesia and akathisia induced by ethosuximide. *American Journal of Diseases of Children*, *132*, 527–528.

Engelhardt, D.M., & Polizos, P. (1978). Adverse effects of pharmacotherapy in childhood psychosis. In M.A. Lipton, A. DiMascio, & K.E. Killam (Eds)., *Psychopharmacology: A generation of progress* (pp. 1463–1469). New York: Raven Press.

Fann, W.E., Smith, R.C., Davis, J.M., & Domino, E.F. (Eds.). (1980). *Tardive dyskinesia: Research and treatment*. Jamaica, NY: Spectrum.

Fann, W.E., Sullivan, J.L., & Richman, W. (1976). Dyskinesias associated with tricyclic antidepressants. *British Journal of Psychiatry*, *128*, 490–493.

Faurbye, A., Rasch, R.J., Peterson, P.B., Brandborg, G., & Pakkenberg, H. (1964). Neurologic symptoms in pharmacotherapy of psychosis. *Acta Psychiatrica Scandinavica*, *40*, 10–27.

Fog, R., & Pakkenberg, H. (1980). Theoretical and clinical aspects of the Tourette syndrome (chronic multiple tics). *Journal of Neurological Transactions*, *16*, 211–215.

Gardos, G., Cole, J.O., & LaBrie, R. (1977). The assessment of tardive dyskinesia. *Archives of General Psychiatry*, *34*, 1206–1212.

Goetz, C.G., & Klawans, H.L. (1984). Tardive dyskinesia. *Neurologic Clinics*, *2*, 605–614.

Golden, G.S. (1985). Tardive dyskinesia in Tourette syndrome. *Pediatric Neurology*, *1*, 192–194.

Gualtieri, C.T., Barnhill, J., McGimsey, J., & Schell, D. (1980). Tardive dyskinesia and other movement disorders in children treated with psychotropic drugs. *Journal of the American Academy of Child Psychiatry*, *19*, 491–510.

Gualtieri, C.T., Breuning, S.E., Schroeder, S.R., & Quade, D. (1982). Tardive dyskinesia in mentally retarded children, adolescents, and young adults: North Carolina and Michigan studies. *Psychopharmacology Bulletin*, *18*, 62–65.

Gualtieri, C.T., & Guimond, M. (1981). Tardive dyskinesia and the behavioral consequences of chronic neuroleptic treatment. *Developmental Medicine and Child Neurology*, *23*, 255–259.

Gualtieri, C.T., Quade, D., Hicks, R.E., Mayo, J.P., & Schroeder, S.R. (1984). Tardive dyskinesia and other clinical consequences of neuroleptic treatment in children and adolescents. *American Journal of Psychiatry*, *141*, 20–23.

Gualtieri, C.T., Schroeder, S.R., Hicks, R.E., & Quade, D. (1986). Tardive dyskinesia in young mentally retarded individuals. *Archives of General Psychiatry*, *43*, 335–340.

Guy, W. (1976). *ECDU Assessment Manual for Psychopharmacology (Rev. 1976).* Washington, DC: U.S. Public Health Service.

Howrie, D.L., & Crumrine, P.K. (1985). Phenytoin-induced movement disorder associated with intravenous administration for status epilepticus. *Clinical Pediatrics, 24,* 467–469.

Kalachnik, J.E. (1983). Tardive dyskinesia. *Minnesota Pharmacist, 37,* 6–13.

Kalachnik, J.E. (1984). Tardive dyskinesia and the mentally retarded: A review. In S.E. Breuning, J.L. Matson, & R. Barrett (Eds.), *Mental retardation and developmental disabilities* (Vol. 2, pp. 329–356). Greenwich, CT: JAI Press.

Kalachnik, J.E., Harder, S.R., Kidd-Nielsen, P., Errickson, E., Doebler, M., & Sprague, R. (1984). Persistent tardive dyskinesia in randomly assigned neuroleptic reduction, neuroleptic nonreduction and non-neuroleptic history groups. *Psychopharmacology Bulletin, 20,* 27–32.

Kalachnik, J.E., Kidd-Nielsen, P., & Harder, S.R. (1983). Number of nonassessable items and cooperation level of the retarded during systematic dyskinesia examinations. *Psychopharmacology Bulletin, 19,* 16–19.

Kalachnik, J.E., Larum, J.G., & Swanson, A. (1983). A tardive dyskinesia monitoring policy for applied facilities. *Psychopharmacology Bulletin, 19,* 277–282.

Kane, J.M., & Smith, J.M. (1982). Tardive dyskinesia: Prevalence and risk factors, 1959–1979. *Archives of General Psychiatry, 39,* 473–481.

Kanner, L. (1943). Autistic disturbances of affective contact. *Nervous Child, 2,* 217–250.

Kaplan, S.R., & Murkofsky, C. (1978). Oral-buccal dyskinesia symptoms associated with low-dose benzodiazepine treatment. *American Journal of Psychiatry, 135,* 1558–1559.

Kirschberg, G.J. (1975). Dyskinesia: An unusual reaction to ethosuximide. *Archives of Neurology, 32,* 137–138.

Klawans, H.L., Falk, D.K., Nausieda, P.A., & Weiner, W.J. (1978). Tourette syndrome after long-term chlorpromazine therapy. *Neurology, 28,* 1064–1066.

McAndrew, J.B., Case, Q., & Treffert, D.A. (1972). Effects of prolonged phenothiazine intake on psychotic and other hospitalized children. *Journal of Autism and Childhood Schizophrenia, 2,* 75–91.

Mizrahi, E.M., Holtzman, D., & Tharp, B. (1980). Haloperidol-induced tardive dyskinesia in a child with Gilles de la Tourette's disease. *Archives of Neurology, 37,* 780.

Mueller, J., & Aminoff, M.H. (1982). Tourette-like syndrome after long-term neuroleptic drug treatment. *British Journal of Psychiatry, 141,* 191–193.

Paulson, G.W., Rizvi, C.A., & Crane, G.E. (975). Tardive dyskinesia as a possible sequel of long-term therapy with phenothiazines. *Clinical Pediatrics, 14,* 953–955.

Perry, R., Campbell, M., Green, W.H., Small, A.M., Die Trill, M.L., Meiselas, K., Golden, R.R., & Deutsch, S.I. (1985). Neuroleptic-related dyskinesias in autistic children: A prospective study. *Psychopharmacology Bulletin, 21,* 140–143.

Polizos, P., Engelhardt, D.M., Hoffman, S.P., & Waizer, J. (1973). Neurological consequences of psychotropic drug withdrawal in schizophrenic children. *Journal of Autism and Childhood Schizophrenia, 3,* 247–253.

Richardson, M.A., Haugland, G., Pass, R., & Craig, T.J. (1986). The prevalence of tardive dyskinesia in a mentally retarded population. *Psychopharmacology Bulletin*, *22*, 243–249.

Rutter, M., & Bartak, L. (1971). Causes of infantile autism: Some considerations from recent research. *Journal of Autism and Childhood Schizophrenia*, *1*, 20–32.

Schonecker, V.M. (1957). Ein eigentumliches syndrom im oralen Bereich bei Megaphen applikation. *Nervenartz*, *28*, 35.

Schooler, N.R., & Kane, J.M. (1982). Research diagnoses for tardive dyskinesia. [Letter]. *Archives of General Psychiatry*, *39*, 486–487.

Schroeder, S.R., & Gualtieri, C.T. (1985). Behavioral interactions induced by chronic neuroleptic therapy in persons with mental retardation. *Psychopharmacology Bulletin*, *21*, 310–315.

Seeman, M.V., Patel, J., & Pyke, J. (1981). Tardive dyskinesia with Tourette-like syndrome. *Journal of Clinical Psychiatry*, *42*, 357–358.

Silverstein, F., & Johnston, M.V. (1985). Risks of neuroleptic drugs in children with neurological disorders. *Annals of Neurology*, *18*, 392–393.

Simpson, G.M., Lee, J.H., Zoubok, B., & Gardos, G. (1979). A rating scale for tardive dyskinesia. *Psychopharmacology*, *64*, 171–179.

Sprague, R.L. (1982). An analysis of institutionalized retarded residents using DIS–CO. *Psychopharmacology Bulletin*, *18*, 60–61.

Stahl, S.M. (1980). Tardive Tourette syndrome in an autistic patient after long-term neuroleptic administration. *American Journal of Psychiatry*, *137*, 1267–1269.

Tarsy, D. (1983). History and definition of tardive dyskinesia. *Clinical Neuropharmacology*, *6*, 91–99.

Thach, B.T., Chase, T.N., & Bosma, J.F. (1975). Oral facial dyskinesia associated with prolonged use of antihistamine decongestants. *New England Journal of Medicine*, *293*, 486–487.

Winsberg, B.G., Hurwic, M.H., Sverd, J., & Klutch, A. (1978). Neurochemistry of withdrawal emergent symptoms in children. *Psychopharmacology*, *56*, 157–161.

Wiznitzer, M., & Younkin, D. (1984). Phenobarbital-induced dyskinesia in a neurologically-impaired child. *Neurology*, *34*, 1600–1601.

10
Issues in Behavioral Pharmacology Implications for Developmental Disorders

JOHN L. EVENDEN

Abstract

The aim of this chapter is to introduce some of the concepts of behavioral pharmacology to readers whose primary interest is in developmental disorders. There is a large gulf between experimental studies of the effects of drugs and the use of these drugs in the clinic. Nowhere is this better exemplified than in the use of drugs that act on the dopaminergic system in the treatment of developmental disorders. There is little evidence of any specific role for dopamine dysfunction as the biological basis of behavioral disorders such as in the hyperactive child syndrome or in mental retardation. Yet dopaminergic stimulant drugs, such as amphetamine or methylphenidate, are the preferred treatment for hyperactive children, and antipsychotic drugs, which block dopaminergic neurotransmission, are the drugs most frequently administered to mentally retarded people. In both examples, it is the observable effects on behavior rather than a biological rationale that led to these drugs being used. This chapter outlines the relationship of behavioral disorder and central nervous system dysfunction, discusses experimental studies of the effects of some commonly used drugs and the relevance of these to the clinic, and introduces some of the general concepts underlying experimental behavioral pharmacology.

What Is Behavioral Pharmacology?

It is a fact of life that drugs can affect behavior. Drunk driving and the difficulties of giving up smoking testify to the ways in which drugs can either disrupt normal behavior or maintain a form of behavior that otherwise would not occur. Behavioral pharmacology is the scientific study of the way in which drugs can affect behavior, and it has a wide-ranging relevance to our daily life. Most often, behavioral pharmacology is carried out in the laboratory with animal subjects. The two examples given above illustrate two topics of research: the way in which drugs used in society, either recreationally, like alcohol, or medicinally, like antihistamines, can affect the ability to perform everyday tasks; and the addictive effects of drugs, again including those recreational drugs already known to be addictive, and the potential addictive side effects of therapeutic drugs. Another important area in which behavioral pharmacology is involved is the development and testing of drugs that may be useful in the treatment of various behavioral or psychological problems (e.g., antianxiety or antipsychotic drugs). Often there are doubts as to the real effectiveness or therapeutic efficacy of these drugs and one of the roles of the behavioral pharmacologist is to collaborate with clinicians to examine these problems.

In behavioral pharmacology, experiments generally fall into two categories, depending upon whether they are testing a behavioral or a pharmacological hypothesis (National Institute of Mental Health, 1984). For example, an experiment may be designed primarily to compare the effects of two different drugs on behavior and perhaps to relate differences in their effects to the chemical structure or physical characteristics of the compounds. This type of experiment (Type I) is really an experiment in pharmacology, using behavior as a measure of drug effect rather than, say, using heart rate or blood pressure. The second type of experiment (Type II) places more emphasis on behavior. In such experiments, drugs are used as tools to explore the way in which the nervous system influences behavior, the functions of different parts of the brain, and what happens when the brain is injured. Both types of experiment are important in the development of drug therapies for behavioral problems. Type II experiments are performed to improve understanding of the neural basis of the disorder, and are likely to result in the development and refinement of animal models of clinical disorders. Pharmacologists can then employ this model in Type I experiments to discover drugs that can ameliorate the clinical problem without having too many adverse side effects. Sometimes, however, a breakthrough in pharmacology may lead to dissatisfaction with the current animal model of a disorder, and in those circumstances, having ensured that the drug is not toxic, it may be necessary to jump straight from the pharmacologist's laboratory to treatment of patients in the clinic. This is a risky business, since what may appear a useful drug "in the test tube" may be of little use in the more complex physiological environment of a living organism.

Unfortunately, there is often a problem of communication between the behavioral pharmacologist and the clinician. In part this stems from the fact that much research in behavioral pharmacology uses animals (pigeons, mice, rats, and monkeys) as subjects. There are obvious difficulties in comparing the behavior of animals in a restricted laboratory environment with that of humans going about their daily lives, even if there is a great deal in common in terms of neuroanatomy, physiology, and biochemistry. For example, much of behavioral pharmacology is carried out within the atheoretical framework of the "Experimental Analysis of Behavior" as originated by Skinner (Ferster & Skinner, 1957), and involves "Skinner boxes," schedules of reinforcement, and all the technical language of that discipline. It is certainly unfashionable, with a few exceptions, to apply this framework

directly to human behavior, although the scientific use of training procedures, token economies, and so on is derived from the behaviorist tradition. Recently, animal researchers have tried to assimilate the conceptual
framework of cognitive psychology—talking about memory, attention,
planning, and so forth. However, in humans a great deal of cognitive performance involves the use of language. As animals do not have language,
can we be sure that their cognitive processes have any resemblance to
ours? Many cognitive psychologists are very sceptical about this, and such
theoretical arguments are, in any case, unlikely to be resolved to everyone's satisfaction. In the end, the utility of the conceptual approaches will
decide which is accepted. In this chapter, I demonstrate that it is possible
to take ideas from animal experiments and apply them usefully in clinical
situations.

Before describing the effects of drugs on behavior, for those unfamiliar
with neuroanatomy and neuropharmacology, a few background notes are
provided on pharmacological actions of some of the drugs used in the behavioral studies, and on the neuroanatomy of transmitter systems on which
they act. These are intended for readers who are not familiar with these
subjects, and should be skipped by those who are.

Some Basic Neuroanatomy and Neuropharmacology

Communication between neurons occurs via chemicals. The transmitting
neuron releases a chemical, the neurotransmitter, which is detected by receptors, of which there may be several types, on the receiving neuron.
Different neurons use different chemicals. Drugs that act on neurons
releasing dopamine or detecting the release of dopamine will form the
main examples discussed in this chapter. Other neurotransmitters include
chemicals related to dopamine (such as noradrenaline and serotonin) and
others that are not (acetylcholine and various amino acids and peptides).
Much of neuroscience is concerned with understanding which neurons
release which neurotransmitter and which regions of the brain they
innervate. The material discussed later in the chapter primarily concerns
drugs that affect the dopamine systems. Figure 10.1, shows that, in the
rat, neurons using the transmitter, dopamine, originate in discrete areas in
the midbrain and innervate more anterior regions. The main area of innervation is the striatum, in the basal ganglia, an area of the brain thought
to be involved in the control of movement (Marsden, 1982). In its turn, the
striatum is divided into two areas, the caudate nucleus (and putamen in
primates) and the nucleus accumbens. The nucleus accumbens also re-
ceives input from the limbic system, and is often assumed to mediate the
way in which emotional stimuli (particularly rewards) influence behavioral
output. The dopamine systems also innervate other areas, such as areas of
frontal cortex (thought to be involved in the planning of sequences of

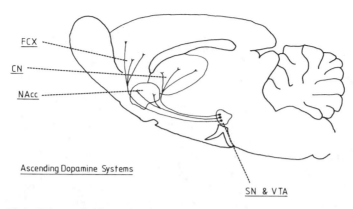

FIGURE 10.1. Schematic diagram of the sites of origin and the terminal regions of the ascending dopamine systems. Sites of origin: SN, substantia nigra; VTA, ventral tegmental area. Terminal regions: FCX, frontal cortex; CN, caudate nucleus; NAcc, nucleus accumbens. Neurons arising in the substantia nigra mainly innervate the caudate nucleus, whereas neurons arising more medially, in the ventral tegmental area, mainly innervate the nucleus accumbens and frontal cortex.

actions), the amygdala, and septum. There are large areas of the brain that do not receive any substantial input from the dopamine cells. The neuroanatomical connections of the dopamine system in primates and humans are essentially the same as those in rats. In all species these connections differ radically from those of the noradrenaline-using and other systems.

There are several ways in which drugs can act on a specific neurotransmitter system. Drugs can block the synthesis of the neurotransmitter itself, disrupt its storage, and release or mimic the actions of the neurotransmitter at the receptor. Amphetamine and apomorphine are dopamine agonists. That is, they have effects similar to dopamine itself. However, their modes of action are different. Amphetamine increases the release of preexisting dopamine, whereas apomorphine mimics the effects of dopamine on the dopamine receptor. On the other hand, most neuroleptics, such as haloperidol and chlorpromazine, are dopamine antagonists. They block the effects of endogenous dopamine (and also the effects of agonist drugs) by occupying receptors ordinarily activated by dopamine without stimulating the receiving neuron. The various neuroleptics are differentially effective at occupying the different types of dopamine receptor.

This is only a brief summary of the topography of the dopamine systems and the actions of a small number of drugs upon it. A more detailed description of this system and the other neurotransmitter systems, together with some of the drugs that act upon them, can be found in the Iversen and Iversen (1981).

Drug Treatment and Psychiatric Disorder

Evidence from behavioral pharmacology suggests that, in the absence of any specific biological link between a syndrome of psychological or behavioral disorder and drug, it may be misleading to assume, simply because a drug alters the disordered behavior, that it is directly affecting a disordered biological mechanism underlying that syndrome. The relationships between drug treatments and psychiatric disorders fall into four categories.

1. In certain disorders a biochemical basis has been established; Parkinson's disease is the best example of this. It is now known that patients with Parkinson's disease have reduced levels of the neurotransmitter dopamine, and that this transmitter can be replaced by treatment with L-dopa, the precursor of dopamine.
2. In most syndromes, such direct evidence for a link between brain chemistry and the psychiatric disorder is lacking. For example, it is generally assumed that overactivity in the dopamine system underlies schizophrenia, but this is not universally accepted (Rupniak, Jenner, & Marsden, 1983). Direct evidence for a link between dopamine overactivity and schizophrenia is far from as solid as the evidence for dopamine underactivity and Parkinson's disease. Some changes in dopamine receptors have been described in schizophrenia (Crow, Cross, Johnstone, & Owen, 1981), but the dopamine hypothesis of schizophrenia still largely rests upon the efficacy of neuroleptics (dopamine blockers) as a treatment and apparent similarities between schizophrenic psychosis and amphetamine-induced psychosis (Rylander, 1971). In a rather similar way, it has been noted that, postmortem, patients with Alzheimer's disease often have low levels of cholinergic activity in the cortex. Research into treatment has concentrated on replacing that acetylcholine by agonist or precursor therapy, although as yet with little success (Sahakian, in press). The relation between pharmacotherapy with tricyclic antidepressants and the biological theories of depression is a third example. Some evidence supports a link with noradrenaline, but there have been sugestions that other neurotransmitters, such as serotonin (Deakin, 1983), may be involved.
3. In other syndromes, there may be evidence of brain trauma, but probably not related to a specific chemical system. The syndrome of dementia is an example. Signs of dementia, forgetfulness, inattention, and confusion may arise from several causes. These are symptoms of senile dementia of the Alzheimer's type (SDAT) but what appears to be dementia can also arise from multiple brain infarcts (multiple infarct dementia, MID), increased intracerebral pressure, or depression, to list only three other causes. The symptoms arising from each disorder are practically indistinguishable, but when the brain of the patient is examined postmortem, or under computerized tomography and similar

scanning techniques, these four causes of dementia-like symptoms can be differentiated. Patients with senile dementia show a general shrinkage of the cortex, patients with MID show several localized areas of brain damage with complete sparing of others, patients with high intracerebral pressure have enlarged ventricles, and depressed patients show no abnormalities at all. Nevertheless, the imperfections in scanning techniques means that misdiagnosis is still quite common and SDAT can only be confirmed with certainty *post mortem*. However, the most appropriate treatment may crucially depend upon diagnosis. When depressed patients are treated with antidepressant drugs or patients with high intracerebral pressure with a shunt, the symptoms of dementia may recede completely. However, because the cerebral cortex is also innervated by dopamine, noradrenaline, and serotonin, as well as by the cholinergic system, and intracortical connections employ a range of excitatory and inhibitory neurotransmitters, all of which are lost to a greater or lesser extent, successful pharmacological treatment of Alzheimer's disease or MID may be almost impossible.

Even in animal studies complete restoration of behavior impaired by a known localized brain lesion is frequently difficult to achieve. For example, recent work on a model of Parkinson's disease in rats has demonstrated that it is possible to reinstate levels of locomotor activity reduced by the dopamine-depleting neurotoxin 6-hydroxydopamine (a model of Parkinson's disease) and to remove symptoms of sensorimotor neglect employing transplants of fetal dopamine neurons. However, restoration of normal feeding has proved impossible (Dunnett, Bjorklund, Schmidt, Stenevi, & Iversen, 1983).

Mental retardation may be brought about by a number of biological mechanisms, including genetics, brain injury, infections, or toxins (Crome & Stern, 1972). Those forms of mental retardation that have an obvious organic cause fall into this third category. However, there is a tendency in studies of mental retardation for all subjects, whatever the etiology of their disorder, to be lumped together. Whereas it may be useful to overlook neurological differences and concentrate on behavioral similarities when developing behavioral therapies (Baumeister & MacLean, 1979), it is difficult to justify such an approach when evaluating pharmacotherapy, especially if one intends to do more than modify overt behavior. Grouping regardless of etiology would obviously be inappropriate in the case of dementia, and, indeed, would lead to the rejection of some therapies because they were ineffective in the majority of patients, thus depriving a subpopulation of an effective and appropriate treatment. There is perhaps a great danger of the same happening in the field of mental retardation.

4. Finally, there are disorders, such as the hyperactive child syndrome, for which there is negligible evidence of any biological problem at all (Campbell & Werry, 1986). In this syndrome, it has been established

empirically that stimulant drugs make behavior more socially acceptable, but until a clear biological cause of hyperactivity is found, it should be assumed that it is only the observable behavior that is being altered rather than a disorder being "cured."

There are also a number of behavioral disorders that arise from primarily social factors which may also fall into this category. An instance would be antisocial behavior displayed by individuals with a history of family problems. Again it may be thought appropriate to treat these individuals with drugs, but until a great deal more is known about the neurobiological basis of, say, aggressive behavior, the possibility again arises that it is the behavioral symptoms that are being treated.

Drugs and Pattern of Behavior

Two approaches to studying behavior are used in behavioral pharmacology. The first of these, the observational approach, is to treat the animal with the drug and observe the effect it has on its spontaneous behavior. Many drugs or classes of drugs have characteristic effects. For example, amphetamine and apomorphine cause hyperactivity at lower doses and stereotyped sniffing and gnawing at higher doses. Many antianxiety drugs, such as the benzodiazepines, chlordiazepoxide (Librium), or diazepam (Valium), are sedatives and muscle relaxants on first administration. Mice treated with morphine carry their tails in a particularly striking manner (the Straub tail) and become unresponsive to painful stimuli. Novel compounds may have the same or opposite effects as known compounds, or may block the effect of a known compound. To test the latter, the animal would be treated with a dose of the known compound expected to produce a clear effect on behavior together with a dose of the novel drug, with the result, it is hoped, that the pharmacological effects of the two drugs cancel one another out, and behavior is unaffected. In the assessment of potentially therapeutic drugs, treatment with a known compound is often used as a way of artificially simulating psychiatric or neurological disorders. The destruction of the ascending dopamine projections by the catecholamine-specific neurotoxin 6-hydroxydopamine has already been mentioned as a model for Parkinson's disease. In a complementary way, potential anti-psychotic drugs are tested for their ability to block amphetamine- or apomorphine-induced locomotor activity or stereotyped behavior. Indeed, it has been shown that the relative effectiveness of different neuroleptics in antagonizing apomorphine-induced locomotor activity correlates with their clinical potency (Seeman, 1980).

One difficulty with measuring very simple behaviors is that many different drugs may have similar effects. Stereotyped behavior is an abnormal behavior pattern that is often a serious clinical problem in developmental disorders. Indeed, in its various forms, stereotypy is so common that it has been taken as a diagnostic sign of organic brain damage (Lezak, 1976), and the fact that it may be used as a general "sign" indicates that stereotyped behavior is not diagnostic for any particular syndrome. A large proportion of retarded individuals show stereotyped behavior, but it is also found in autism, schizophrenia, and the frontal lobe syndrome. Stereotyped speech is shown by aphasic individuals, and stereotyped motor performance by apraxic individuals. Stereotypy is also found in dementia and in sensory and social deprivation. In animal studies, stereotyped behavior of different forms may be seen after treatment with drugs that act on the dopaminergic, cholinergic, and serotonergic systems. Among developmentally disabled persons, it is likely that stereotypy is as much a product of psychological processes as of changes in brain physiology or biochemistry.

Observational Studies

Experimental Studies of Amphetamine Stereotypy

Assessment of the degree of stereotypy of behavior is often difficult since form and degree are frequently confounded. This can be illustrated by reference to amphetamine-induced stereotypy. The effects of amphetamine on spontaneous behavior are frequently assessed by a rating scale. Typical of these scales is the Creese-Iversen scale (Creese & Iversen, 1973), which scores stereotypy on a 7-point scale from 0 (asleep or stationary) through 3 (stereotyped activity such as sniffing along a fixed path) to 6 (continual gnawing or licking of the cage bars). It is indisputable that as the score on such a scale rises, so behavior becomes more stereotyped. However, it is questionable whether an animal that scores 3 is half as stereotyped as one that scores 6 on the scale, since the behaviors being measured are completely different. Such scales are used widely and are undoubtedly empirically useful (in the same way that clinical ratings of symptoms are a useful quick check of the degree of behavioral disorder), but they are less useful in studying how a drug can change normal, flexible, responsive behavior into inflexible, unresponsive, stereotyped behavior. To do this it is necessary to examine the animal's normal and disturbed behavior patterns much more carefully.

One of the first studies of this type was by Norton (1973). In this study the behavior of rats was analyzed using time-lapse photography and the frequency and duration of all the different behavioral acts were measured. As expected, under amphetamine the relative frequency of different types of behavior was altered, but, more importantly, across all behaviors the duration of each act was reduced. Norton (1973) suggested that it was this increased rapidity in changing from one act to another that led to amphetamine-induced hyperactivity.

Lyon and Robbins (1975) extended this suggestion by noting that complicated chains of behavior shown by untreated rats (such as grooming, social behavior, and feeding) tended to become truncated and to disappear at relatively low doses of amphetamine. In contrast, less complicated behaviors such as lever pressing continued, often at higher frequencies than in the absence of the drug. At higher doses still, lever pressing and locomoter activity also disappeared, leaving only sniffing in a restricted location, the typical stereotyped behavior of rats under high doses of dopaminergic agonists. Lyon and Robbins (1975) summarized these changes in behavior under the drug as demonstrating that the animal performed a reduced number of categories of behavior at an increased rate. Categories of behavior that involved pauses or that required the successful completion of a complex chain of behavior extended over a long period of time tended to disappear, leaving brief, repetitive behaviors, which evolved into stereotypy.

To test this proposition, experiments become complicated by the need to record almost all of what the animals are doing. With modern computers this is possible, although still time consuming, and the data provided are complex. Lyon and Magnusson (1982) described a method in which an observer recorded precisely each individual item of behavior performed by rats in a brief open field test. They then analyzed the sequence of items to find patterns that recurred even if the individual items of behavior that made them up were separated in time or by other items. In doing this, they confirmed that long chains of behavior made up of several response units did disappear under amphetamine, while the occurrence of exactly the same individual response units in shorter chains increased.

As studying the behavior of rats in an unstructured environment is both complex and somewhat open to subjective observer effects, it would obviously be convenient to study response sequences in a more restricted environment, with more objective measures. This can be done by using schedules of reinforcement in an operant chamber, where the behavior of the animal can be measured easily by automatic equipment. Robbins and Watson (1981) investigated the effects of amphetamine on the pattern of behavior using a method developed by Morgan (1974). Two levers on which the animal could respond were provided in the chamber. Food was available for responding on only one of the levers at any one time, but no signal was given to the animal indicating which lever was correct. After each delivery of food the lever designated "correct" was reselected at random by the computer. Under this procedure there is a simple response unit, the response on a given lever, which can occur in chains, and it is clear when a chain has ended since the rat will switch to the other lever. Also, of course, the units that make up each chain are very similar. Robbins and Watson (1981) recorded the frequency of switching between the two levers and could follow the changes in response chain length using this probabilistic measure which is independent of the rate of responding. With amphetamine they found that the probability of switching increased (i.e., the rats made fewer consecutive responses on a particular lever before switching, reflecting reduced chain length). However, this finding also has a counterintuitive aspect: an increase in response switching indicates an increase in the variability of responding as response choice becomes more random under amphetamine, not increased stereotypy as one might expect.

Recently, this author examined the performance of pigeons responding under a similar schedule (Evenden, 1986), in an experiment that showed that different drugs produce behavior that loses the normal pattern produced by environmental contigencies in a similar way, but is still characteristically different. In this experiment pigeons were reinforced for switching between two keys, but only after they had made 31 key-peck responses. The bird could distribute the responses that made up this FR31 on either key in any order. In fact, under this schedule, pigeons tend to make very few switches at the start of the ratio, but the probability of switching increases toward the end. This changing pattern of behavior as the pigeons peck out the ratio is an indication of the control over behavior exerted by the schedule (i.e., the environmental contingencies). After training, these pigeons were treated with three drugs: amphetamine, chlorpromazine, and scopolamine. Chlorpromazine is a dopamine antagonist and scopolamine acts as a cholinergic antagonist by competing with acetylcholine.

Figure 10.2 shows the effects of these three drugs on a single pigeon. The doses of each drug shown in the figure reduced the rate of responding to a similar extent. When treated with the drugs the pigeon tended to switch with a constant probability throughout the ratio, but the level of switching shown by the same pigeon under each of the three drugs was quite different. Under amphetamine the pigeon consistently switched between the two levers with a probability greater than .5 but less than 1. When treated with chlorpromazine the pigeon switched throughout the ratio with a probability less than .2, and when treated with scopolamine the pigeon switched with a probability between the baseline and random performance.

In more general terms, control of behavior by the schedule of food reinforcement broke down in the same way under all three drugs, but only under scopolamine did the pigeons really choose at random. Under amphetamine, which facilitates dopaminergic neurotransmission, this non-random pattern consisted of a high proportion of switches between the levers, whereas under chlorpromazine, which blocks dopamine transmission, the opposite pattern prevailed. Under these latter two drugs, the pigeon showed "stereotyped" behavior, both in the sense that its behavior was no longer controlled by the environment and it had an invariant pattern, but the exact forms of the invariance reflected their different causes.

These experiments show that amphetamine-induced stereotypy involves quite complicated changes in both spontaneous and conditioned patterns of behavior. The stereotyped behavior pattern may only be one, very obvious, symptom of an underlying more general change in psychological or behavioral processes that could even result in more variable behavior

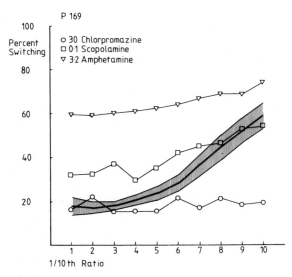

FIGURE 10.2. The effects of chlorpromazine, scopolamine, and amphetamine on switching between two keys by a pigeon responding under a fixed-ratio switch schedule. The vertical axis shows the percentage of switches made in each 10th of a FR 30 which could be completed by responding on either of two keys. The baseline and day-to-day variation (+/− 2 SEM) are shown by the continuous line and shaded area, respectively. The doses of each drug shown in the figure reduced the rate of responding to an equivalent extent. However, the effects on switching were quite different. Chlorpromazine reduced the percentage of switches when the baseline was highest; amphetamine increased switching, particularly at the start of the ratio when the baseline percentage was lowest; and under scopolamine the percentage switching tended toward an intermediate level.

under other circumstances. Furthermore, invariance in behavior may indicate loss of control by normal contingencies, but it is also necessary to characterize the exact way in which it is expressed, as different changes in brain biochemistry can produce different patterns of invariance.

Clinical Implications of Drug Effects on Behavior Patterns

The similarity between observational studies of drug effects and assessment of symptoms has already been mentioned. Treating an animal with a drug and observing how its behavior changes is similar in principle to observing the abnormal behavior of a person with a developmental disorder. However, it is possible to observe the animal subject in both a drugged and undrugged state (a within-subject comparison), whereas it is often only possible to compare a disabled person with an appropriately selected control subject (a between-subjects comparison).

There have been a number of experiments similar to the operant studies described above involving autistic children or schizophrenic adults. Frith (1970a, 1970b, 1972) published a series of studies on the ability of autistic children to recall or generate patterned sequences of responses. In one study (Frith, 1970a), the subjects were required to recall sequences of words of the form "spoon horse spoon horse horse spoon," which were either predominantly repeating or predominantly alternating. Normal children would tend to base their recall on the predominant pattern (i.e., they would make alternation errors if the pattern was predominantly alternating and vice versa), whereas autistic children tended to repeat even if the predominant pattern was alternation. Frith also showed that this was not dependent on memory processes. If normal and autistic children were presented with cards dealt from a shuffled pack and asked to guess whether the next would be black or red, normal children generated a variable sequence of guesses (the sequence of cards was, of course, randomized), whereas autistic children tended either to repeat or to alternate. This latter, guessing test is very similar to that used by Robbins and Watson (1981), described above, and the behavior of the subjects bears an obvious resemblance to that of the drugged animals.

A similar method has been used by Frith and Done (1983) in an experiment involving schizophrenic adults as subjects. Frith and Done (1983) found that the choice patterns of both acute and chronic schizophrenics were less random than controls, but that acute schizophrenics showed more switching than controls, whereas chronic schizophrenics showed less. This experiment is particularily interesting in view of the apparent comparability of amphetamine-induced and schizophrenic psychoses. The animal study by Robbins and Watson (1981) suggested that *mild* dopamine overactivation would lead to increased switching, whereas a later study using the same procedure (Evenden & Robbins, 1983b) indicated that *severe* dopamine overactivation using higher doses of amphetamine did not produce increased switching, but perhaps even an increase in repetitive responding. Comparison with the animal model suggests that, as far as choice patterns are concerned, acute and chronic schizophrenics may fall on a continuum of dopamine overactivity, with the chronic patients being more overactive, rather than having to appeal to other factors such as institutionalizaton or neuroleptic treatment to account for the differences. Thus the animal models of stereotypy presented earlier may help to explain in neurochemical terms some of the abnormalities observed in developmental and psychiatric disorders (see Lyon, Mejsholm, & Lyon, 1986).

All of the experiments in this section were essentially observational, even those investigating switching in the choice procedures in animals and man. This is because of one feature common to most of the procedures: there is no correct or incorrect way of doing the task. This is most obvious in the human card- or position-guessing tasks. Obviously, the subject gets about 50% correct regardless of whether he or she alternates between the available choices. In this way we can observe changes in the behavior of the subjects, human or animal, without their being penalized by poor performance. However, in most tasks both in everyday life and in experimental studies, a stereotyped behavior is penalized by reduced reinforcement. This can either be diminished social reinforcement in a retarded individual, or less food for a hungry rat. Sometimes "poor performance" can be a problem when one is trying to achieve a better understanding of a drug effect or disorder, since attention is focused on the subject's inability to complete the task, rather than on what they are actually doing.

Behavioral Testing

Drug Effects on "Cognitive" Performance

In contrast to observational studies, the second class of experiment is more specifically designed to assess deficits in particular aspects of a subject's abilities. In this way, such experiments resemble the different types of subtests that make up a test battery such as the Wechsler Adult Intelligence Scale (WAIS). A test is designed to measure an aspect of performance in which normal subjects are competent but which may be disrupted by neurological, psychological, or drug-induced disturbance. Generally there will be some theoretical reason for testing a particular aspect of behavior. For example, from animal studies has come the idea that noradrenaline may be involved in attention, so it is of interest to find out whether disturbance of the noradrenaline systems affects attention, and if so, under what circumstances (Carli, Robbins, Evenden, & Everitt, 1983). Similarly, from both human and animal work has come the proposition that the acetylcholine systems may be involved in memory, and hence there have been several recent studies examining whether destruction of the acetylcholine innervation of cortex impairs animals' ability to remember, with the hope of increasing our understanding of Alzheimer's disease (Murray & Fibiger, 1985). In the previous section, emphasis is placed upon the role of the dopamine systems. These systems have been implicated in two aspects of performance, motor control (cf. Parkinson's disease) and reward, and a large number of experiments of this second type have been used to study the role of dopamine in reward and to separate this role from its role in motor control.

Role of Dopamine in Reward Enhancement

Hill (1970) found that animals treated with amphetamine continued to respond for longer in extinction than untreated rats, and that they continued for longer still if stimuli associated with the reinforcer (conditioned reinforcers, e.g., the sound of the delivery mechanism) were still presented. He suggested that psychomotor stimulant drugs exert their effects by enhancing the reward value of conditioned reinforcers. More recently Robbins and colleagues (Robbins, 1976, 1978; Robbins, Watson, Gaskin, & Ennis, 1983; Taylor & Robbins, 1984) have used a more elegant method to examine this problem. In Hill's experiment the rats already had a long experience of lever pressing before the reinforcer was taken away, so that the continued responding may have been partially a result of an exaggeration of habit.

Robbins (1978) used a paradigm in which the conditioned reinforcer was established by classical conditioning, through pairing it with deliveries of water, with no opportunity to press levers. Only during the extinction phase was the conditioned reinforcer made contingent upon pressing the lever. The animals had a choice between two levers. Responses on one lever produced the conditioned reinforcer (CR) while responses on the other were recorded but had no scheduled consequences. Robbins (1978) found that the rats had a tendency to respond preferentially on the lever that produced conditioned reinforcers, and that the number of responses made on this lever was greatly increased under the psychomotor stimulant drugs, methylphenidate and pipradrol. Taylor and Robbins (1984) found that responding on the CR lever was also increased if amphetamine was infused directly into the nucleus accumbens, but not if it was infused into the ventrolateral caudate nucleus or into the thalamus. These authors concluded that amphetamine enhanced the control over behavior exerted by conditioned reinforcers. Descriptively, this was clearly true, but is a subtly different proposition from that put forward by Hill (1970), since this conclusion does not specifically imply that the reinforcing effectiveness of the CR was enhanced. The reason for caution on the part of Taylor and Robbins (1984) was that some results have been obtained which show an enhancement of responding under amphetamine simultaneously with a breakdown of control by conditioned reinforcers. Robbins (1976) used the same training procedure as outlined above, but then in extinction required the rats to switch between the two levers before the CR was presented. If amphetamine genuinely enhanced the efficacy of the CR as a reinforcer then the rats should have switched since this was the only reliably reinforced behavior pattern. Instead, Robbins (1976) found that under the methylphenidate-like stimulant, pipradrol, the rats sometimes responded many times on one lever even if this led to very few CRs being delivered. In other words, pipradrol did not enhance the efficacy of the CR to reinforce a chain of behavior, and by inference, amphetamine would not be expected to either.

Another property of reinforcers is that animals tend to approach them. Evenden and Robbins (1985) trained rats to track a light that could switch between two positions above each of two levers. Only if the rat responded on the lever under the light did it obtain food. By association with food during pretraining and during the experiment, the light becomes a conditioned reinforcer, and on the baseline the rats become very efficient at tracking it, making few responses on the unlit lever. Under amphetamine, they actually became more efficient, so apparently the drug enhanced the tendency of the rats to approach the CR. However, switching between the two levers was also analyzed. Rats rarely switched from the lit lever to the unlit lever on the baseline, but under the drug they did so *more* frequently, so that their discrimination performance measured by when they switched was worse. Thus, at certain doses of the drug, by the criterion of tracking, all the rats became more efficient, whereas by a second, switching, most of them became less so.

Earlier it was shown that rats switch more under amphetamine in the absence of any discriminative stimuli or CRs. Clearly, the most parsimonious way of explaining data obtained by Evenden and Robbins (1985) is to suppose that, under the discriminated switching schedule, amphetamine also increased switching. The increased number of switches improved tracking but were also made at inappropriate times. Amphetamine has a general effect of increasing switching when rats have a history of switching (Evenden & Robbins, 1983b), and, in some circumstances, this is consistent with improvements in performance and, in others, it is deleterious to performance. The same analysis can be applied to the experiments by Robbins (1976). If animals have no history of switching between the levers, amphetamine still can increase low rates of the more simple response of pressing a single lever. Newly learned lever pressing only occurs at a low rate and is a prime candidate to be increased under the drug. Rats respond preferentially on the CR lever in the absence of the rate-increasing effect of the drug so that it is possible that the increase in rate becomes apparent only after the animal has chosen. Hence responding on the CR lever is increased preferentially.

To summarize, the overall conclusion of this section is that the drug appears to act directly on behavioral output and the nature of the behavioral output is determined by the prevailing contingencies and the experimental history of the subjects. In certain experiments, particularly those involving the extinction of a previously reinforced stimulus, the additional behavior that results from the drug treatment can be "captured" by stimuli that would control behavior even in the absence of the drug. Because animals treated with stimulant drugs like amphetamine emit more behavior, it appears that the reinforcing effects of these stimuli are themselves enhanced. However, if the underlying control by the stimuli breaks down, the additional behavior is then channeled into unreinforced forms of behavior, such as perseverative responding or stereotyped behavior, and the independence of behavioral activation and the reinforcing stimuli is exposed.

Role of Dopamine in Blockade of Reward

Hill's (1970) hypothesis suggested that amphetamine enhances the effectiveness of conditioned reinforcers. Complementary to this, there have been suggestions that drugs that block the actions of the dopamine system reduce the effectiveness of reinforcers by blocking reward. For example, there are similarities between treatment with neuroleptics and extinction of previously reinforced operant responses.

Wise, Spindler, de Wit, and Gerber (1978) conducted one of several experiments supporting what is known as the "anhedonia" hypothesis. In the Wise et al. (1978) experiment, rats were trained to press a lever for food, and were then divided into six groups. One group had 4 test days with food present, and these rats continued to press the levers normally. The rats in two more groups were treated with two doses of the neuroleptic, pimozide, for 4 days. Rats in these two groups responded more and more slowly on each succeeding drug test day. To ensure that this was not simply due to increasing levels of drug within the rats, a fourth group had the first injections of pimozide in the home cage and were not tested on those days. On the fourth day they were treated with drug before testing and responded as quickly as had the other two drug groups on the first day. A fifth group of rats had 4 test days in which they were placed in the test apparatus, but lever pressing was not reinforced by food. Again, the rate of lever pressing decreased gradually over the 4 test days. The final condition provided the critical comparison. These rats had 3 days of extinction, but on the fourth day lever pressing was reinforced. In addition, the rats were treated with the high dose of pimozide. Their response rate was almost the same as those rats given no food on the fourth day and those that had had 4 days of drug treatment. Wise and his colleagues argued that removal of the food and treatment with the drug had similar effects and that *the drug reduced response rate by blocking the rewarding effects of the food.*

This claim is probably too general, however, and the similarities between extinction and neuroleptic treatment may be restricted only to paradigms similar to that employed by Wise et al. (1978). Ettenberg, Koob, and Bloom (1981) trained rats both to press a lever or to poke their noses into a small hole, both responses being reinforced by electrical stimulation of the brain. They then treated the rats with 0.1–0.8 mg/kg of alpha-flupenthixol. When treated with the higher doses, the rats would not press the levers at all, but continued to perform the nose poke response. Their evidence suggested that the rate-reducing effect of neuroleptics cannot entirely be due to reduction in reinforcer efficacy, because the reinforcer was the same in both cases. Instead, the data imply that the type of response employed plays an important part in the neuroleptic effect.

There is also evidence that, although the effects of extinction and neuroleptics on the rate of responding may be similar, when other measures of behavior are used, the two treatments have quite different effects. For example, Salamone (1986) used a fixed-interval 30-sec schedule in which the response was simply to sit near the place where the food was delivered in a large open apparatus. He then either stopped the food or treated the rats with a dose of the neuroleptic, haloperidol, higher than that which he had shown previously reduced rates of lever-press responding. He found that in extinction the rats quickly gave up sitting and spent much of their time exploring other parts of the apparatus. In contrast, the neuroleptic-treated rats still spent as much time sitting near the food delivery point as did controls. In other words, they behaved as if the food was still a reinforcer.

Evenden and Robbins (1983a) obtained a similar dissociation. They compared the effects of extinction and alpha-flupenthixol treatment on both response rate and choice of lever in the random reinforcement paradigm used by Robbins and Watson (1981). Morgan (1974) and Robbins and Watson (1981) had noted that rats tended to repeat a reinforced response choice even though this "win-stay" strategy was not itself differentially reinforced. Evenden and Robbins (1983a) found that if the food was explicitly omitted the rats tended to avoid the "unlucky" lever for their next response, the result being a strategy of win-stay/lose-shift. They found that both extinction and neuroleptic treatment resulted in a reduction in response *rate*, but, whereas removal of the food did reduce the tendency for the rats to show the win-stay/lose-shift strategy, treatment with neuroleptics did not. In other words, the neuroleptic did not affect the rats' perception of whether or not they had been reinforced.

These experiments suggest that neuroleptics have an effect opposite to that of amphetamine, in that they generally reduce behavioral output, but the degree to which they do so depends upon what the animal is doing. And, as with activation, whether this impairs performance or appears to reduce the effectiveness of the reinforcer depends upon the scheduled contingencies.

Clinical Implications

The series of studies described above has two main implications for clinical work. The first of these is to emphasize how difficult it is, in general, to interpret the results of the "testlike" experiments, particularly if the treatment or the effects of the treatment are relatively nonspecific. Before dealing with this, the second and more specific aspect of these studies, namely the information they provide about the effects of neuroleptics, will be discussed. This is of particular importance since this class of drugs is the one most frequently used in mental retardation (see Chapter 1).

As was emphasized earlier there is no evidence specifically linking mental retardation to dopamine hyperactivity in the way that is suspected in schizophrenia, and thus there is no biologically based rationale for treating retarded patients with this type of drug. Such patients are treated with the drug to abolish aggressive, destructive, hyperactive, antisocial, and self-injurious behaviors, and possibly to reduce stereotypies (Aman & Singh, 1983). In other words, they are used to suppress inappropriate or unwanted behavior. The animal studies cited above indicated that neuroleptics do indeed block behavioral output. However, they do so regardless of whether it is appropriate or inappropriate. How effectively they block it also depends upon the form of behavior. Aman and Singh (1983) concluded that in controlled studies, with the exception of stereotyped behavior (which, as suggested earlier, may have a genuine dopaminergic component), the effectiveness of neuroleptics in blocking antisocial behavior has not been well established (see also Chapter 4). This is probably because, according to experimental studies, it appears that neuroleptics primarily block the outward display of emotional or motivated behavior, not the underlying emotional or motivational states.

This conceptualization of neuroleptic effects based on behavioral pharmacology research has two main implications for the clinical use of these drugs. The first of these is that if the maladaptive behavior does not have a predominantly motor component (perhaps if it is verbal) it is unlikely to be suppressed, but in contrast, if the maladaptive behavior is primarily motoric in nature, as is stereotyped or hyperactive behavior, then the drugs may be effective. Methodologically satisfactory evidence from studies on mental retardation appears to fit this division (Aman & Singh, 1983). The second implication is that, providing that incapacitating doses of drug are not used in the treatment, there should be no adverse effects on "cognitive" processes. Recently, there have been isolated reports that use of neuroleptic drugs in mental retardation might actually impair the effectiveness of behavioral therapy (see Aman & Singh, 1986). If substantiated, the clear implication of these reports is similar to that of Wise (1982), namely that neuroleptics block the effectiveness of rewarding behavior. The limitations of this suggestion have already been discussed.

Certainly there are paradigms in which neuroleptics and nonreward have similar effects in animals, but these similarities are limited and generally only occur at doses of the drugs that affect rate and patterns of responding in ways that changes in reinforcer effectiveness do not. In other studies no proof of an impairment in the *control* of behavior was noted, even when the *rate* of responding was severely reduced by the drug. Furthermore, there is little evidence that neuroleptics affect learning per se, although they may affect the expression of that learning through motor performance. For example, Beninger and Phillips (1980) found that pimozide only slightly impaired transfer of a classically conditioned tone-food association to instrumental performance, and Beninger, Mason, Phillips, and Fibiger (1980) found no impairment in transfer of an association between a tone and shock produced by classical conditioning. Similarly, there is little support for the proposition that neuroleptics selectively impair instrumental discrimination performance, even in the paradigm used by Evenden and Robbins (1985) which required a good deal of locomotion to maintain performance accuracy. In more conventional paradigms, disruption of discrimination performance may be seen, but only at doses higher than those that disrupt the probability or speed of responding (Appel & Dykstra, 1977; Ksir & Slifer, 1982). At present it is not clear whether this is because the change in motor performance itself produces the impairment in discrimination (perhaps as some form of speed-error trade-off), whether both are independent effects of the drug's action at one particular site in the brain, or whether they reflect the actions of the drug at two separate sites. However, when given peripherally, neuroleptics appear to affect motor performance or actions at doses lower than those producing impairments in the effectiveness of discriminative or reinforcing stimuli.

Clark, Geffen, and Geffen (1986) have recently demonstrated that this also applies to human behavior. They examined the effects of the dopamine antagonist droperidol on attentional performance in normal adults. They found small impairments on attentional performance using a dose of the drug that had very marked effects on spontaneous behavior. They suggested that the drug affected the effort necessary to allocate attention to the task. However, once effort had been directed to the task, performance was relatively normal. A similar suggestion, that modulation of the dopamine systems affects the effort required to perform a task, based upon animal studies, has been made by Neill and Justice (1981).

Finally, I would like to return to the more general point arising from the behavioral pharmacology studies cited here. When performing experiments in behavioral pharmacology, the experimenter has under his or her control the biological manipulation that is the object of the study. Even so, interpreting the results of any particular experiment can be very difficult. Changes in general aspects on which I have concentrated, like changes in the pattern of responding or in motor performance, can affect performance in quite subtle ways on tests that are intended to investigate more specific processes.

Studies of this type help to bring together experiments involving both animal and human subjects, since the same methods may be used to examine similar cognitive capacities across species. Experience with methods that provide a good measure of the cognitive abilities of animals may assist in the development of tests for human subjects. Recently I have become involved in a program studying cognitive performance in aging and demented individuals (Morris, Evenden, Sahakian & Robbins, 1987). In this program, all the tests involve very simple responses such as pressing a key and, mostly, pointing to a touch-sensitive VDU screen, and simple training procedures have been incorporated into the tests to ensure that everyone can complete them at a simple level, even if they are unable to when the tests are made more difficult. Some have been based upon quite well-known neurological tests that are probably too difficult to use with nonhuman subjects, whereas others have been developed from work with rats or monkeys. In many cases the problems of demented subjects, like those of developmentally disabled individuals, resemble the problems discussed in this chapter, such as slowness of responding, inappropriate sequencing of different responses, general inattention, and so on, rather than the specific type of deficit commonly cited as being shown by neurological patients. As pointed out by Aman and White (1986), severely and profoundly retarded individuals, by the very nature of their handicap, are exceedingly difficult to assess. Clinical psychopharmacology of developmentally disabled persons may be able to benefit by borrowing some of the technology developed in behavioral pharmacology. By doing this, it may be possible to test both human and nonhuman subjects on similar tasks, and their successful performance and the difficulties that they experience may be similar. Animal experimenters can exert better control over the social and biological history of their subjects and can evaluate a wider range of potential therapies than those undertaken with human beings, since they do not have to follow so strictly the ethics of medical care, such as the witholding of potentially beneficial treatment, that may limit clinical studies. Through both animal and human experimentation, using similar procedures, it should be possible to draw parallels that may bridge the large and divisive gap that presently exists between the two areas, and hopefully to develop better therapies.

Acknowledgments. I should like to thank M.G. Aman, T.W. Robbins, A.C. Roberts, and C.N. Ryan for their advice and helpful comments on the manuscript. The work was funded by the Medical Research Council of Great Britain.

References

Aman, M.G., & Singh, N.N. (1983). Pharmacological intervention. In J.L. Matson & J.A. Mulick (Eds.), *Handbook of mental Retardation* (pp. 317–337). New York: Pergamon Press.

Aman, M.G., & Singh, N.N. (1986). A critical appraisal of recent drug research in mental retardation: The Coldwater studies. *Journal of Mental Deficiency Research, 30*, 203–216.

Aman, M.G., & White, A.J. (1986). Measures of drug change in mental retardation. In K.D. Gadow (Ed.), *Advances in learning and behavioral disabilities*, (Vol. 5, pp. 157–202). Greenwich, CT: JAI Press.

Appel, J.D., & Dykstra, L.A. (1977). Drugs, discrimination and signal detection theory. In T. Thompson & P.B. Dews (Eds.), *Advances in behavioral pharmacology* (Vol. 1, pp. 139–166). New York: Academic Press.

Baumeister, A.A., & MacLean, W.E. (1979). Brain damage and mental retardation. In N.R. Ellis (Ed.), *Handbook of mental deficiency: Psychological theory and research*. New York: Erlbaum.

Beninger, R.J., Mason, S.T., Phillips, A.G., & Fibiger, H.C. (1980). The use of conditioned suppression to evaluate the nature of neuroleptic-induced avoidance deficits. *Journal of Pharmacology and Experimental Therapeutics, 213*, 623–627.

Beninger, R.J., & Phillips, A.G. (1980). The effects of pimozide on the establishment of conditioned reinforcement. *Psychopharmacology, 68*, 147–154.

Campbell, S.B., & Werry, J.S. (1986). Attention deficit disorder (hyperactivity).

In H.C. Quay & J.S. Werry (Eds.), *Psychopathological disorders of childhood* (3rd ed., pp. 111–155). New York: Wiley.

Carli, M., Robbins, T.W., Evenden, J.L., & Everitt, B.J. (1983). Effects of lesions to the ascending noradrenergic neurones on performance of a 5-choice serial reaction task: Implications for theories of dorsal noradrenergic bundle function based on attention and arousal. *Behavioural Brain Research, 9*, 361–380.

Clark, C.R., Geffen, G.M., & Geffen, L.B. (1986). Role of monoamine pathways in the control of attention: Effects of droperidol and methylphenidate in normal adult humans. *Psychopharmacology, 90*, 28–34.

Creese, I., & Iversen, S.D. (1973). Blockage of amphetamine induced motor stimulation and stereotypy in the adult rat following neonatal treatment with 6-hydroxydopamine. *Brain Research, 55*, 369–382.

Crome, L., & Stern, J. (1972). *Pathology of mental retardation.* Edinburgh: Churchill Livingstone.

Crow, T.J., Cross, A.J., Johnstone, E.C., & Owen, F. (1981). Schizophrenia: Dopaminergic and non-dopaminergic dimensions of pathology. In F.C. Rose, (Ed.), *Metabolic disorders of the nervous system* (pp. 486–496). London: Pitman.

Deakin, J.F.W. (1983). Roles of serotonergic systems in escape, avoidance and other behaviors. In S.J. Cooper (Ed.), *Theory in psychopharmacology*, (Vol. 2, pp. 149–194). London: Academic Press.

Dunnett, S.B., Bjorklund, A., Schmidt, R.H., Stenevi, U., & Iversen, S.D. (1983). Intracerebral grafting of neuronal cell suspensions: V. Behavioural recovery in rats with bilateral 6-OHDA lesions following implantation of nigral cell suspensions. *Acta Physiologica Scandinavica, 522* (Suppl.), 39–47.

Ettenberg, A., Koob, G.F., & Bloom, F.E. (1981). Response artifact in the measurement of neuroleptic-induced anhedonia. *Science, 222*, 1253–1254.

Evenden, J.L. (1986). Contrasting baseline-dependent effects of amphetamine, chlorpromazine and scopolamine on response switching in the pigeon. *Psychopharmacology, 89*, 421–428.

Evenden, J.L., & Robbins, T.W. (1983a). Dissociable effects of d-amphetamine, chlordiazepoxide and alpha-flupenthixol on choice and rate measures of reinforcement in the rat. *Psychoparmacology, 79*, 180–186.

Evenden, J.L., & Robbins, T.W. (1983b). Increased response switching, perseveration and perseverative switching following d-amphetamine in the rat. *Psychopharmacology, 80*, 67–73.

Evenden, J.L., & Robbins, T.W. (1985). The effects of d-amphetamine, chlordiazepoxide and alpha-flupenthixol of food-reinforced tracking of a visual stimulus by rats. *Psychopharmacology, 85*, 361–366.

Ferster, C.B., & Skinner, B.F. (1957). *Schedules of reinforcement.* New York: Appleton-Century-Crofts.

Frith, C.D., & Done, D.J. (1983). Stereotyped responding by schizophrenic patients on a two-choice guessing task. *Psychological Medicine, 13*, 779–786.

Frith, U. (1970a). Studies in pattern detection in normal and autistic children: I. Immediate recall of auditory sequences. *Journal of Abnormal Psychology, 76*, 413–420.

Frith, U. (1970b). Studies in pattern detection in normal and autistic children: II. Reproduction and production of color sequences. *Journal of Experimental Child Psychology, 10*, 120–135.

Frith, U. (1972). Cognitive mechanisms in autism: Experiments with colour and tone sequence production. *Journal of Autism and Childhood Schizophrenia, 2,* 160–173.

Hill, R.T. (1970). Facilitation of conditioned reinforcement as a mechanism of psychomotor stimulation. In E. Costa & S. Garattini (Eds.), *Amphetamines and related compounds* (pp. 781–795). New York: Raven Press.

Iversen, S.D., & Iversen, L.L. (1981). *Behavioural Pharmacology* (2nd ed.). New York: Oxford University Press.

Ksir, C., & Slifer, B. (1982). Drug effects on discrimination performance at two levels of stimulus control. *Psychopharmacology, 76,* 286–290.

Lezak, M.D. (1976). *Neuropsychological assessment.* New York: Oxford University Press.

Lyon, M., & Magnusson, M. (1982). Central stimulant drugs and the learning of abnormal behavioural sequences. In M.Y. Spiegelstein & A. Levy (Eds.), *Behavioral models and the analysis of drug action* (pp. 135–153). Amsterdam: Elsevier.

Lyon, M., & Robbins, T.W. (1975). The action of central nervous stimulant drugs. In W.B. Essman & L. Valzelli (Eds.), *Current developments in psychopharmacology* (Vol. 2, pp. 80–163). New York: Spectrum Publications.

Lyon, N., Mejsholm, B., & Lyon, M. (1986). Stereotyped responding by schizophrenic outpatients: Cross-cultural confirmation of perseverative switching on a two-choice task. *Journal of Psychiatric Research, 20,* 137–150.

Marsden, C.D. (1982). The mysterious motor function of the basal ganglia: The Robert Wartenburg lecture. *Neurology, 32,* 514–539.

Morgan, M.J. (1974). Effects of random reinforcement sequences. *Journal of the Experimental Analysis of Behavior, 22,* 529–538.

Morris, R.G., Evenden, J.L., Sahakian, B.J., & Robbins, T.W. (1987). Computer-aided assessment of dementia: Comparative studies of neuropsychological deficit in Alzheimer-type dementia and Parkinson's disease. In S.M. Stahl, S.D. Iversen, & E. Goodman (Eds.), *Cognitive neurochemistry* (pp. 21–36). Oxford: Oxford University Press.

Murray, C.L., & Fibiger, H.C. (1985). Learning and memory deficits after lesions of the nucleus basalis magnocellularis: Reversal by physostigmine. *Neuroscience, 14,* 1025–1032.

National Institute of Mental Health. (1984). *The neuroscience of mental health* (DHSS Publication No. (ADM) 85–1363). Washington: U.S. Department of Health and Human Services.

Neill, D.B., & Justice, J.B. (1981). An hypothesis for a behavioral function of dopaminergic transmission in nucleus accumbens. In R.B. Chronister & J.F. De France (Eds.), *The neurobiology of the nucleus accumbens.* Brunswick: Haer Institute for Electrophysiological Research.

Norton, S. (1973). Amphetamine as a model for hyperactivity in the rat. *Physiology and Behavior, 11,* 181–186.

Robbins, T.W. (1976). Relationship between reward-enhancing and stereotypical effects of psychomotor stimulant drugs. *Nature, 264,* 57–59.

Robbins, T.W. (1987). The acquisition of responding with conditioned reinforcement: Effects of pipradrol, methylphenidate, d-amphetamine and nomifensine. *Psychopharmacology, 58,* 79–87.

Robbins, T.W., & Watson, B.A. (1981). Effects of d-amphetamine on response repetition and win-stay behaviour in the rat. In C.M. Bradshaw, E. Szabadi, &

C.F. Lowe (Eds.), *Quantification of steady-state operant behaviour* (pp. 441–444). Amsterdam: Elsevier/North Holland Biomedical Press.

Robbins, T.W., Watson, B.A., Gaskin, M., & Ennis C. (1983). Contrasting interactions of pipradrol, d-amphetamine, cocaine and cocaine analogues, apomorphine and other drugs with conditioned reinforcement. *Psychopharmacology, 80*, 113–119.

Rupniak, N.M.J., Jenner, P.G., & Marsden, C.D. (1983). Long-term neuroleptic treatment and the status of the dopamine hypothesis of schizophrenia. In S.J. Cooper (Ed.) *Theory in psychopharmacology* (Vol. 2, pp. 195–238). London: Academic Press.

Rylander, G. (1971). Stereotype behaviour in man following amphetamine abuse. In S. de C. Baker (Ed.), *The correlation of adverse effects in man with observations in animals* (pp. 26–31). Amsterdam: Excepta Medica.

Sahakian, B.J. (in press). Cholinergic drugs and human cognitive performance. In L.L. Iversen, S.D. Iversen, & S.H. Snyder (Eds.), *Handbook of Psychopharmacology* (Vol. 20). New York: Plenum Press.

Salamone, J.D. (1986). Different effects of haloperidol and extinction on instrumental behaviours. *Psychopharmacology, 88*, 18–23.

Seeman, P. (1980). Brain dopamine receptors. *Pharmacological Reviews, 32*, 229–313.

Taylor, J.R., & Robbins, T.W. (1984). Enhanced behavioural control by conditioned reinforcers following microinjections of d-amphetamine into the nucleus accumbens. *Psychopharmacology, 84*, 405–412.

Wise, R.A. (1982). Neuroleptics and operant behaviour: The anhedonia hypothesis. *The Behavioural and Brain Sciences, 5*, 39–87.

Wise, R.A., Spindler, J., de Wit, H., & Gerber, G.J. (1978). Neuroleptic-induced "anhedonia" in rats: Pimozide blocks the reward quality of food. *Science, 201*, 262–264.

11
Conclusions

JOHN S. WERRY

Abstract

The content of this book is surveyed, and some conclusions are drawn about the state of psychopharmacology of the developmental disabilities. These are then related to the field of psychopharmacology in general and some directions for the future are outlined.

This book is a timely composite of knowledge about psychopharmacology of mentally retarded or developmentally disabled persons. In their preface, the editors draw attention to the robust state of the field and the need to have it collated in one readily available source that should, as much as practicable, be comprehensible to all members of the multidisciplinary team that is now necessary to deal effectively not only with developmentally disabled individuals, but with all disabled persons. To attempt this task, they have selected as content all drugs in common use, their patterns of application (or their epidemiology), legal and ethical aspects of their application, how to measure their effects and their side effects, their pharmacological features, and finally a look at the relevance of animal research or behavioral pharmacology. All that now remains is to pull all these threads together in some general statements and to relate these to the field of psychopharmacology as a whole and, in so doing, to point out some directions for future developments and research.

General Conclusions

First, it does no harm to repeat what has appeared in almost every chapter—that psychotropic drugs have been, and are, widely used in developmentally disabled persons, especially in those who are institutionalized. This fact has been known since Lipman's pioneering 1966 study (see Lipman, 1970) but is now much better documented.

Second, the doses used have tended to be high and medical supervision has been less than exemplary. This lack of high-quality medical involvement has a number of implications that are discussed at several points below.

Third, the mentally retarded population are a neglected, dispossessed people who have had to resort, in the United States at least, to the courts to force those responsible for their care to invest enough resources to ensure a minimially humane level of care and to set down guidelines for ethical and adequate standards of pharmacological treatment. This is not a pretty picture and one that does no great credit to the public or helping professions.

Fourth, the range of drugs used is large, though one class of drugs predominates—that is, antipsychotics or neuroleptics, and two drugs in this group in particular, thioridazine and chlorpromazine. Both these drugs were among the first of their type to be introduced and both belong to the small subclass that has the additional property of being strongly anticholinergic. It is of interest to ask why these two have predominated and what are their peculiar effects and side effects. I have hypothesized elsewhere (Werry, 1980) that their popularity may be related to their anticholinergic sedative action which adds to, or even dominates over their ataractic dopamine-blocking action. While, as pointed out in Chapter 10, blocking dopamine does not appear to interfere with learning in animals, this is definitely not true of anticholinergic drugs, which have a most disruptive effect (see Werry, 1980). Paradoxically then, in a population that already has impaired learning, two potentially "learning-disruptive" drugs are among the most popular. Unfortunately, little good research has looked at their effects on cognitive function (see Chapters 1 and 4).

This leads to a fifth conclusion regarding measurement of drug effects. It is true that problems of comprehension and social adaptation make assessment in this field very difficult, but mensuration of drug effects on behavior and adaptive function is considerably less advanced in the developmentally disabled population than in other fields of psychopharmacology. Measurement of effects on learning and cognitive function (surely of critical importance) is literally light years behind that conducted with children of normal intelligence having Attention Deficit Disorder with Hyperactivity (see Aman & White, 1986; Werry, 1988). Much of what is known there and the measurement techniques used could be adapted to the field of developmental disabilities, but so far few authors, except some of those involved with this book, seem to have been willing to try. Surely, the field of psychopharmacology of the developmental disabilities should be leading here, not following far behind.

Sixth, as pointed out in a number of places in this text, the greatest use of psychotropic drugs in mental retardation has been nonspecific, empirical, and aimed at the suppression of undesirable behavior. This nonspecific use was never as true of adult psychiatry where most of these drugs first appeared. There, the separation of drugs into specific therapeutic groups of antipsychotic, antidepressant, antianxiety, antimanic, stimulant, and so on occurred soon after their introduction. Such use of these drugs for the general suppression of undesired behavior as there may have been in the early days (1950–1960s) in adult psychiatry has now largely disappeared and/or is discredited. However, it continues to be true to some extent of pediatric and geriatric psychopharmacology, but even there the thrust is toward *therapeutic specificity*. It is probably fair to say that generalized suppression of behavior can be equated with clinical desperation and is only one small advance on physical restraint. This is not to say that such may not still be needed sometimes to prevent a worse outcome, but simply that we recognize it for what it is and strive for a better way of conceptualizing and using drugs.

The chapters on antiepileptic (anticonvulsant) drugs (Chapter 5) and tardive dyskinesia (Chapter 9) suggest a seventh conclusion. Just because a drug may have a bona fide specific function (for example, in the case of neuroleptics, the most common use is for schizophrenia, which affects 1% of the total adult population), does not mean that it cannot have disastrous effects upon other functions. This underlines the plea in some of the chapters for more attention to overall quality of life as the most important measure of effects of drugs in developmentally disabled persons. Paraphrasing the comment about generals and war, one can say that the effect of drugs upon the quality of life of the patient is too important to be left solely to the medical profession.

However, an eighth conclusion is that most of the methodologically adequate psychopharmacological research with persons with developmental disabilities (as, incidentally is also the case with children of normal IQ) has been done by nonmedical professionals, notably psychologists. Although this area is too important to be left entirely to the medical profession, it can no longer proceed adequately without them. In the last decade, psychopharmacology has moved away from being largely empirical to becoming one of the more exciting areas of neuroscience. This is made clear in a number of chapters, but nowhere more so than in Chapter 10. Nearly all of the original major psychotropic drugs were discovered serendipitously—the incidental observation of certain effects in some patients for whom the drugs were not originally intended. But that was 30 years ago, and in the intervening period basic research on these drugs has unlocked a whole new science based upon their cellular actions and the systems in which those cells are to be found or impact. New drugs are now being deliberately synthesized, not for an organismic effect but for a *cellular action* such as blocking a particular neurotransmitter, and most lately, for only one kind of receptor for that neurotransmitter. If pharmacotherapy of developmentally disabled persons is to go in the same direction, then involvement of biomedical investigators is absolutely essential. Continuing with the tiresome homily, it could be said that pharmacotherapy of retarded persons is now too important to be left solely to psychologists.

Finally, Chapter 8 on diet and vitamins carries its own message. In any serious, chronic handicapping disorder beyond the reach of modern medical cure, there is always the risk of "false prophets," most with the best of intentions, offering panaceas to those whose hope of cure never quite disappears. The history of the Feingold diet, megavitamin treatment, and cell therapy are examples. Also, like all expert high-status groups in our society, medicine is victim to populist anti-intellectualism, which holds that medicine's sole concern is self-enrichment and aggrandizement. It is now over 30 years since C.P. Snow drew attention to the fact that science is now an integral part of literacy and that traditional "culture" of the arts is only half the story. However, few of the well-educated general public, including journalists, have any real understanding of the scientific method as a tool for evaluating knowledge and preventing the corrupting self-deception of ordinary experience. Thus, not only does hope of cure spring eternal in the consumer's breast, but the public and much of the media begin with a paranoid set toward medicine and other experts. Yet, both public and media often lack the fundamental tools to evaluate the worth of what they are enthusiastically embracing. If we have learned anything in the last 30 years in psychopharmacology, it should be that there is no place for uncontrolled clinical trials of treatments—except as a first step to see whether to proceed with research or in those rare instances where outcome is fixed and known (e.g., rabies, which is uniformly fatal). For example, Sulzbacher (1973) reviewed all clinical trials of psychotropic drugs in children as of that date and found that of those that had no proper (placebo) controls, almost all reported a marked beneficial result from the medication tested, whereas the (then) few controlled studies were mostly negative or far from spectacular. While good journals now will not accept uncontrolled trials, the public and press are not so discriminating. So, rebuffed by the proper vehicle to promulgate new findings, these false prophets seek and gain a public platform through a credulous, sensationalist media and an ever-hopeful public. For too long, those who know what constitutes good research have been far too passive in allowing nonsense to go unchallenged. This task is unenviable, being usually unrewarded and unpopular. Anyone who doubts this should read Conners's (1980) brilliant description of his debate with Feingold before an audience largely composed of parents of hyperactive, learning disabled children. His message of caution fell on deaf and restless ears.

What of the Future?

I shall now try to summarize what I see as the implications for the future, though much of this is implicit in the aforementioned conclusions. For this reason, they will be mostly merely itemized without too much further elaboration.

1. Traditional studies of the epidemiology of prescription of psychotropic drugs for developmentally disabled persons and of their gross clinical effects on behavior should continue since these are, in a way, arbiters of the quality of care.
2. These studies need greater attention to measures of learning and cognitive function, but also more sophisticated measures of the "quality of life" or the net gain to the patient in all areas of function and personal comfort.
3. The editors' plea for more attention to the majority of developmentally disabled persons who do not live in institutions should be heeded. Not only are they vastly more numerous, but the push toward community care will make institutions (and, hence, the bulk of the current findings) increasingly obsolete.
4. While the need for drugs that regulate behavior in general will still exist for the foreseeable future, much more attention must be given to defining specific clinical requirements and therapeutic goals. Some of this may use as a starting point the diagnostic indications of adult and child psychiatry, since the available evidence suggests not only that psychiatric disorders such as depression and schizophrenia are to be found among the developmentally disabled population, but they should be more common than in nondisabled groups—certainly in those disabled persons who are institutionalized (Menolascino, Levitas, & Greiner, 1986). For example, recent research (Lewis, Reveley, Reveley, Chitkara, & Murray, 1987) suggests that there are probably two broad types of schizophrenia: hereditary and acquired. A primary cause of the acquired form seems to be brain damage occurring early in life, which is also a prime cause of mental retardation in its more severe forms. Similarly, autism has been shown to be a nonspecific concomitant of severe brain damage, proof of which can be seen in the relationship between autism and accidents of pregnancy and the quite common development of epilepsy in autism (Coleman & Gillberg, 1985).

Another thrust must come from greater attention to psychopharmacology as an evolving basic neuroscience. More effort must be made to look at the cellular action of drugs, including new ones as they are clarified, and to ask quite deliberately whether there are any implications for persons with developmental disabilities. Nowhere is this more cogent than in one of the most urgent public health problems of the next century—senile dementias. Such is the magnitude of this problem that it is likely to result in huge investments in research. It is probable that what is learned about the biology and pharmacology of memory and other cognitive functions in the aged will have important implications for those born with "dementia" (defined as loss of intellectual function), which is what developmental disabilities really are in functional terms. Since it is unlikely that the aging process is exactly similar to the effects of congenital, mostly anoxic, brain impairment (except in isolated areas such as trisomy 21), the fallout for developmental disabilities seems more likely to be in the area of cognitive facilitator drugs, rather than dramatically curative agents.

5. It follows from item 4 above that there is a need for a much stronger rapprochement between the field of developmental disabilities and psychiatry, and also with medicine in general. Pediatrics is already strongly involved with developmental disabilities, but this must be complemented by interest from other branches of medicine with a rather more direct interest in behavior, whole brain function, cognition, and psychopharmacology.

6. Movements of services for developmentally disabled persons away from huge, remote "pork barrel" institutions for the retarded must continue. Not only are these large facilities impediments to independence and humane care of people with developmental disabilities, but they continue the isolation from mainstream medicine and human biology with its rapidly developing high-technology diagnostic panoply. Regular blood level estimations of drugs, telemetric video/EEG recording, and organ imaging techniques such as positron emission tomography (PET scans) and nuclear magnetic resonance (NMR) have a potentially major role to play in research and therapeutic psychopharmacology of persons with mental retardation.

7. While much emphasis has been given to the medical areas, similar remarks might be made about nonmedical research and professions such as neuropsychology and physiological, experimental, and developmental psychology which are no less critical to the advance of psychopharmacology of the developmentally disabled population. They must provide much of the theory and technology of measurement of behavior and cognition and, as ever, maintain a strong interface between whole and higher organismic function and underlying structure. Like medical personnel, they are more likely to be found proximate to, and increasingly in, academic general hospitals than remote, downstate institutions.

8. Consumer and social action groups and the legal profession have a continuing role to play in their efforts to improve care and swing the change from institutional to community care. This is also just as critical to development of psychopharmacology of the developmental disabilities as are the biomedical and psychosocial sciences and professions.

9. Those who have the technical knowledge to evaluate claims for new psychopharmacological and related chemical/nutritional treatments for developmental disabilities have a peculiar obligation to act as advocates for those who cannot protect themselves against every therapeutic Pied Piper who comes through town, by prompt and accurate public criticism of these claims. To some this may smack of paternalism but in some ways, especially in the United States, consumerism is at times a

caricature of itself, which denies the expertise of the helping professions and thus harms those whom it seeks to protect. For example, despite what is commonly believed, the medical profession is not conservative about treatment for the sake of conservatism, but because it has knowledge of its own sorry history of centuries of poisoning, mutilation, and exsanguination, all ostensibly in the name of helping the patient. Only the scientific method can prevent this terrible saga of self-deception from being continued.

10. While this book illustrates just how far we have come in three decades, it also shows how far there is yet to go in the psychopharmacology of the developmental disabilities.

References

Aman, M.G., & White A.J. (1986). Measures of drug change in mental retardation. In K.D. Gadow (Ed.), *Advances in learning and behavioral disabilities* (Vol. 5, pp. 157–202). Greenwich, CT: JAI Press.

Coleman, M., & Gillberg, C. (1985). *The biology of the autistic syndromes*. New York: Praeger.

Conners, C.K. (1980). *Food additives and hyperactive children* (pp. 12–13). New York: Plenum Press.

Lewis, S.W., Reveley, A.M., Reveley, M.A., Chitkara, B., & Murray R.M. (1987). The familial-sporadic distinction as a strategy in schizophrenia research. *British Journal of Psychiatry*, *151*, 306–313.

Lipman, R.S. (1970). The use of psychopharmacological agents in residential facilities for the retarded. In F.J. Menolascino (Ed.), *Psychiatric approaches to mental retardation* (pp. 387–398). New York: Basic Books.

Menolascino, F.J., Levitas, A., & Greiner, C. (1986). The nature and types of mental illness in the mentally retarded. *Psychopharmacology Bulletin*, *22*, 1060–1071.

Sulzbacher, S.I. (1973). Psychotropic medication with children: An evaluation of precedural bias in reported studies. *Pediatrics*, *51*, 513–517.

Werry, J.S. (1980). Anticholinergic sedatives. In G.D. Burrows & J.S. Werry (Eds.), *Advances in human psychopharmacology* (Vol. 1, pp. 19–42). Greenwich, CT: JAI Press.

Werry, J.S. (1988). Drugs, learning and cognition in children: An update. *Journal of Child Psychology and Psychiatry*, *29*.

Glossary of Psychoactive Drug Classes, Generic Names, and Trade Names

Drug and class	Trade name(s)
NEUROLEPTICS (Antipsychotics, "Major tranquilizers")	
Phenothiazines	
chlorpromazine	Largactil, Thorazine
fluphenazine	Prolixin
mesoridazine	Serentii
peracetazine	Quide
pericyazine	Neulactil
perphenazine	Trilafon
prochlorperazine	Compazine
promazine	Sparine
thioridazine	Mellaril
trifluoperazine	Stelazine
Thioxanthenes	
chlorprothixene	Taractan, Tarasan
thiothixene	Navane
Butyrophenones	
haloperidol	Haldol, Serenace
pipamperon	Dipiperon
Diphenylbutylpiperidine	
pimozide	Orap
Rauwolfia Alkaloids	
reserpine	Rauloydin, Reserpoid, Sandril
ANTICONVULSANTS	
carbamazepine	Tegretol
clonazepam	Clonopin
diazepam*	Valium
ethosuximide	Zarontin
lorazepam*	Ativan
phenobarbital (phenobarbitone)	Luminal, Gardenal
phenytoin, (diphenylhydantoin, DPH)	Dilantin
primidone	Mysoline
sodium valproate	Depakene, Epilim
sulthiame	Ospolot
SEDATIVE-HYPNOTICS	
Antihistamines	
dyphenhydramine	Benadryl
hydroxyzine	Atarax
promethazine**	Phenergan
trimeprazine	Temaril, Vallergan
Benzodiazepines ("Minor Tranquilizers")	
alprazolam*	Xanax

Drug and class	Trade name(s)
diazepam*	Valium
chlordiazepoxide	Librium
flurazepam	Dalmane
lorazepam	Ativan
oxazepam	Serax
prazepam	Verstran
temazepam	Restoril
triazolam	Halcion
Other	
chloral hydrate	Noctec
meprobamate	Equanil, Miltown
secobarbital	Seconal

ANTIDEPRESSANT/ANTIMANIC DRUGS

Tricyclic Antidepressants	
amitriptyline	Elavil, Amitril, Endep
desipramine	Norpramin, Pertofrane
doxepin	Sinequan, Adapin
imipramine	Tofranil, Janimine, Dumex
nortriptyline	Arentyl, Nortab, Pamelor
Monoamine Oxidase Inhibitors (MAOIs)	
isocarboxazid	Marplan
phenelzine	Nardil
tranylcypromine	Parnate
Atypical Antidepressants	
alprazolam*	Xanax
amoxapine	Asendin
maprotiline	Ludiomil
nomifensine	Merital
Antimanic Drugs	
lithium carbonate	Eskalith, Lithane, Lithobid

CNS STIMULANTS

amphetamine sulfate	Benzedrine
deanol (2-dimethylaminoethanol)	Deaner
dextroamphetamine (d-amphetamine)	Dexedrine
levoamphetamine (l-amphetamine)	Cydril
methylphenidate	Ritalin
pemoline	Cylert

ANTIPARKINSON DRUGS***

benztropine mesylate	Cogentin
diphenhydramine hydrochloride	Benadryl
trihexyphenidyl hydrochloride	Artane

Drug and class	Trade name(s)
MISCELLANEOUS	
Clonidine HCl	Catapres, Combipres
(alpha adrenergic blocker)	
fenfluramine	Pondimin, Ponderax
(serotonin depleter)	
5-hydroxytryptamine	
(serotonin)	
naloxone	Narcan
(endorphin antagonist)	
naltrexone	Trexan
(endorphin antagonist)	
propranolol	Inderal
(beta adrenergic blocker)	
glutamic acid	Prostade, Selerex
(amino acid)	
essential fatty acid supplement	Efamol
(linoleic & gammalinoleic acid)	
pyridoxine	Nature's Bounty,
(vitamin B_6)	Hexa-Betalin, Meg-B

* Drug belongs to more than one clinical group.
** More correctly classed as a phenothiazine but often used as an hypnotic in children.
*** Commonly used to counter extrapyramidal side effects of neuroleptic drugs. Not ordinarily used as psychotropic drugs.

Author Index

Subject Index